Spirulina
in
Human Nutrition
and
Health

Edited by

M. E. Gershwin
Amha Belay

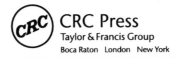

CRC Press
Taylor & Francis Group
Boca Raton London New York

CRC Press is an imprint of the
Taylor & Francis Group, an informa business

This book is for educational purposes only and is not intended to diagnose, treat, cure or prevent any disease.

CRC Press
Taylor & Francis Group
6000 Broken Sound Parkway NW, Suite 300
Boca Raton, FL 33487-2742

© 2008 by Taylor & Francis Group, LLC
CRC Press is an imprint of Taylor & Francis Group, an Informa business

No claim to original U.S. Government works
Printed in the United States of America on acid-free paper
10 9 8 7 6 5 4 3 2 1

International Standard Book Number-13: 978-1-4200-5256-5 (Hardcover)

Library of Congress Cataloging-in-Publication Data

Spirulina in human nutrition and health / editors, M.E. Gershwin and Amha Belay.
    p. ; cm.
"A CRC title."
Includes bibliographical references and index.
ISBN-13: 978-1-4200-5256-5 (hardcover : alk. paper)
ISBN-10: 1-4200-5256-X (hardcover : alk. paper)
    1. Spirulina--Therapeutic use. I. Gershwin, M. Eric, 1946- II. Belay, Amha.
[DNLM: 1. Spirulina. 2. Diet Therapy. 3. Dietary Supplements. QW 131 S759 2007]

RM666.S663S65 2007
615.8'54--dc22   2007016306

Visit the Taylor & Francis Web site at
http://www.taylorandfrancis.com

and the CRC Press Web site at
http://www.crcpress.com

Contents

Preface

Foods provide nutrients such as vitamins, minerals, proteins, carbohydrates, and fats and a host of other nonessential nutrients that may confer health benefits. Research into the mechanisms of action of foods and their components have led to a virtual cottage industry of nutraceuticals that, in some cases, have been suggested to boost the immune system, enhance cognitive function, and perhaps even have the potential to slow the aging process. On the basis of these findings, some manufacturers have even begun the creation of functional foods by fortifying, bioengineering, or otherwise modifying foods so that they contain higher than normal concentrations of these components. Others market the extracts of certain foods such as garlic, parsley, and cranberries in the form of pills, capsules, tablets, or liquids. In addition, individual phytochemicals are available in health food stores and even in mainstream supermarkets. Indeed, many food extracts and plant components are sold as dietary supplements, and the market has exploded, fueled in part by claims that select botanicals can do everything from curing colds to facilitating weight loss. This change in market is reflected by the incredible consumer interest in dietary supplements. Unfortunately, all too often the use of dietary supplements comes without the rigorous scientific data required for health claims and there is very little systematic research on not only many nutraceuticals but also the interactions of these materials between prescription or even over-the-counter drugs. One indication of this complexity is that isolated plant ingredients or even the isolation of a bioactive constituent often have different effects than the whole plant extract. One major exception to these myriad problems is the use of Spirulina. Spirulina, essentially an extraordinarily simple extract of blue-green algae, has been extensively studied and is now in widespread usage throughout the world as a food product and as a dietary supplement. Despite this wealth of data in individual experimental papers, there has not hitherto been an attempt to combine this body of knowledge into a monograph that is useful for scientists, physicians, workers in the food industry, and, of course, consumers. This volume, which is edited by a professor of immunology and an expert in nutrition and immunology, as well as a basic scientist with extensive background in Spirulina, aims to fill this gap. We are particularly appreciative of our contributors who worked arduously to meet deadlines and to set their pen to paper on an important subject in a readable fashion. We are especially grateful to Kathy Wisdom, our editorial assistant, who has followed, tracked, and made the writing process ever so much easier. We are also grateful to our editors at CRC Press for their encouragement and advice.

M. Eric Gershwin

Amha Belay

Editors

M. Eric Gershwin, MD is a distinguished professor of medicine as well as the Jack and Donald Chia professor of medicine. He is also chief of the division of allergy and clinical immunology at the University of California School of Medicine in Davis. Dr. Gershwin graduated from Stanford Medical School in 1971 and subsequently trained in internal medicine and then immunology at Tufts University-New England Medical Center and the National Institutes of Health. He joined the UC Davis faculty in 1975 and has been division chief since 1982. Dr. Gershwin has been continuously funded by NIH since 1975 and currently has published more than 20 books, 600 experimental papers, and 200 book chapters or review articles. He is editor of the *Journal of Autoimmunity and Clinical Reviews in Allergy and Immunology* and on the editorial board of multiple other journals. His major contributions revolve around the theme of autoimmune disease. Dr. Gershwin was the first individual to clone an autoantigen and identified the mitochondrial autoantigens of PBC in 1986; this antigen was identified as the E2 component of pyruvate dehydrogenase. Subsequently, his lab has focused entirely on PBC and his diagnostic reagents have become the standard throughout the world. More importantly, however, he has dissected the CD4, CD8 and B cell response in PBC and demonstrated that the autoepitope is nearly identical in each case. Further, his research has helped to explain why only small bile duct cells are involved and this thesis has led to our understanding of the pathophysiology of biliary damage as an orchestrated response that begins with adaptive immunity and ends with innate immunity. This work has been published in the *Journal of Immunology*, the *Journal of Clinical Investigation*, and the *Journal of Experimental Medicine*. He has sat and chaired on committees for NIH, NSF, USDA, FTC and the FDA. Dr. Gershwin has been studying nutrition and immunology for more than three decades.

Amha Belay, PhD is a highly respected and leading expert in microalgal biotechnology in general and Spirulina (*Arthrospira*) in particular. He has an extensive experience in the use of algae in health management, and in a wide variety of applications such as food, feed, nutraceuticals, and environmental management. His other areas of expertise include nutraceutical and functional foods development, quality assurance, and regulation.

Dr. Belay is currently senior vice president and scientific director of Earthrise Nutritionals, the largest Spirulina-producing company in the world. He oversees algal production and quality assurance, quality management systems, product development, and regulatory affairs.

Before joining Earthrise in 1989, he was associate professor and head of the Biology Department at Addis Ababa University, Ethiopia. He was also a senior research fellow at the Institute of Hydrobiology, Pallanza, Italy, under the auspices of the Third World Academy of Sciences, a visiting researcher at the Freshwater Institute in Windermere, UK, under the auspices of the British Council, and a senior Fulbright fellow at the University of California, Santa Barbara.

Dr. Belay has published numerous articles in peer-reviewed journals and has presented several invited scientific presentations worldwide. He has served as editor and editorial advisory board member of many scientific journals. He is a founding and executive member of the International Society for Applied Phycology, and a member of several professional associations including the American Association for the Advancement of Science, the American Nutraceutical Association, the American Herbal Products Association, the Institute of Food Technologists, the Natural Products Association (formerly the NNFA), the Phycological Society of America, and the Asia-Pacific Society for Algal Biotechnology to mention a few.

Dr. Belay was born in Ethiopia (the land of the Spirulina lakes). He earned his first degree at the now Addis Ababa University in Ethiopia and his PhD at the Universities of London and North Wales, UK, under the late Professor G. E. Fogg, F.R.S. He lives in La Quinta, California with his wife and two children.

Contributors

Adam Bachstetter
Department of Molecular Pharmacology &
Physiology
University of South Florida College of
Medicine
Tampa, Florida

Blanca Lilia Barrón
Escuela Nacional de Ciencias Biológicas
Instituto Politécnico Nacional
Casco de Santo Tomás, Mexico

Amha Belay
Earthrise Nutritionals LLC
Irvine, California

Paula C. Bickford
Department of Neurosurgery, and
Department of Molecular
Pharmacology and Physiology
University of South Florida College of
Medicine
Tampa, Florida
and
James A. Haley VA Medical Center
Tampa, Florida

Mahendra Bishnoi
University Institute of Pharmaceutical
Sciences
Punjab University
Chandigarh, India

Andrea T. Borchers
Department of Rheumatology
University of California
Davis, California

Germán Chamorro-Cevallos
Escuela Nacional de Ciencias Biológicas
Instituto Politécnico Nacional
Casco de Santo Tomas, Mexico

Kanwaljit Chopra
University Institute of Pharmaceutical
Sciences
Punjab University
Chandigarh, India

Meltem Conk Dalay
Department of Bioengineering
Ege University
Bornova, Izmir, Turkey

Swati A. Dhruv
Department of Foods and Nutrition WHO
Collaborating Centre
The maharaj Sayajirao University of Baroda
Vadodara, India

Takashi Ebihara
Department of Microbiology and
Immunology
Hokkaido University
Kita-ku Sapporo, Japan

Carmelina Gemma
Department of Neurosurgery, and
Department of Molecular Pharmacology
and Physiology
University of South Florida College of
Medicine
Tampa, Florida
and
James A. Haley VA Medical Center
Tampa, Florida

M. Eric Gershwin
Department of Rheumatology
University of California
Davis, California

Osamu Hayashi
Department of Health and Nutrition
Kagawa Nutrition University
Sakado, Saitama, Japan

Kaoru Hazeki
Division of Molecular Medical Science
Hiroshima University
Minami-ku, Hiroshima, Japan

Ja-an Annie Ho
Department of Chemistry
National Tsing Hua University
Hsinchu, Taiwan

Kyoko Ishii
Department of Health and Nutrition
Kagawa Nutrition University
Sakado, Saitama, Japan

Uma M. Iyer
Department of Foods and Nutrition WHO
    Collaborating Centre
The maharaj Sayajirao University of Baroda
Vadodara, India

Toshimitsu Kato
Health Care Foods Division
Dainippon Ink and Chemicals Inc.
Ichihara, Japan

Carl L. Keen
Department of Nutrition
University of California at Davis
Davis, California

Mahmood Khan
Davis Heart and Lung Research Institute
Department of Internal Medicine
The Ohio State University
Columbus, Ohio

Ken Kodama
Osaka Medical Center for Cancer and
    Cardiovascular Diseases
Higashinari-ku Osaka, Japan

Periannan Kuppusamy
Davis Heart and Lung Research Institute
Department of Internal Medicine
The Ohio State University
Columbus, Ohio

Vijay Kumar Kutala
Davis Heart and Lung Research Institute
Department of Internal Medicine
The Ohio State University
Columbus, Ohio

Indirani U. Mani
Department of Foods and Nutrition and
    WHO Collaborating Centre
The Maharaja Sayajirao University of
    Baroda
Vadodara, India

Uliyar V. Mani
Department of Foods and Nutrition
MS University of Baroda
Gujarat, India

Misako Matsumoto
Department of Microbiology and
    Immunology
Hokkaido University
Kita-ku Sapporo, Japan
and
Osaka Medical Center for Cancer and
    Cardiovascular Diseases
Higashinari-ku Osaka, Japan

Iyyapu Krishna Mohan
Davis Heart and Lung Research Institute
Department of Internal Medicine
The Ohio State University
Columbus, Ohio

Guven Ozdemir
Department of Biology
Ege University
Bornova, Izmir, Turkey

Narasimham L. Parinandi
Division of Pulmonary, Allergy, Critical
    Care, and Sleep Medicine
Davis Heart and Lung Research Institute
Department of Internal Medicine
The Ohio State University
Columbus, Ohio

Tsukasa Seya
Department of Microbiology and
   Immunology
Hokkaido University
Kita-ku Sapporo, Japan
and
Osaka Medical Center for Cancer and
   Cardiovascular Diseases
Higashinari-ku Osaka, Japan

Kavita S. Sharma
Department of Foods and Nutrition and
   WHO Collaborating Centre
The Maharaja Sayajirao University of
   Baroda
Vadodara, India

Ingrid Strömberg
Department of Integrative Medical Biology
Umeå University
Umeå, Sweden

J. Martín Torres-Valencia
Centro de Investigaciones Químicas
Universidad Autónoma del Estado de
Hidalgo
Carretera Pachuca-Tulancingo, Cd.
   Universitaria
Pachuca, Hidalgo, México

Jorge Vázquez-Sánchez
Escuela Nacional de Ciencias Biológicas,
Instituto Politécnico Nacional
Carpio y Plan de Ayala S/N
Casco de Santo Tomás, Mexico

Jennifer Vila
Center of Excellence for Aging and Brain
   Repair
Department of Neurosurgery, and
   Department of Molecular
Pharmacology and Physiology
University of South Florida
College of Medicine
Tampa, Florida

Yun Wang
National Institute on Drug Abuse
Intramural Research Program
Baltimore, Maryland

Li-chen Wu
Department of Applied Chemistry
National Chi-Nan University
Puli, Natou, Taiwan

Armida Zúñiga-Estrada
Centro de Investigaciones Químicas
Universidad Autónoma del Estado de
Hidalgo
Carretera Pachuca-Tulancingo, Cd.
   Universitaria
Pachuca, Hidalgo, Mexico

1 *Spirulina* (*Arthrospira*): Production and Quality Assurance

Amha Belay

CONTENTS

INTRODUCTION

The microscopic, filamentous prokaryote, *Arthrospira (Spirulina)*, has been the subject of intense investigation mainly owing to its use as food, feed, dietary supplement, and functional food. Its recorded historical use as food spans centuries and it has been commercialized as food for the past 30 years. Though there are numerous studies on its mass production outdoors, these are mainly from studies involving small experimental outdoor ponds. There is therefore only limited information from large-scale commercial facilities that produce *Spirulina* in large outdoor ponds. Small-scale production in experimental ponds is limited in its scope since it does not deal with effects of harvesting and recycling of nutrients on a continuous basis that affect both the yield and quality of the product. This chapter presents information on the production and quality of *Spirulina (Arthrospira)* grown in large outdoor ponds, drawing examples from the Earthrise Farms located in southern California.

WHAT IS *SPIRULINA?*

In its commercial use, the common name, *Spirulina*, refers to the dried biomass of the cyanobacterium, *Arthrospira platensis*, and is a whole product of biological origin. The source strain, cultivated by producers in the United States was obtained from the University of Texas at Austin Algae Culture Collection (UTEX). This strain, designated UTEX 1926, was originally isolated from an alkaline salt flat near Del Mar, California, by R. Lewin in 1969.

In its taxonomic use, *Spirulina* is a name used to describe mainly two species of Cyanobacteria, *A. platensis* and *A. maxima*, that are commonly used as food, dietary supplement, and feed supplement. These and other *Arthrospira* species were once classified by Geitler[1] who combined all species forming helical trichomes into a single genus, *Spirulina*. Before Geitler, Gomont[2] had in fact placed the two genera as separate on the basis of the presence of septa or divisions in the trichomes, the *Spirulina* species being without septa and the *Arthrospira* species with septa. Recent detailed studies of morphological, physiological, and biochemical examination of representatives of these genera have shown that these two genera are distinctively different and that the edible forms commonly referred to as *Spirulina platensis* have little in common with other much smaller species such as *Spirulina major*.[3–5] This distinction has also been borne out by results from the complete sequence of the 16S rRNA gene and the internal transcribed spacer (ITS) between the 16S and 23S rRNA genes determined for two *Arthrospira* strains and one *Spirulina* strain showing that the two *Arthrospira* strains formed a close cluster distant from the *Spirulina* strain.[6]

The various Arthrospira species found in nature and in culture collection appear to be very closely related. Scheldeman et al.[7] carried out an ARDRA (Amplified

Ribosomal DNA Restriction Analysis on the ITS of 37 cultivated clonal strains from four continents. The data showed that all these strains were closely related. Only two different major restriction patterns were discernible defining two clusters, I and II, with two strains from cluster I falling in a small subcluster. No clear relationship could be observed between this division into two clusters and the geographic origin of the strains, their designation in the culture collection, or their morphology. Subsequent studies by Baurain et al.,[8] using amplification and determination of the full ITS, also showed a remarkable conservation of the ITS sequences of 21 of the 37 *Arthrospira* clonal strains from the four continents and assigned to four different species (*A. platensis, A. maxima, A. fusiformis, A. indica*) in the culture collections. Using 28 morphological characters or character states, Mühling et al.[9] have also found these strains to be grouped into two loose clusters. It is therefore evident that these strains are very closely related and the assignment of binomial is therefore difficult at this stage of our knowledge of their taxonomy.

It should be pointed out that the name *Spirulina* is used commonly as a name of commerce and will continue to be used since many companies have devoted a lot of money in the marketing of *Arthrospira* with the trade name of *Spirulina*. This chapter will use these names interchangeably with the understanding that all the edible forms that are under commercial cultivation and sold as "*Spirulina*" actually belong to the Genus *Arthrospira*.

The botanical nomenclature is also used often because *Spirulina* and *Arthrospira* are considered plants (blue-green algae) by botanists who look at the photosynthetic ability of these organisms as a major determinant of their classification. However, the most recent comprehensive treatise on the subject identifies *Arthrospira* as follows[10]:

Phylum BX. Cyanobacteria
Subsection III. (formerly Order Oscillatoriales)
Form-genus I. *Arthrospira*

MORPHOLOGICAL FEATURES

Arthrospira (Spirulina) species show great plasticity in morphology. This is attributed to environmental factors like temperature and other physical and chemical factors and possibly also due to genetic change. In nature and in culture, *Arthrospira* forms helical trichomes of varying size and degree of coiling from tightly coiled morphology to an even straight uncoiled form. The trichomes in *Arthrospira* species show distinct transverse cross-walls under the light microscope. The filaments are solitary and reproduce by binary fission. The cells of the trichomes are broader than long and the width can vary from 3 to 12 μm though it can reach 16 μm occasionally. The cell organization is that of a typical prokaryote with a lack of membrane-bound organelles.[4]

EVOLUTIONARY HISTORY

The cyanobacteria are believed to have evolved 3.5 billion years ago. Fossils discovered in the 3.5-Ga-old Apex chert in northwestern Western Australia[11] bear filamentous cyanobacteria with strikingly similar morphologies to present-day filamentous cyanobacteria (Oscillatoriacea). The occurrence of aerobic respiration and oxygenic photosynthesis, photosynthetic carbon dioxide fixation like that of extant cyanobacteria, cell division more similar to the extant cyanobacterial and recent rRNA analyses showing that the Oscillatoriacea are among the earliest evolved also lend further evidence to the fossil record.[12] *Arthrospira* belongs to the Class Oscillatoriacea and therefore has a very old lineage. Despite their old lineage, the fossil cyanobacteria are morphologically very similar to their extant forms, suggesting a slow evolutionary process.[13]

The cyanobacteria are the first group of bacteria that evolved that could fix atmospheric carbon dioxide into organic carbon compounds using water as an electron donor and thereby evolving oxygen. We owe the present oxygen-rich environment partially to the millions of years of photosynthetic activity by Cyanaobacteria that made it possible for other life forms that are oxygen dependent to evolve. Indeed it is this same ability to fix carbon dioxide and produce organic matter that we are presently utilizing in the mass cultivation of these organisms for food.

DISTRIBUTION IN NATURE

Species of the genus *Arthrospira* have been isolated from alkaline brackish and saline waters in tropical and subtropical regions. Among the various species included in the genus *Arthrospira*, *A. platensis* is the most widely distributed and is mainly found in Africa but also in Asia. *Arthrospira maxima* is believed to be found in California and Mexico. It should be noted that the taxonomic distinction between these two species is based mainly on ultrastructural and morphological differences, some of which are hardly a distinctive feature in view of the morphological elasticity of these species under different growth and stress conditions. The recent 16s rRNA sequence data on 52 strains collected from various regions have revealed only two clusters with species from the various geographical areas represented in both clusters.

HISTORY OF HUMAN USE AS FOOD

Algae, especially the macroalgae, have been used as food since prehistoric times and still play a prominent role in the food traditions of many countries, particularly in Asia. The use of microalgae as food is fairly recent. Jasby[14] cites numerous examples of traditional use of microalgae as food spanning over four continents though the majority of the cases are from Asia as in the case of seaweeds or macroalgae.

The first recorded history of the use of *Arthrospira* (*Spirulina*) as food comes from Bernal Diaz del Castillo, a member of Hernan Cortez's troops who reported in 1521 that *Spirulina maxima* (*A. maxima*) was harvested from Lake Texcoco, dried, and sold for human consumption in a Tenochtitlan (today Mexico City) market. Bernal Diaz de Castillo described what he saw in the market as "… small cakes made from some sort of a ooze which they get out of the great lake, and from which they make a bread having a flavor something like cheese." A few years later a Franciscan friar, Bernardino da Sahagun, described the food, then called Tecuitlatl, as "neither grass nor earth, rather like hay ... of clear blue color ... ."[15] There was no mention of Tecuitlatl after the sixteenth century, though perhaps not surprisingly, the first commercial production of *Spirulina* started in Lake Texcoco in the 1970s. An interesting description of the history of *Spirulina* during the Aztec civilization is given by Farrar.[16]

The present Republic of Chad in Africa, about 10,000 km away from Lake Texcoco, provides additional evidence for the use of *Spirulina* as food. People have probably being using it for centuries, though it is not clear exactly since when. The recent historical evidence goes back to 1940 when the French phycologist, Dangeard[17] published a paper about a cake called "dihe" and consumed by people of the Kanembu tribe, near Lake Chad in Africa. This report, which stayed unnoticed until the 1960s, described dihe as "a true filamentous, spiral shaped blue alga."[15] The alga described was *Arthrospira (Spirulina) platensis* that was also known to Dangeard to grow abundantly in the East African Rift Valley lakes where they represented the main source of food for the lesser flamingoes. Dihe was rediscovered 25 years later in 1966 by J. Leonard, who was attracted by a "curious substance green bluish, sold as dried biscuits" around Fort Lamy.[15] Leonard confirmed that dihe was composed almost exclusively of dried mats of *S. platensis (A. platensis)*. It was collected from the waters of the alkaline lakes in the Kanem area, northeast of Lake Chad.[18-19] *Arthrospira* still makes a large portion of the daily protein diet of the Kanembu tribe in the Lake Chad area and contributes significantly to the local economy.[20] It was at about the same time that the French Petroleum Institute got interested in some samples of *Spirulina (S. maxima)* that grew abundantly in Lake Texcoco near Mexico City. The subsequent studies by the French group culminated in the establishment of the first commercial production of *Spirulina* in the world in the 1970s.

SPIRULINA PRODUCTION: NATURE TO NURTURE

Most of the information that is used to grow *Spirulina* in outdoor culture is derived from observations made on natural blooms of these algae in natural lakes. Of special significance is their adaptation to highly alkaline (up to 400 meq/l) and very high pH (up to 11) of tropical and subtropical regions of the world. This harsh chemical environment essentially prohibits the growth of other algae. It is therefore not uncommon to find almost unialgal populations of *Arthrospira* in these lakes. The crater lakes around the Great African Rift Valley are good examples of these. These lakes support high-standing crops of *Spirulina* (up to 2.0 g Chl a l^{-1}) and support huge populations of flamingoes (Figure 1.1). It is estimated that adult and juvenile flamingoes consume on the average about 66 g of *Spirulina* per day on a dry weight basis. This means that the whole flamingo population, about a million individuals at the time, extracted 50–94% of the daily primary production or 0.4–0.6% of the algal biomass.[21]

The productivity of these natural ecosystems has not been studied to any great extent. However, there have been some studies looking into photosynthetic productivity[22] (Belay, unpublished). On the basis of these studies some of these soda lakes are among the most productive natural systems. The photosynthetic productivity reported for these lakes is the highest ever recorded for any natural systems and are comparable to those observed in some waste treatment ponds or mass culture

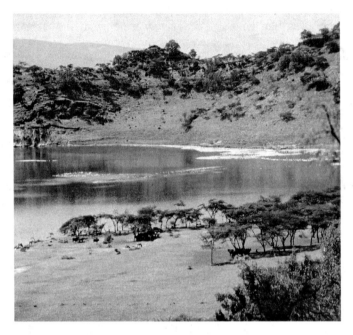

FIGURE 1.1   Unialgal population of *Arthrospira* in Lake Chitu, Ethiopia: courtesy Biology Department, Addis Ababa University.

facilities. The values of 43–57 g m^{-2} d^{-1} recorded by Talling for Lake Arenguadie in Ethiopia are among the highest ever recorded for natural systems. Comparable values have also been recorded recently for this same lake (Belay, unpublished). The high productivity of these soda lakes is a result of (a) high algal contents in the euphotic zone, (b) high photosynthetic capacity favored by high temperature, and (c) a surplus of dissolved inorganic phosphate and an especially huge reserve of CO_2. Maximal photosynthetic rates (mg C l^{-1} h^{-1}) and photosynthetic efficiency (mg C [mg Chl a]$^{-1}$ h^{-1}) obtained at light saturation in a continuous culture replete with nutrients were comparable to those obtained in these highly productive lakes.[23] Aerial biomass concentrations (mg Chl a m^{-2}) for Lakes Arenguadie and Kilole have been found to be close to the maximum possible on theoretical grounds (180–300 mg Chl a m^{-2}).[22]

LARGE-SCALE, COMMERCIAL PRODUCTION OF *SPIRULINA*

Although the development of the technology of outdoor mass production of *Spirulina* dates back to the 1970s, it is very recently that its production and utilization has expanded beyond a few countries or producers. This is because of the many constraints that had to be surmounted. These relate to some environmental, physical, chemical, and biological problems encountered in commercial production of algae. It is not within the scope of this chapter to provide details of these constraints. The relevant

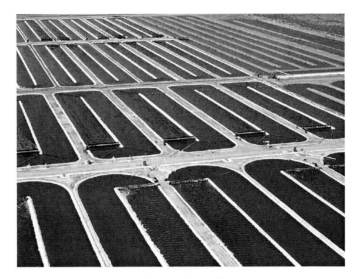

FIGURE 1.2 Aerial view of an outdoor mass culture of *Arthrospira*.

information can be found in other reviews.[24–28] This chapter will highlight the various processes involved in the production and quality assurance of *Spirulina*, drawing information mainly from the experiences of Earthrise Nutritionals LLC, the largest *Spirulina* producer in the world located in California, USA (Figure 1.2).

ENVIRONMENTAL CONDITIONS FOR OUTDOOR MASS PRODUCTION OF *SPIRULINA*

Arthrospira requires an abundant supply of light and nutrients and a relatively high temperature. As a result production facilities are located in tropical or subtropical regions of the world where both the intensity and duration of sun light are high and where the temperature is high enough to enable production year round. Such locations are hard to find but are mandatory for economic production of high-quality *Spirulina*. The optimum temperature for the growth of *Spirulina* is 35–38°C while the minimum temperature required to sustain growth is 15–20°C. There is virtually no facility in the world that is located in an area where the optimum temperature is experienced throughout the year. As a result facilities operate between 7 and 12 months. Another condition for *Spirulina* growth is minimal precipitation. Unfortunately, those areas where production can take place throughout the year usually have seasonal rains that may affect the condition of the culture adversely. Even though weather conditions vary over the year, it is possible to manipulate pond and culture parameters in order to minimize or counteract such effects on the yield and quality of the culture. Another problem associated with such a dry and hot climatic condition is the evaporation from the ponds that must be replenished with fresh water, thereby limiting further where the facility can be operated. Desert climates usually offer constancy of climatic conditions that result in higher yield and consistent quality of the product.

COMMERCIAL PRODUCTION OF *SPIRULINA*: OVERVIEW

Commercial production of *Spirulina* involves four stages: (a) culturing, (b) harvesting, (c) drying, and (d) packaging. All these steps can affect the final yield and/or quality of the product. Careful and routine monitoring of these processes is therefore essential to the successful economic production of high-quality *Spirulina* that meets the often strict quality and safety requirements of the food and supplement industry.

The production process involves a closed-loop system where material is recycled continuously and the only loss of material is through evaporation. The recycling of the growth medium takes place over the entire production season. A semicontinuous culture system is employed where each pond is harvested to the extent that it has grown over the last 24 h. The medium is recycled back to the same pond where it came from for optimizing growth and for traceability of the production lot in case there is a problem. Make-up nutrient is supplied routinely to replenish uptake by the harvested algae. Nutrients are monitored and adjusted by laboratory chemists who conduct daily tests to assure consistency and optimal conditions. Ponds are harvested daily. The culture is transferred with a pump through PVC pipes into a dedicated processing building where it is transferred to stainless-steel screens to rinse and concentrate the biomass. The biomass slurry is then transferred to a vacuum belt, which further dehydrates the biomass as a paste and subjects it to a final washing step. The *A. platensis* paste is then pumped into a spray dryer to remove the moisture, resulting in the free-flowing fine powder known commonly as *Spirulina*. The entire process from pond to powder takes less than 15 min. Samples of the powder are collected in sterilized bags, labeled, and transferred to the Quality Control Laboratory for microbiological assays and other quality-control analyses. The laboratory staff logs all data collected onto written sheets and into a database on the computer network. The Quality Control Department releases the product for packaging and inventory once the analysis shows that the product meets quality and safety requirements.

OUTLINE OF THE PRODUCTION SYSTEM AND FACTORS AFFECTING PRODUCTION

Algae can be produced either in open ponds or in closed bioreactors. The latter are believed to be more productive but a recent side-by-side comparison study has shown that there is virtually no difference in aerial productivity using the two systems (Paola Pedroni, personal communication). Since there is very little, if any, commercial production of *A. platensis* or *A. maxima* in closed bioreactors, the following discussion deals with open-pond systems only. A schematic diagram of a typical production system is given in Figure 1.3.

Production Ponds

Mass culture of *Spirulina* is often conducted in large raceway ponds made of concrete or lined with reinforced plastic approved for use for potable water. This raceway design for outdoor mass cultivation of photosynthetic microorganisms was developed

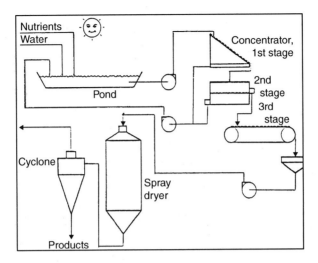

FIGURE 1.3   A schematic diagram of a *Spirulina* production system.

in the 1950s and is used widely in the industry.[29–30] A detailed description of the design of the ponds is given by Shimamatsu.[31] The ponds used in several facilities vary in size from about 2000 m^2 to the largest ponds of 5000 m^2 and may contain anyway between 400 and 1000 m^3 of culture depending on the pond depth used. The depth can vary between 15 and 40 cm depending on season, desired algal density, and, to a certain extent, the desired biochemical composition of the final product. Mixing of the culture is mandatory in outdoor mass culture in order to facilitate light distribution and minimize self-shading in an otherwise buoyant alga-like *Spirulina*. Mixing is facilitated by paddle wheels. Mixing also facilitates diffusion of nutrients and maintenance of uniform temperature with depth. Generally, the higher the mixing rate and hence light availability, the higher the growth rate. Mixing also avoids scum formation. Algal mass culture is often referred to as "scum." This is a misconception derived from observations in natural lakes and ponds where lack of mixing results in the accumulation and aggregation of floating biomass. This situation does not occur under controlled outdoor production where the algal culture is being mixed continuously by paddle wheels (Figure 1.2).

The Composition of the Culture Medium

The culture medium used in *Spirulina* mass culture mimics that of the natural system. The medium that is commonly used is based on the original medium of Zarouk[32] and is typically composed of water, sodium carbonate/bicarbonate, a source of nitrogen, phosphorus, iron, and other trace minerals. *Arthrospira platensis* is cultivated in an alkaline aqueous medium rich in nutrient salts. The high pH and alkalinity of the growth medium inhibits the growth of potentially contaminating organisms, resulting in a virtual monoculture of *A. platensis* (Figure 1.4). Nutrients are supplied by reliable manufacturers that include specifications for heavy metals and other possible

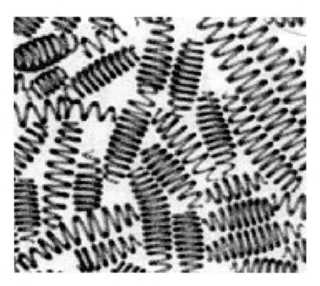

FIGURE 1.4   A microscopic view of a sample of an outdoor *Spirulina* culture.

contaminants. No solvents, pesticides, herbicides, or toxic substances are used during any cultivation or manufacturing step of the product.

Scale-Up of Culture and Maintenance of Unialgal Culture of *A. platensis*

The maintenance of a unialgal population of *Arthrospira* in outdoor ponds requires a good understanding of the physiology and ecology of the algae. Optimization of the productivity and quality of the culture requires the appropriate climatic environment, pond design, chemistry, and routine monitoring to fit the physiological and ecological requirements of the algae. Even though the medium used for growing *Spirulina* prevents contamination by other algae owing to its high pH and alkalinity, suboptimal operation of the culture control process can lead to contamination by other algae. This is particularly true during the scale-up process when the biomass concentration of *Arthrospira* is low. However, this problem is surmounted through careful manipulation of the nutrient content and through an ecosystem approach. Culture can be scaled up either from laboratory culture or from culture overwintered in green house or open ponds. The latter makes the expansion process a lot faster. However, not all production facilities have the know-how to maintain a healthy culture during the cold winter months.

The maintenance of unialgal culture calls for continuous analysis of various pond parameters. The most important of these is daily microscopic examination of the culture from each pond to monitor contamination by other algae, and to detect any abnormal morphological changes that provide signs of culture deterioration. In addition to microscopic examination, various methods are employed to observe the physiological state of the algae. Routine monitoring of nutrient concentration is also essential in order to avoid nutrient limitation that can affect both the yield and the quality of the final product. Since the maintenance of high alkalinity and pH are also important for successful pond management, these are measured routinely as are depth and circulation of the ponds. Some facilities have developed simple bioassay techniques that enable them to find out causes for culture deterioration within a few hours and apply quick corrective measures in order to avoid excessive culture renewal. It is clear from the forgoing discussion that the maintenance of a unialgal culture of *Spirulina* outdoors is not an easy task. For more detailed information on this subject the reader is referred to other reviews.[24,25,33]

HARVESTING THE BIOMASS

The frequency of harvesting depends on the daily growth rate, which is dependent upon light and temperature conditions. For example, the production facility at Earthrise harvests close to 3 metric tons of *Spirulina* a day during the peak season. As described above, the culture is transferred with a pump through PVC pipes into a dedicated processing building, where it is passed over a series of stainless-steel screens to rinse and concentrate the biomass. The filtrate is transferred back to the pond while the paste from the final stage of the filtration process is pumped into a spray dryer to remove the moisture, resulting in the free-flowing fine powder.

DRYING AND PACKAGING

Proper and quick drying is an essential step of high-quality *Spirulina* production. Various types of drying systems are used in the industry for drying *Spirulina*. For economic reasons, the dryer of choice in large-scale *Spirulina* production facilities is the spray dryer. Freeze drying would give better overall product quality, but the cost is rather prohibitive. *Spirulina* droplets are sprayed into the drying chamber just long enough to flash evaporate the water. The powder is exposed to heat for a few seconds as it falls to the bottom. No preservatives, additives, or stabilizers are used in drying. This quick spray-drying process guarantees preservation of heat-sensitive nutrients, pigments, and enzymes. Efficient control of drying temperature is very important because the drying temperature can affect the moisture content, and the latter in turn affects the growth of bacteria and molds.

Proper packaging is also important for high-quality *Spirulina* production. The dried powder is weighed and vacuum-sealed into oxygen-barrier bags to minimize exposure to air and prevent possible oxidation of phytonutrients. The bags are then packed into cardboard boxes, sealed with tape, and labeled to reflect the package weight and lot numbers for tracking purposes. All reasonable precautions are taken to assure that production procedures do not contribute contamination such as filth, harmful chemicals, undesirable microorganisms, or any other objectionable material to the processed product. Under this packaging condition, the product can stay up to four years with little change in biochemical composition or nutritional properties (Tables 1.1 and 1.2).

TABLE 1.1
Nutritional Profile of *Spirulina* Powder

Composition[a]	per 100 g	Composition[a]	per 100 g
1. *Macronutrients*		2. *Vitamins*	
Calories	373	Vitamin A (as 100% β-carotene)[b]	352,000 IU
Total fat	4.3 g	Vitamin K	1090 mcg
Saturated fat	1.95 g	Thiamine HCl (Vitamin B1)	0.5 mg
Polyunsaturated fat	1.93 g	Riboflavin (Vitamin B2)	4.53 mg
Monounsaturated fat	0.26 g	Niacin (Vitamin B3)	14.9 mg
Cholesterol	<0.1 mg	Vitamin B6 (Pyridox. HCl)	0.96 mg
Total carbohydrate	17.8 g	Vitamin B12	162 mcg
Dietary fiber	7.7 g	3. *Minerals*	
Sugars	1.3 g	Calcium	468 mg
Lactose	<0.1 g	Iron	87.4 mg
Protein[b]	63 g	Phosphorus	961 mg
Essential amino acids (mg)		Iodine	142 mcg
Histidine	1000	Magnesium	319 mg
Isoleucine	3500	Zinc	1.45 mg
Leucine	5380	Selenium	25.5 mcg
Lysine	2960	Copper	0.47 mg
Methionine	1170	Manganese	3.26 mg
Phenylalanine	2750	Chromium	<400 mcg
Threonine	2860	Potassium	1,660 mg
Tryptophan	1090	Sodium	641 mg
Valine	3940	4. *Phytonutrients*	
Nonessential amino acids (mg)		Phycocyanin (mean)[b]	17.2%
Alanine	4590	Chlorophyll (mean)[b]	1.2%
Arginine	4310	Superoxide dismutase (SOD)	531,000 IU
Aspartic acid	5990	Gamma linolenic acid (GLA)	1080 mg
Cystine	590	Total carotenoids (mean)[b]	504 mg
Glutamic acid	9130	β-carotene (mean)[b]	211 mg
Glycine	3130	Zeaxanthin	101 mg
Proline	2380		
Serine	2760		
Tyrosine	2500		

[a] Most data are based on recent analysis by third-party laboratory.
[b] In-house data.
Source: Data from Earthrise 2006 production.

QUALITY ASSURANCE

Process Control

The maintenance of the quality and safety of the product depends on how the entire process from pond to powder is controlled. Process control is a very important aspect of *Spirulina* production. *Spirulina* powder is manufactured in accordance with current

TABLE 1.2
Stability and Shelf Life of *Spirulina* Powder

Lot	Initial level of carotenoids (mg/100 g)	Final level of carotenoids (mg/100 g)	Loss (%)	Time final level was measured (years)
1	479	380	21	4.5
2	495	374	25	4.5
3	452	397	22	4.5
4	498	411	17	4.4
5	520	470	10	4.3
6	471	449	5	4.3
7	477	424	12	4.3
8	486	463	5	4.3
9	464	444	4	4.2
10	493	425	14	4.2
11	487	417	15	4.2
12	521	493	5	4.1
Mean	487	429	13	4.3
STD	21	36	7	0.1
N	12	12	12	12

Note: Bulk *Spirulina* product specifications: Carotenoids >370 mg/100 g.
Source: Data from Earthrise.

good manufacturing practices (cGMPs) promulgated under the United States Federal Food, Drug, and Cosmetic Act and applicable state statutes and regulations. These laws assure that the facilities, methods, practices, and controls used in the manufacture, processing, packing, or holding of food products are in conformance with or are operated in conformity with good manufacturing practices (GMPs) to assure that the food products are safe for consumption and have been prepared, packed, and held under sanitary conditions.

All operations in receiving, inspecting, transporting, packaging, segregating, preparing, processing, and storing of the product are conducted in accord with adequate sanitation principles. Raw materials and ingredients are inspected and segregated as necessary to assure that they are clean, wholesome, and fit for processing and are stored under conditions that will protect against contamination and minimize deterioration. Packaging materials do not transmit contaminants or objectionable substances to the product, and provide adequate protection from contamination.

The quality assurance director (QCD) has the responsibility and authority to approve or reject all raw materials, in-process materials, packaging materials, and final product and labeling, and the authority to review production records to assure that no errors have occurred or, if errors have occurred, that they have been fully investigated. The QAD has the responsibility for approving or rejecting all procedures or specifications impacting on the identity, strength, quality, and purity of the final product. Adequate laboratory facilities for the testing and approval (or rejection) of raw materials, in-process materials, packaging materials, and final product are available to the QAD. The manufacturing facility is also audited and inspected for violations of GMP on a regular basis by the Quality Systems Manager (QSM). *Spirulina* facilities in the United States are subjected to periodic unannounced inspections from federal, state, and local regulatory agencies. Audits are also conducted by third-party registrars as part of an ISO 9001:2000 or equivalent programs. External laboratories are used to standardize methods and for independent verification of analytical results.

PRODUCT QUALITY AND CONSISTENCY

One aspect of high-quality *Spirulina* production is that the product must have a consistent chemical and physical property. Table 1.1 provides data on a typical chemical and physical analysis of *Spirulina* powder produced at Earthrise. The analysis was done on a blend of 21 lots of product made up of three samples taken approximately on the 10th, 20th, and 30th of each month, during the entire seven-month production season. As shown in Table 1.1, *Spirulina* contains high levels of protein, phycoyanin, total carotenoids, chlorophyll, gamma linolenic acid (GLA), iron, and vitamin B12, the latter as measured by the microbiological method. Its amino acid profile is comparable to that recommended by FAO/WHO with the exception of the sulfur amino acids and lysine.[34]

Seasonal and yearly variations in product quality are observed. However, when one considers the open nature of the production system, the consistency of biochemical composition is remarkable (Figure 1.5). This shows that while it is possible that product quality and consistency may be better in algae grown in closed bioreactors, the variation in product quality of algae grown in well-maintained open ponds is not as high as one would expect from such open systems. Data on the quality of products from closed bioreactors are lacking, making comparison difficult. Good culture and product management conditions are prerequisites for product quality, uniformity of biochemical composition, and safety.[24]

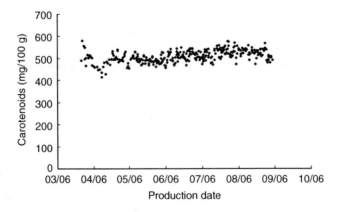

FIGURE 1.5   Seasonal variation in carotenoid content of *Spirulina* (Earthrise 2006 data).

PRODUCT SAFETY

Food safety has occupied center stage in the past few years owing to the outbreak of many pathogenic organisms, particularly in fresh produce. Problems of hygiene associated with conventional foods also apply to algae. *Spirulina* is a dry product and, drying takes care of some of the microbiological content. Despite this, good process control as part of an overall GMP is important to guarantee not only the quality and stability of the product but also its safety. The major areas of concern for safety are microbiological load, heavy metal content, pesticides, extraneous matter, and cyanobacterial toxins.

Microbial Contamination

A potential problem of open-pond *Spirulina* production is that the water may be contaminated with pathogenic organisms. Handling of the product during processing can also result in microbial contamination. The final microbial load of the product will therefore depend on how carefully the culture and product are handled at the various stages of production. Only GMPs and direct analysis of microbial flora and concentration in each lot of product can guarantee the safety of the product. The final product should meet microbiological standards set by the various national and international standards (Table 1.3) Standard plate counts (SPC) and confirmed coliform counts are used in the food industry to monitor and inspect mal-handling of food products during processing.[35] Analysis of hundreds of *Spirulina* samples from modern commercial farms in Thailand, Japan, Taiwan, and Mexico show that coliforms are rarely present,[36] indicating the generally good sanitary conditions of growth, harvest, drying, and packaging. Apparently, failure to meet microbiological standards has forced some producers to irradiate their products as evidenced by very low bacterial load, which are difficult to achieve under natural conditions. Irradiation is allowed by regulation for some foods by the FDA. However, such foods, when sold in bulk, should bear information specifying that the product has been irradiated.

Heavy Metal Contamination

As in other agricultural products, lead, mercury, cadmium, and arsenic are potential contaminants in algal products since they are components of industrial pollution and occur in trace amounts in certain agricultural fertilizers. It is known that certain microalgae are effective accumulators of heavy metals.[37] The production of high-quality *Spirulina* therefore requires the use of high-grade nutrients and a meticulous and routine analysis of heavy metals in the culture medium and the product. This is particularly important in situations where food-grade *Spirulina* is to be produced from earthen ponds or natural lakes. The soil in certain regions may have a high content of heavy metals that can easily be accumulated by the algae.

Table 1.4 shows some examples of regulatory standards for heavy metals in dietary supplements and foods.

It is important to clear a controversy that has been created by reports of questionably high mercury levels in commercial *Spirulina* products in two papers published

TABLE 1.3
Microbiological and Related Regulatory Standards

Organization	Total plate count	Total yeast + mold	Total coliforms	Fecal coliforms	Salmonella	Escherichia coli	Enterobacteria	Staphylococcus	Insect fragments	Rodent hair
AHPA[a]	10,000,000 cfu/g	100,000 cfu/g	10,000 cfu/g	No data	Absent in 10 g	Absent in 1 g	No data	No data	No data	No data
EU[b]	100,000 cfu/g	10,000 cfu/g	No data	No data	Absent in 10 g	Absent in 1 g	1000 cfu/g	Absent in 1 g	No data	No data
Canada[c]	100,000 cfu/g	10,000 cfu/g	No data	No data	Negative	Negative	No data	<100 cfu/g (cyanobacteria)	No data	No data
WHO[d]	100,000 cfu/g	1,000 cfu/g	No data	No data	Negative	10 cfu/g	1,000 cfu/g	No Data	No data	No data
NNFA[e]	50,000 cfu/g	1,000 cfu/g	10 cfu/g	Negative	Negative	Negative	No data	MPN <10 cfu/g	No data	No data
USP: dietary supp ingredients and products	<1,000 cfu/g	<100 cfu/g	No data	No data	No data	Negative (10 g)	No data	No data	No data	No data
USP: dried or powdered botanicals	<100,000 cfu/g	<1,000 cfu/g	No data	No data	Negative (10 g)	Negative (10 g)	No Data	No data	No data	No data
USFDA[f]	No data	No data	No data	No data	No data	No Data	No Data	No data	150/50 g	1/150 g
Japan pharmacopoeia	<100,000 cfu/g	<1,000 cfu/g	No data	No data	Negative	Negative	1,000 cfu/g	No data	No data	No data

[a] American Herbal Products Association: Botanicals—These are the specific recommended limits for dried raw agricultural commodities, including cut and powdered commodities that are used as botanical ingredients in dietary supplements. www.ahpa.org/guidelines.htm

[b] European Union Pharmacopoeia: Botanicals—Page 14 of Kneifel W et al (2002). Microbial contamination of medicinal plants—a review. *Planta Med* 68:5–15.

[c] Health Canada Compendium of Monographs: Plants, cyanobacteria, alga, enzymes, probiotics—Table 1A. http://www.hc-sc.gc.ca/dhp-mps/alt_formats/hpfb-dgpsa/pdf/prodnatur/compendium_mono_e.pdf

[d] World Health Organization: Botanicals—Page 5 of http://www.fda.gov/ohrms/dockets/dailys/03/Aug03/081803/96N-0417_emc-000239-01.pdf

[e] National Nutritional Food Association (now Natural Products Association) recommendations for herbal materials.

[f] United States Food and Drug Administration.

TABLE 1.4
Heavy Metal Regulatory Standards

	Arsenic	Cadmium	Lead	Mercury (Total)
USA California proposition 65[a]	10 mcg/person/day (carcinogen)	4.1 mcg/person/day (reproductive toxicity)	0.5 mcg/person/day (reproductive toxicity)	No data
USA HHS/FDA[b]	No data	55 mcg/person/d	25 mcg/person/d (pregnancy) 75 mcg/person/d (adults)	1 ppm (action level for methyl Hg)
USA ATSDR[c]	0.3 mcg/kg/d (chronic)	0.2 mcg/kg/d (chronic)	Not determined	0.3 mcg/kg/d (chronic)
Health Canada: *Spirulina*[d]	<0.14 mcg/kg bw/d	<0.09 mcg/kg bw/d	<0.29 mcg/kg bw/d	<0.29 mcg/kg bw/d
UN (WHO/FAO): JECFA[e]	2 mcg/kg bw/d	1 mcg/kg/day	3.6 mcg/kg/d	0.23 mcg/kg/d (methyl Hg) 0.1 mcg/kg/d (methyl Hg in pregnancy) 0.71 mcg/kg/d (total Hg)
EU (foodstuff) commission regulations[f]	No legislation in force (UK: 1 ppm in food)	<1 mcg/kg/d (UN)	<3.6 mcg/kg/d (UN)	0.23 mcg/kg/d (methyl Hg)

[a] California Proposition 65 Safe Harbor Levels. www.oehha.ca.gov/prop65/pdf/Aug2006StatusReport.pdf

[b] United States Food & Drug Administration (FDA): www.fda.gov The Cd and Pb values are suggested daily maximum intakes.

[c] The Agency for Toxic Substances and Disease Registry (ATSDR) is a federal public health agency of the U.S. Department of Health and Human Services. The data refer to the Minimum Risk Levels (MRLs) for chronic exposure. www.atsdr.cdc.gov/

[d] Health Canada Compendium of Monographs Table 1A: Specifications template for finished products of a plant, plant material, alga, fungus, or bacterium. www.hc-sc.gc.ca/dhp-mps/alt_formats/hpfb-dgpsa/pdf/prodnatur/compendium_mono_e.pdf

[e] United Nation's Joint FAO/WHO Expert Committee on Food Additives (JECFA) has established Provisional Tolerable Weekly Intakes (PTWI) for various heavy metals. The values in this table have been converted to daily amounts. www.who.int/ipcs/food/jecfa/en/

[f] European Union: http://ec.europa.eu/food/food/chemicalsafety/contaminants/cadmium_en.htm

by Johnson and Shubert.[38,39] A subsequent but rarely quoted study by Slotton et al.[40] has shown that the prior studies by Johnson and Shubert using inductively coupled plasma detection technology (ICAP) were faulted because of interference from iron. Using cold vapor atomic absorption and graphite furnace atomic absorption techniques that avoid iron interference, Slotton et al. found that the mercury levels reported by Johnson and Shubert were two orders of magnitude higher, whereas those reported for lead were an order of magnitude higher. Unsafe mercury levels in *Spirulina* have never been reported by any other researchers or independent testing laboratories.

Pesticides

No pesticides or herbicides should be used during the cultivation of *Spirulina*. Even though the medium's high pH discourages the persistence of many pesticide compounds,[36] it is imperative to monitor for pesticides periodically in the product. Measurements of pesticides in source water and culture water and conducting pesticide bioassays are normally used to monitor pesticide levels. Periodic analysis of more than 30 different pesticides in independent laboratories has failed to show any detectable levels of these compounds.

Extraneous Material

According to AOAC (Association of Official Analytical Chemists),[41] extraneous material is the name given to "any foreign matter in product associated with objectionable conditions or practices in production, storage, or distribution." If the extraneous matter is contributed by insects, rodents, birds, or other animal contamination, it is referred to as *filth*. The major components of extraneous matter in food products are insect fragments, rodent hair, and feather fragments. A standardized analytical method exists for counting insect fragments (AOAC[41,42]). Although the sample preparation and counting techniques are very well standardized, a lot is to be desired for the identification process. The author has sent the same preparations to three different laboratories and found results varying by two orders of magnitude. Most of the literature on identification of insect fragments is based on agricultural or storage insects and not on aquatic insects that are normally present in outdoor ponds. In addition, it is often difficult to distinguish between insect parts and plant parts, resulting in an overestimation of "unidentified insect" parts. Researchers at Earthrise Nutritionals and the University of Texas at Austin have developed a method to quantify insect fragment biomass in microalgal products using a myosin enzyme-linked immunosorbant assay (ELISA) technique.[43] This new method provides an improvement on the standard method that registers insect fragment counts irrespective of the large differences in insect fragment size that are commonly observed.

The presence of rodent hair in microalgal products is considered to be an indicator of potential contamination. It is very rare to observe rodent hair when proper pest control measures are taken (Table 1.3). Feathers, plant fragments, and any other extraneous material are normally strained during pond netting and preharvest screening.

Cyanobacterial Toxins

Reports of widespread poisoning of animals and humans[44] call for due attention to be given to the control of cyanobacterial contaminants. There is no report of cyanobacterial toxins in *Arthrospira* species to date. Although inadvertent harvest of these toxic species is a risk when harvesting algae from natural bodies of water with mixed phytoplankton populations, it is very unlikely to be a problem in properly controlled and properly managed monoculture of *Arthrospira*. Nevertheless, it is essential to monitor these cyanobacterial toxins in the product. To this effect, in 1995–1996, a group of leading microalgae and cyanobacteria producers including Cyanotech Corporation and Earthrise Nutritionals LLC sponsored research conducted by phytoplankton toxicologists. The result was a Technical Booklet for the Microalgae Biomass Industry (MBI) as a guide to the use of a very sensitive ELISA and a protein phosphate inhibition assay (PPIA) for the detection of toxic microcystins and nodularins. These methods enable the detection, monitoring, and controlling of cyanotoxins, so producers can assure a safe product for human food supplements.[45]

REGULATORY STATUS OF *SPIRULINA*

GRAS (GENERALLY RECOGNIZED AS SAFE) STATUS

Cyanotech Corporation of Hawaii and Earthrise Nutritionals LLC of California are the only *Spirulina* producers in the world that have determined their *Spirulina* as GRAS through scientific procedures and FDA review. "GRAS" is an acronym for the phrase "Generally Recognized As Safe." Under sections 201(s) and 409 of the Federal Food, Drug, and Cosmetic Act, any substance that is intentionally added to food is a food additive that is subject to premarket review and approval by FDA, unless the substance is generally recognized, among qualified experts, as having been adequately shown to be safe under the conditions of its intended use, or unless the use of the substance is otherwise excluded from the definition of a food additive. Under sections 201(s) and 409 of the Act, and FDA's implementing regulations in 21 CFR 170.3 and 21 CFR 170.30, the use of a food substance may be GRAS either through scientific procedures or, for a substance used in food before 1958, through experience based on common use in food. Under 21 CFR 170.30(b), general recognition of safety through scientific procedures requires the same quantity and quality of scientific evidence as is required to obtain approval of the substance as a food additive and ordinarily is based upon published studies, which may be corroborated by unpublished studies and other data and information. The GRAS determination by the two US companies was based on an extensive review of the published information on the safety of *Spirulina* and on a thorough description of their process and their GMP and Quality Assurance Program (QAP).

FOOD AND DIETARY SUPPLEMENT GMPS

Spirulina is regulated as food and as a dietary supplement. The latter is a subset of food and falls under FDA's regulation. As discussed earlier, *Spirulina* is produced under FDA GMPs for food. The FDA has recently released a separate regulation for dietary supplement GMP. Nevertheless, some companies have already attained dietary supplement GMP certification through the industry's (Natural Products Association) certification program. The two facilities in the United States are subject to inspection by federal, state, and local regulatory bodies.

DIETARY SUPPLEMENT HEALTH AND EDUCATION ACT (DSHEA)
AND *SPIRULINA*

Spirulina is sold in health food stores and similar outlets as a dietary supplement. There appears to be a lack of understanding about their regulatory status. Until 1994 dietary supplements were regulated as foods by FDA. However, with passage of the Dietary Supplement Health and Education Act of 1994 (DSHEA), Congress amended the food regulations to include several provisions that apply only to dietary supplements and dietary ingredients of dietary supplements. As a result of these provisions, dietary ingredients used in dietary supplements are no longer subject to the pre-market safety evaluations required of other new food ingredients or for new uses of old food ingredients. They must, however, meet the requirements of other safety provisions. FDA defines a dietary supplement as "a product (other than tobacco) that is intended to supplement the diet that bears or contains one or more of the following dietary ingredients: a vitamin, a mineral, an herb or other botanical, an amino acid, a dietary substance for use by man to supplement the diet by increasing the total daily intake, or a concentrate, metabolite, constituent, extract, or combinations of these ingredients." Under DSHEA a dietary supplement is adulterated if it or one of its ingredients presents "a significant or unreasonable risk of illness or injury" when used as directed on the label, or under normal conditions of use. If a dietary supplement contains a new dietary ingredient (i.e., an ingredient not marketed for dietary supplement use in the United States before October 15, 1994), it may be considered adulterated when there is inadequate information to provide reasonable assurance that the ingredient will not present a significant or unreasonable risk of illness or injury. DSHEA was enacted to meet the concerns of consumers and manufacturers to help ensure that safe and appropriately labeled products remain available to those who want to use them, and taking into consideration "that there may be a positive relationship between sound dietary practice and good health, and that, although further scientific research is needed, there may be a connection between dietary supplement use, reduced healthcare expenses, and disease prevention." The DSHEA provides for the use of various types of claims or statements on the label of dietary supplements, although claims may not be made about the use of a dietary supplement to diagnose, prevent, mitigate, treat, or cure a specific disease. A disclaimer must be placed on the label to this effect. Claims related to effects of a dietary supplement on the structure and function of the body are allowed. In this regard there are several structure and function claims made for *Spirulina* by manufacturers. The structure and function claims that are made for *Spirulina* point mainly to its immunomodulation, and antioxidant/anti-inflammatory effects. These claims are made on the basis of the review of the scientific evidence to support such a claim. DSHEA stipulates that there is evidence to support the claim but FDA does not require submission of such information for approval of a substance as a dietary supplement. Health Canada, the Canadian equivalent of the US FDA, does require submission of the evidence before approval for marketing of products and because of this allows similar or stronger claims to be made without any disclaimer. For more information on DSHEA the reader is referred to the following FDA website: www.cfsan.fda.gov/~dms/dietsupp.html

ENVIRONMENTAL ASPECTS OF *SPIRULINA* PRODUCTION

There are some environmental advantages of growing *Spirulina* that are worth mentioning. These features of *Spirulina* become especially important if developments in technology bring cost of production to make it a protein source competitive enough with the current cheap sources of protein like soya beans. *Spirulina* production is not associated with some of the environmental degradations like soil erosion, water contamination, and deforestation that are so commonly encountered in conventional crop production.[46] The following features of *Spirulina* production are important in this respect:

1. *Spirulina* is grown in marginal land unsuitable for conventional agriculture. It can also be grown in sea water, and thus there is a vast potential to grow it in the coastal areas of the tropical and subtropical areas of the world where again the land is not useful for conventional agriculture.
2. *Spirulina* requires lower land area utilization on a protein production basis (20 times less land than soybeans).
3. More efficient water use on a protein basis (one-third of the water needed for soy, one-fifth of that of corn).
4. *Spirulina* production is energy efficient (3.5 times more efficient than soy production).
5. Unlike most conventional crops and other feed or food products, the biomass produced is wholesome, with all components being used as food and no biomass waste to deal with.
6. The cell wall of *Spirulina* is not composed of indigestible cellulose as in other plants. It is composed of more than 60% protein on dry weight basis, the rest being composed of carbohydrates and fats. As such it is easily digested and wholly utilized.
7. The culture system is a closed-loop system where the nutrients are recycled completely with minimal discharge to the environment.
8. Owing to the fast growth rate of the algae (turnover time of about 4–5 days), nutrients are stripped off the medium at a very fast rate, leaving virtually no detectable levels at the end of the growth season.
9. Although *Spirulina* production currently uses carbon dioxide from commercial sources, it can conceivably use carbon dioxide from power plants, thus contributing to CO_2 mitigation.
10. No pesticides or herbicides are needed for its production, thus minimizing environmental pollution.

WORLDWIDE PRODUCTION OF *SPIRULINA* AND ITS CURRENT USE

Arthrospira (*Spirulina*) is currently grown commercially in several countries. The major producers of *Spirulina* are the DIC group of companies, Earthrise Nutritionals in California, USA; Hainan DIC Marketing in Hainan Island, China; and Siam Algae Company in Bangkok, Thailand. Together these facilities produce about 1000 metric tons of *Spirulina* annually. The other major producer is Cyanotech Corporation of Hawaii with an annual production of 300 tons of *Spirulina*. There are also many producers mainly from the Asia-Pacific region, especially in China and India.[47] According to Wu,[48] there were once between 100 and 120 producers of *Spirulina* in China with annual production ranging from 15 to 300 tons. Total production during that period was estimated to be about 500 tons. Current production of *Spirulina* in China is estimated to be about 1500 tons. It is difficult to know the total worldwide production of *Spirulina*. It is probably in the order of 3000–4000 metric tons (personal communication with producers and researchers).

Currently *Spirulina* is used in various food application such as juice smoothies, confectionary, food bars, baked desserts, doughnuts, muffins, pasta, salad dressing, frozen desserts, snack foods, popcorn, corn chips, crackers, breakfast cereals, liquid or instant meals, instant soup, gnocchi, and even specialty beer. *Spirulina* is also widely used as an animal feed supplement.[49] The increasing scientific and clinical evidence for its nutritional and potential health benefits[50] is also attracting its use as a functional food in addition to its already established use as a dietary supplement.

CONCLUDING REMARKS

Spirulina has been used as food for centuries. Several toxicity tests including some sponsored by the United Nations have proven its safety. Moreover, it has been produced commercially over the past 30 years and consumed by thousands of people without problem. Recently, two companies in the United States have affirmed their *Spirulina* as GRAS by scientific procedures and after FDA review. In addition, the production process and the product are regulated by applicable laws and regulations to make sure that the product is safe and meets label specifications. Numerous studies show that it has a good nutritional profile in addition to containing some phytonutrients that have potential health benefits as discussed in the reviews in this book.

The technology of *Spirulina* production has also advanced in the past 30 years, resulting in better quality of product at relatively lower cost. *Spirulina* has attracted the attention of researchers for many years, as shown by the thousands of publications in its various aspects. More and more information is being made available about its biology, biotechnological application, and health application and even in what seem to be remote applications like biofuel production and as a life support system in space exploration. This interest will no doubt continue. Research along these lines will be rewarding both socially and professionally.

ACKNOWLEDGMENTS

I am grateful to Brian Wood who introduced me to the algae early in my college life and to my mentor, the late Professor G. E. Fogg, FRS. My thanks also go to past Earthrise associates, Yoshimichi Ota, Robert Henrikson, and Hidenori Shimamatsu for their constant encouragement. I am indebted to Juan Chavez and all current associates at

Earthrise for their support and inspiration. I thank Jackie Montes and Mohammed Youssefi for their assistance during the preparation of this manuscript.

REFERENCES

1. Geitler, L. (1932) Cyanophyceae. In: *Rabenhorst's Kryptogamenflora von Deutschland, Ostereiich nd der Scheweiz*, Vol. 14, pp. 916–931, Akad Verlag, Leipzig.
2. Gomont, M. (1892) Monographie des Oscillatoriees. *Annales des Sciences Naturelles (Botanique)*. Series 7, 15: 91–264.
3. Guglielmi, G., Rippka, R. and Tandaeau De Marsac, N. (1993) Main properties that justify the different taxonomic position of *Spirulina* spp. and *Arthrospira* spp. among cyanobacteria. *Bull. Inst. Oceanogr. Monaco*, 12: 13–23.
4. Tomaselli, L. (1997) Morphology, ultrastructure and taxonomy of *Arthrospira (Spirulina) maxima* and *Arthrospira (Spirulina) platensis*. In: Vonshak, A. (Ed) *Spirulina platensis (Arthrospira): Physiology, Cell Biology,and Biotechnology*, pp. 1–19, Taylor and Francis Ltd. London.
5. Cohen, Z. and Vonshak, A. (1991) Fatty acid composition of *Spirulina* and *Spirulina-like* cyanobacteria in relation to their chemotaxonomy. *Phytochemistry* 30: 205.
6. Nelissen, B., Wilmotte, A., De Baere, R., Haes, F., Van De Peer, Y., Neefs, J. M. and De Wachter, R. (1992) Phylogenetic study of cyanobacteria on the basis of 16S ribosomal RNA sequences. *Belg. J. Bot.* 125: 210–213.
7. Scheldeman, P., Baurain, D., Bouhy, R., Scott, M., Whitton, BA, Belay, A. and Wilmotte, A. (1999) *Arthrospira (Spirulina)* strains from four continents are resolved into only two clusters, based on amplified ribosomal DNA restriction analysis of the internally transcribed spacer. *FEMS Microbiol. Lett.* 172(2): 213–222.
8. Baurain, D., Renquin, L., Grubisic, S., Scheldeman, P., Belay, A. and Wilmotte, A. (2002) Remarkable conservation of internally transcribed spacer sequences of *Arthrospira* ("*Spirulina*") (Cyanophyceae, Cyanobacteria) strains from four continents and of recent and 30-year-old dried samples from Africa. *J. Phycol.* 38: 384–393.
9. Mühling, M., Sommerfield, P. J., Harris, N., Belay, A. and Whitton, B. A. (2006) Phenotypic analysis of *Arthrospira (Spirulina)* strains (Cyanobacteria). *Phycologia* 45: 148–157.
10. Boone, D. R. and Castenholz, R. W. [Eds] (2001) The *Archaea* and the deeply branching and phototrophic Bacteria. *Bergeys Manual of Systematic Bacteriology*, 2nd ed., Vol. 1, Springer Verlag, New York.
11. Schopf, J. W. (1993) Microfossils of the early Archean Apex chert: new evidence of the antiquity of life. *Science* 260: 64–646.
12. Schopf, J. W. (2000) The fossil record: tracing the roots of the cyanobacterial lineage. In: Whitton, B. and Potts, M. (Eds) *The Ecology of Cyanobacteria Their Diversity in Time and Space*, pp. 13–35, Kluwer Academic Publishers, The Netherlands.
13. Castenholz, R. W. (1992) Species usage, concept and evolution in the cyanobacteria (blue-green algae). *J. Phycol.* 28: 737–745.
14. Jassby, A. (1988a) *Spirulina*: A model for microalgae as human food. In: Lembi, C. A. and Waaland, J. R. (Eds) *Algae and Human Affairs*, pp. 149–179, Cambridge University Press, Cambridge.
15. Cifferi, 0. (1983) *Spirulina*, the edible microorganism. *Microbiol. Rev.* 47: 551.
16. Farrar, W. V. (1966) Tecuitlatl: a glimpse of Aztec food technology. *Nature* 211: 341–342.

17. Dangeard, P. (1940) Sur une algue bleue alimentaire pour l'homme: *Arthrospira platensis* (Nordst.) *Gomont. Actes Soc. Linn. Boreaux Extr. Proces-verbaux*, 91: 39.

18. Leonard, J. (1966) The 1964–1865 Belgian Trans-Saharan expedition. *Nature* 209: 126–128.

19. Leonard, J. and Compare, P. (1967) *Spirulina platensis* (Gom) Geitl., algue bleue de grande valeur alimentaire par sa richeseen proteins. *Bull. Jard. Bot.nat. Belg.* 37: 3–23.

20. Abdulquader, G., Barsanti, L. and Tredici, M. (2000) Harvest of *Arthrospira platensis* from Lake Kossorom (Chad) and its household usage among the Kanembu. *J. Appl. Phycol.* 12: 493–498.

21. Vareschi, E. (1978) The ecology of Lake Nakuru (Kenya) I. Abundance and feeding of the lesser flamingo. *Oecologia* 32: 11–35.

22. Talling, J. F., Wood, R. B., Prosser, M. V. and Baxter, R. M. (1973) The upper limit of photosynthetic productivity by phytoplankton: evidence from Ethiopian soda lakes. *Freshwater Biol.* 3: 53–56.

23. Kebede, E. and Ahlgren, G. (1996) Optimum growth conditions and light utilization efficiency of *Spirulina platensis* (= *Arthrospira fusiformis*) (Cyanophyta) from Lake Chitu, Ethiopia. *Hydrobiologia* 332: 99–109.

24. Belay, A. (1997) Mass culture of *Spirulina* outdoors: The Earthrise Farms experience. In: Vonshak, A. (Ed) *Spirulina platensis (Arthrospira): Physiology, Cell-Biology and Biotechnology*, pp. 131–158, Taylor & Francis Ltd, London.

25. Richmond, A. (2004) Biological principles of mass cultivation. In: Richmond, A. (Ed) *Handbook of Microalgal Culture*, pp. 125–177, Blackwell Publishing, Ames, USA.

26. Lee, Y. K. (2001) Microalgal mass culture systems and methods: Their limitation and potential. *J. Appl. Phycol.* 13: 307–315.

27. Shimamatsu, H. (2004) Mass production of *Spirulina*, an edible microalga. *Hydrobiologia* 512: 39–44.

28. Borowitzka, M. (2005) Culturing microalgae in outdoor ponds. In: Anderson, R. (Ed) *Algal Culturing Techniques*, pp. 205–218, Elsevier Academic Press, New York.

29. Dodd, J. C. (1986) Elements of pond design and construction. In: Richmond, A. (Ed), *CRC Handbook of Microalgal Mass Culture*, pp. 265–283. CRC Press, Boca Raton, Florida.

30. Oswald, W. J. (1988) Large-scale algal culture systems (engineering aspects). In: Borowitzka, M. A. and Borowitzka, L. J. (Eds) *Micro-algal Biotechnology*, pp. 357–398, Cambridge University Press, Cambridge.

31. Shimamatsu, H. (1987) A pond for edible *Spirulina* production and its hydraulic studies. *Hydrobiologia* 151/152: 83–89.

32. Zarouk, C. (1966) Contribution a l'etude d'une cyanophycee. Influence de divers facteurs physiques et chimiques sur la croissance et la photosynthese de *Spirulina maxima* (Setch. et Gardner) Geitler, PhD thesis, University of Paris, France.

33. Vonshak, A. (1997) Outdoor mass production of *Spirulina*: The basic concept. In: Vonshak, A. (Ed) *Spirulina platensis (Arthrospira): Physiology, Cell Biology, and Biotechnology*, pp. 79–99, Taylor and Francis Ltd. London.

34. Dillon, J. C. and Phan, P. A. (1993) *Spirulina* as a source of proteins in human nutrition. *Bull. Inst. Oceanogr. Monaco.* 12: 103–107.

35. US FDA (1998) *Bacteriological Analytical Manual.* 8th ed. AOAC International, Gaithersburg, Maryland.

36. Jassby, A. (1988b) *Spirulina:* A model for microalgae as human food. In: Lembi, C. A. and Waaland, J. R. (Eds) *Algae and Human Affairs*, pp. 181–202, Cambridge University Press, Cambridge.

37. Lacquerbe, B., Busson, F. and Maigrot, M. (1970) On the mineral composition of two cyanophytes, *Spirulina platensis* (Gom) Geitler and *S. geitleri J.* de Toni, *C. R. Acad. Sci. Paris. Ser. D* 270: 2130.
38. Johnson, P. E. and Shubert, L. E. (1986a) Availability of iron to rats from *Spirulina*, a blue-green alga. *Nutr. Res.* 6: 85–94.
39. Johnson, P. E. and Shubert, L. E. (1986b) Accumulation of mercury and other elements by *Spirulina* (Cyanophyceae). *Nutr. Rep. Int.* 34: 1063–1070.
40. Slotton, D. G., Goldman, C. R. and Franke, A. (1989) Commercially-grown *Spirulina* found to contain low levels of mercury and lead. *Nutr. Rep. Int.* 40: 1165–1172.
41. AOAC (1990a) *Official Methods of Analysis*, 15th ed, Helrich, K. (Ed) p. 372, Association of Official Analytical Chemists, Inc., Arlington.
42. AOAC (1990b) *Official Methods of Analysis*, 15th ed, First (Suppl), Helrich, K. (Ed), p.17, Association of Official Analytical Chemists, Inc., Arlington.
43. Belay, A., Kato, T. and Ota, Y. (1996) *Spirulina (Arthrospira)*: potential application as an animal feed supplement. *J. Appl. Phycol.* 8: 303–311.
44. Carmichael, W. W. (1994). The toxins of cyanobacteria. *Sci. Am.* 78–86.
45. An, J. and Carmichael, W. W. (1996). *Technical booklet for the microalgae biomass industry: detection of microcystins and nodularins using an enzyme linked immunosorbant assay (ELISA)and a protein phosphatase inhibition assay (PPIA).* Dept. of Biological Sciences, Wayne State University, Dayton, OH.
46. Henrikson, R. (1997) *Earthfood Spirulina*, p. 187, Renore Enterprises, Inc., Kenwood, California.
47. Lee, Y. K. (1997) Commercial production of microalgae in the Asia-Pacific rim. *J. Appl. Phycol.* 9: 403–411.
48. Wu, B., Xiang, W. and Tseng, C. K. (1998) *Spirulina* cultivation in China. *Chin. J. Oceanol. Limnol.* 16 (Suppl): 152–157.
49. Belay, A., Kato, T. and Ota, Y. (1996) *Spirulina (Arthrospira)*: potential application as an animal feed supplement. *J. Appl. Phycol.* 8: 303–311.
50. Belay, A. (2002) The potential application of *Spirulina (Arthrospira)* as a nutritional and therapeutic supplement in health management. *J. Am. Nutraceut. Assoc.* 5(2): 27–48.

2 Toxicologic Studies and Antitoxic Properties of *Spirulina*

Germán Chamorro-Cevallos, Blanca Lilia Barrón, and Jorge Vázquez-Sánchez

CONTENTS

INTRODUCTION

Spirulina sp. (*Arthrospira* sp.) is a photosynthetic, filamentous nondifferentiated, spiral-shaped, multicellular, and blue-green microalga that grows naturally in warm climates.[1,2] The most commonly used species of *Spirulina* are *Spirulina platensis* (*S. platensis*) and *Spirulina maxima*.[3]

Today, there are several companies producing *Spirulina* as a food supplement, which is sold in many health food stores around the world.[4] On the other hand, about 30% of the current world production of 2000 ton is sold for animal food applications.[5] *Spirulina* is being grown in the United States, Hawaii, Thailand, Taiwan, Chile, Vietnam, India, Japan, Cuba, Spain, Argentina, Mexico, India, and other countries.[6]

Biochemical analyses on some *Spirulina* strains have shown that this alga is potentially of considerable importance in human and health nutrition. It is a rich source of proteins, vitamins, essential amino acids, minerals, essential fatty acids including γ-linoleic acid, glycolipids, and sulfolipids[7,8], as well as phycobilins (such as phycocyanin)[9] and other phytochemicals.[10] Likewise, determination in rats of net protein utilization, protein efficiency ratio, and repletion testing have shown its high nutritional value of *Spirulina*.[11,12]

While some pharmacological activities had been previously reviewed in publications by Khan et al.,[3] Belay et al.,[4,10] Chamorro et al.,[13,14] over the past few years, additional pharmacological properties have been reported or confirmed. Thus *Spirulina* shows antiviral,[15] antibacterial,[16] antiplatelet,[17] hypocholesterolemic,[18] anti-inflammatory,[19] and anti-Parkinson[20] activities. It is also involved in preventing cataracts,[21] cerebral ischemia,[22,23] acute allergic rhinitis,[24] and vascular reactivity.[25] Many of the above properties are attributed to the antioxidant activity[26–28] of the alga as a whole, or that of particular ingredients such as phycocyanin.[29–33]

The purpose of this chapter is to provide an overview on the work conducted in relation to the toxicity as well as the antitoxic properties of *Spirulina*, as determined in laboratory animals or other experimental models.

TOXICOLOGICAL STUDIES

Food is an exceedingly complex mixture of nutrients and nonnutrient substance.[34] Hence, before any new food item is considered safe for human consumption, it has to undergo a series of detailed test for toxicology to prove it is indeed safe. The material has to be analyzed for toxic compounds, followed by toxicology evaluations including short, medium and long-term studies.

Toxic compounds can be classified into two categories, that is, biogenic and nonbiogenic toxins. According to this classification, the first group includes all those compounds that are either synthesized by cells or made by the decomposition of metabolic products. The second group involves environmental pollutants and other substances, mostly anthropogenic, entering the algal culture from the outside and absorbed and accumulated by algal cells.[35]

BIOGENIC TOXIC SUBSTANCES

Toxins

The term toxin usually refers to a substance that is highly poisonous to other living organisms, and that comes from a protein or conjugated protein produced by plants, animals, fungi, and pathogenic bacteria.[36,37]

At least 12 different species of Cyanobacteria have been shown to produce different toxins[38] affecting the nervous, hepatic, and dermatologic systems, although the mechanism of action is still unknown.[39] Some *Spirulina* samples have been tested for aflatoxin, ochratoxin A, sterigmatocystin, citrinin, patulin, penicillin acid, zearalenone, diacetoxyscirpenol, and thrichothecene. None of these compounds could be detected in the alga, as can be seen in different animal experiments conducted so far, where no toxicity was found.[40]

Nucleic Acids

Nucleic acids may be considered as biogenic substances and are repeatedly blamed for major limitations in the use of algae and other microorganisms as sources of food.[35]

Because uric acid is produced in humans and other mammals when purines are metabolized and since high levels of this metabolite may result in pathological conditions such as gout while also representing a risk factor for coronary heart disease, the high content of nucleic acid in microbial cells used as food or feed is a constant source of concern.[41] Gout and hyperuricemia usually occur after the age of 30 and are more frequently found in men.[42] Gout affects about 3 out of 1000 people[43] and is characterized by deposits of monosodium urate crystals in tissues.[44]

The normal plasma uric acid concentration in men is 5.1 ± 0.9 mg 100 mL^{-1} and that in women is about 1 mg less. Most authorities agree that 6.0 mg of uric acid per 100 mL plasma is the lower limit for the high-risk population.[35] Thus the daily intake of nucleic acids resulting from single cell protein (SCP) should not be more than 2 g with the total nucleic acid from all sources not exceeding 4 g per day. Accordingly, a maximum daily intake of 30 g algae is recommended in order to have a safety margin.[11]

NONBIOGENIC TOXIC SUBSTANCES

Metals

As a result of industrialization and changes in the environment, heavy metal pollution has become a serious problem for humans and other organisms.[45]

Metals are a unique class of toxicants that occur and persist in nature, but their chemical form may be changed by physical-chemical, biological, or anthropogenic activities.[46] They are neither created nor destroyed by organisms (plants, animals, or humans) because as chemical elements they cannot be degraded beyond their elemental state.[47]

Metals are naturally redistributed in the environment by both geologic and biological cycles, the latter of which include bioconcentration by plants and animals and incorporation into food cycles. Human industrial activity may shorten the time of metals in ore, form new compounds, and greatly enhance worldwide distribution by disposal into land, water, and the atmosphere.[48]

It is a well-known fact that virtually all microorganisms are capable of accumulating heavy metals at concentrations that are several orders of magnitude higher than those present in the surrounding media. Their accumulation in algae is a relatively rapid process.[35] In *Spirulina*, special attention has been paid to the concentration of heavy metals (lead, cadmium, mercury, and arsenic).[11]

On the other hand, various algae strains have shown appropriate properties for heavy-metal removal from wastewater.[49] This biosorption property of *Spirulina* has been used for removing metals such as lead,[50,51] cadmium,[52] and chromium.[53]

Some of the toxic effects of these metals involve hematopathies, neuropathies, nephropathies, and carcinogenesis attributed to lead; pulmonary edema, nausea, vomiting, abdominal pain, prostate, and lung cancer attributed to cadmium; neuropathies, teratogenesis, and mutagenesis attributed to mercury; and both central nervous system (CNS) and peripheral nervouos system (PNS) pathologies, including muscle weakness and loss of sensory perception, attributed to arsenic.[47]

To illustrate the extent of heavy metals found in algal samples, selected analytical data found in the literature are summarized in Table 2.1 and are compared to recommendations on upper limits of heavy-metal contents in different food goods.[54] Estimates differ widely, depending on the origin of the algal samples as well as on the laboratories doing the analyses.[11]

Several concentrations detected in the algal samples can be seen to exceed the recommended limit. The main causes for these high levels are environmental pollutants, owing to unfavorable locations of algal plants as well as to contamination introduced through water and fertilizers. Moreover, under alkaline conditions and in the presence of phosphate and sulfate ions from fertilizers, dissolved cadmium and lead ions in the medium produce slightly soluble compounds that precipitate or can

TABLE 2.1

Heavy-Metal Concentrations in *Spirulina* Compared with International Recommendations (Data Given in p.p.m.)

Sample	As	Pb	Hg	Cd	Reference
Limits in SCP	2.0	5.0	0.1	1.0	92
Spirulina (India)	0.97	3.95	0.07	0.62	93
Spirulina (Mexico)	2.9	5.1	0.5	0.5	94
Spirulina (Chad)	1.8	3.7	0.5	—	94
Spirulina (Chile)	<0.002	<0.002	<0.0005		57

Source: From reference 35, modified.

float when attached to small particles. These particles are harvested together with algal biomass and subsequently found in algal material after processing.[35]

WHO recommends maximum intake levels of heavy metals from SCP sources. Adults weighing 60 kg should take in no more than 3 mg of lead, 0.5 mg of cadmium and 0.3 mg of mercury and 20 mg of arsenic per week.[54]

Organic Compounds

Another group of nonbiogenic hazardous pollutants found in algal samples include organic compounds such as polychlorinated biphenyls. In rat studies these compounds were shown to be involved in carcinogenesis. In addition the liver is quite sensitive to the effects of these compounds, resulting in increased organ weight, hypertrophy, and proliferation of smooth endoplasmic reticulum.[37] Polycyclic aromatic hydrocarbons, on the other hand, are also significant pollutants showing mutagenic and carcinogenic effects on experimental animals.[55] No reports about either of these compounds in *Spirulina* were found.

N-Nitroso Derivatives

Studies of *N*-nitroso derivatives have been carried out in India. Although the concentrations of *N*-nitroso derivatives such as dialkylnitrosamines of dimethyl- and dipentyl nitrosopiperidine, nitrosomorholine, and nitrosopyrrolidine were found in *Spirulina* samples, the levels were below the 0.1 μg kg^{-1} detection limit. Naturally these contaminants differ from place to place and from season to season, resulting in significant variations of the analytical data.[35]

Pesticides

It has been well established that micro algal cells provide a larger surface area for attracting pesticide molecules and that they help to predict the extent of pollution in aquatic systems. Among pesticides, organochlorides are the most persistent substances.[55]

Analyses conducted in samples of Mexican *Spirulina* found only traces (<0.001 parts per million) of certain organochloride pesticides such as p,p'-dichloro,-diphenyl trichloro etane (DDT) and its metabolites, and confirmed that *Spirulina* is free of other pesticides,[56] which are less toxic than the organophosphate type.

SANITARY ANALYSES

Testing for bacterial contamination was performed with fresh cultures and dried *Spirulina* material. Outdoor cultures of this alga had an initial bacterial contamination of 2.0×10^4 CFU mL^{-1}, which increased to 7.0×10^4 mL^{-1} after 10 days. Bacterial contamination is to be expected, as commercial algae cultures have usually been exposed in basins where neither the medium nor the environment is sterile.[35]

However, analyses carried out in Mexico have shown no contamination above the permitted levels according to protein and calorie advisory group (PAG) and

International union of pure and applied chemistry (IUAC) stipulations. This is mainly due to sterilization of the algal powder at 120°C.[11] Besides bacteria, no reports could be found in the literature on contamination by mould, yeast, fungi, and zooplankton in *Spirulina* cultures.[35]

Moreover, in *Spirulina* samples from Chile no insects, insect fragments, hair or excretions were found alimentos esenciales para la humanidad (AEH).

SAFETY EVALUATIONS

In addition to analytical studies on biogenic and nonbiogenic toxic substances found in *Spirulina* algae, safety evaluations have also been conducted involving acute, subchronic, chronic, teratogenic, mutagenic, carcinogenic, and multiple generation effects.

Some studies discussed in this chapter were conducted on *Spirulina* from Sosa Texcoco, a company no longer in existence, and were supported by the United Nations Industrial Development Organization (UNIDO).[58] Other studies have been conducted in various institutions in several countries around the world with different *Spirulina* samples. Sometimes, studies have been conducted with phycocyanin, the main component of *Spirulina* color.

In most safety evaluation studies of *Spirulina*, rats and mice have been used because of several advantages: they are easy to house, require relatively low quantities of test substances, are well understood with ample historical control data, have short life spans as well as good regulatory acceptance, have genetic consistency and a metabolism that tends to be rapid, and present systemic exposure lower than in humans.[59]

Unless specified, most of our short and long-term studies incorporated dried algae into the experimental diets at levels (w/w) of 0 (control), 10, 20, and 30%.[58]

Studies by other authors employed different dose and concentrations and a variance of environmental conditions in the laboratories, where testing was conducted.

ACUTE TOXICITY TESTS

Acute toxicity is defined as adverse effects occurring because of short-term administration of a single dose or multiple doses given within 24 h. The most frequently used acute toxicity test is the determination of the median lethal dose (LD_{50}). LD_{50} has been defined as a statistically derived expression of a single dose of a material that can be expected to kill half of the experimental animals.[55]

Acute toxicity tests give a quantitative estimate of acute toxicity, identify target organs and other clinical manifestations of acute toxicity, establish the reversibility of toxic responses, and provide dose-ranging guidance for other studies.[36] This test is usually a valid predictor of the response seen in humans.[60]

Some authors recommend accompanying this test with a histological analysis similar to the one conducted with phycocyanin. Table 2.2 shows that the LD_{50} value for phycocyanin in one study was >5000 mg/kg, which belongs to the "practically nontoxic" category, according to one of the LD_{50} range tables.[61] This value has not been determined for *Spirulina* and only as much as 800 mg/kg was given to rats with

TABLE 2.2
Spirulina Short- and Long-Term Toxicity Studies*

Study	Animals	Methods and results summary	Reference
Acute	Rats	The oral treatment with as much as 800 mg/kg produced no alterations in body weight or organs. Tissues showed normal histology. Also there was no allergic skin reaction with an application of as much as 2000 mg/kg.	95
	Rats	Phycocyanin isolated from *Spirulina* given orally (0.5–5 g/kg) added with the feed induced no toxicity symptoms or mortality in animals. At terminal autopsy no macroscopic or microscopic changes were seen on vital organs.	96
Subchronic	Rats	The continuous feeding of dried algae to young rats at a dietary level of 10% of *Spirulina* for 3 months did not evoke deleterious effects in general appearance, behavior, mortality, hematology, serum analysis, urine composition, organ weights, and histopathological examination.	63
	Rats	Animals were fed for 2 or 4 months on diets having 60% of their protein replaced by *Spirulina*. There was an increase in kidney, heart, and lung weight and the appearance of a nephrocalcinosis syndrome prevalent in the female rat which was present in the control as well as experimental groups.	64
	Rats	Feeding 10% *Spirulina* for 12 weeks as the only source of protein in the diet resulted in significantly lower weight gains compared to a casein control group. All rats survived the experimental period in apparently good health. All organs were normal macroscopically and microscopically.	40
	Rats	*Spirulina* given for 13 weeks produced no toxic effects on hematology, serum chemistry, semiquantitative analysis of urine or tissues. Body weights of the test animals were slightly lower than in the control in both sexes.	97
	Mice	*Spirulina* given for 13 weeks showed no effects on mouse behavior, food and water intake, growth, or survival. Hematology, clinical chemistry and histopathology values did not reveal differences compared to the control animals.	98
Chronic	Rats	Rat tolerance to a 100-day period of feeding on *Spirulina*-rich diets with a final concentration of 36 and 48% of protein, respectively, was good and no histological abnormalities were found in several organs examined.	99
	Rats	*Spirulina* at the maximum protein portion (14.25%) was given to rats for 18 months, resulting in no obvious toxicity signs.	94
	Rats	Although hematological tests such as Hb and SGPT showed some statistical differences after 6 months, abnormal findings were not detected in growth and external appearance of the whole body or in the shape, weight and histological findings of organs.	100
	Rats	*Spirulina* was given for 86 weeks in experimental diets. No adverse effects on hematology or urine were observed at the different time periods, and no changes on serum biochemistry were found. No differences in macroscopic or histopathological findings were found.	65

* Unless otherwise specified, *Spirulina* was added to the diet at 10, 20, and 30% concentrations, using the corresponding controls.

no toxic effects seen. However, such a value in relation to *Spirulina* is not expected to exceed that of phycocyanin as the latter is on of its components.

SUBCHRONIC TOXICITY TESTS

The primary purpose of a subchronic study as part of the toxicological appraisal of a xenobiotic is the characterization of its physiological impact following repeated administrations over a significant fraction (10%) of the life span of the test species.[62]

Subchronic toxicity studies on *Spirulina* have been conducted by some researchers. There have been some differences, mainly in preparing the feeds given to the animals, the administration time, and the type of analysis conducted. In studies conducted in our laboratory, the consumption of food and water and the weight gain were measured. Hemoglobin concentration, total red blood cell counts, packed cell volume, and total and differential leukocyte counts were analyzed. The biochemical analysis determined the concentrations of asparte-aminotransferase, glucose, urea nitrogen, cholesterol, and proteins. At the end of the study animals were humanely killed and the brain, heart, liver, spleen, kidneys, gonads, and seminal vesicles were weighed. Samples of these organs, stomach, and duodenum were fixed and microscopically examined for morphological effects that may have correlated with other changes seen *in vivo* or in clinical pathology. As summarized in Table 2.2 *Spirulina*, even at very high concentrations, produced no adverse effects, which coincides with the findings of other authors.[40,63,64]

CHRONIC TOXICITY TESTS

Chronic toxicity testing is performed to assess the cumulative toxicity of chemicals, often including a consideration of the carcinogenic potential of chemical.[36] Chronic toxicity studies involve repeated administrations over the entire life-span of the test animals or at least a major fraction thereof.[46]

For this study *Spirulina* was included in the feed at the same concentrations as in the subchronic study. Animals were fed for 84 weeks, during which time the effect on the weight gain was observed and analysis of hematology and serum chemistry were made. Kidney function testing over the different administration stages were examined to determine the ability of this organ to produce concentrated urine.[59] After killing the animals, different organs were weighed and a histopathology study was performed. The survival of animals treated with the alga was equal or slightly higher than that of soy fed controls. This excludes, therefore, the possibility that *Spirulina* contains any toxic agents that would interfere with the normal physiological or biochemical processes in the long run. There were no obvious intergroup differences in macroscopic or histopathological findings, as would be expected in older animals[65] (Table 2.2).

REPRODUCTIVE TOXICITY TESTS

Fertility and General Reproductive Performance

This study is designed to assess the potential toxic effects of a test substance on gonad function and mating behavior in both male and female animals, as well as conception rates, early and late stages of gestation, labor, lactation, and development of offspring.[66]

In our experiments we used rats and mice. Males were fed *Spirulina* for 9 weeks while females were fed for 2 weeks before mating, and feeding continued afterward and throughout gestation. Every day females were housed overnight with males from the same treatment group, until mating was confirmed by the presence of a vaginal plug. During the study, bodyweight, mating performance, and pregnancy rates were recorded. After killing the animals, the ovaries and uteri were examined to determine the number of *corpora lutea* and implantations. The number of dead fetuses and resorptions were also counted. After external examination, fetuses were examined for visceral and skeletal anomalies.

As shown in Table 2.3 treatment was not associated with any adverse effects in any measure of reproductive performance, including male and female fertility and duration of gestation and, except for isolated results with no toxicology significance, did not result in adverse effects on fetus developmental markers.[67,68]

Teratogenicity

Teratogenesis testing is an important aspect of subchronic testing. Teratogenesis may be defined as the onset of developmental abnormalities at any time between zygote formation and postnatal maturation. The embryo development stage most susceptible to adverse influences is organogenesis.[69]

Although mutations occurring in germ cells may lead to abnormalities in neonates, teratogenicity is normally confined to the effect of foreign agents on somatic cells within either the developing embryo or fetus to be distinguished from inherited defects.[70]

The teratogenic study with *Spirulina* was conducted in rats, mice and hamsters. *Spirulina* was given at various stages during gestation and all females were killed 2 days before the day set for the birth of offspring. Live and dead fetuses and embryo resorptions were counted. Fetuses were weighed and examined for external, skeletal, and visceral malformations.[71–73]

As shown in Table 2.3 *Spirulina* given during different gestation periods did not affect embryo development or produce embryo resorptions in any of the species studied.

Peri- and Postnatal Studies

In perinatal and postnatal research the chemical is given during the last third of pregnancy as well as the period of lactation, to detect its effects on late fetus development, labor and delivery, lactation, neonatal viability, and growth of neonates.[74]

Spirulina was given until Day 21 postpartum. After birth, the numbers of live, dead and externally abnormal newborns were counted. Postimplantation loss was calculated and bodyweight and viability were recorded. At approximately 10 weeks of age, the reproductive performance was assessed by mating males and females. Fetuses in the F_2 generation were examined for survival, bodyweight and external, visceral and skeletal anomalies. Uteri were examined for implantations and resorptions and

TABLE 2.3
Spirulina Reproductive Toxicity Studies*

Study	Animals	Methods and results summary	Reference
Fertility	Rats	Fertility and pregnancy were unaffected by treatment of *Spirulina*. For rats allowed to deliver their young, there were no intergroup differences in the number of live or dead pups at birth, survival rate, or weaning rate.	67
	Mice	Fertility and pregnancy were unaffected by treatment of *Spirulina*. There were no significant differences in the number of *corpora lutea*, total implantations, or number of live or dead fetuses. The number of resorptions in the treated group was similar to that in the control group.	68
Teratogenic	Hamsters	Gestating females were given *Spirulina* on Days 7–11, 1–11, or 1–14. Weights did not change compared to the control group during treatment. No fetus malformations or embryo resorptions were found.	71
	Rats	Giving *Spirulina* to gestating animals on Days 7–13, 1–13, and 1–19 resulted in no embryo resorptions or fetuses affected compared to the control group.	72
	Mice	The alga was given in the diet on gestation Days 7–14, 1–14, and 1–21. Maternal and fetal weights were not affected and no fetal toxicity or teratogenicity was found.	73
Peri- and post-natal development	Rats	There is a decrease in the gestation rate but no alterations in other parameters of fertility and post-natal development with diets in which 6% of their protein was substituted by *Spirulina*.	64
	Rats	*Spirulina* was incorporated into the diet of male and female rats. There were no clinical signs of toxicity related to treatment. Pregnancy and duration of gestation were unaffected by consumption of *Spirulina*. External examination of the offspring did not reveal any malformations.	67
	Mice	Pregnancy was unaffected and dams delivered their litters between Day 19–20. However, a significant decrement in body weights and in survival rate on 0–4 postnatal days was observed by 30% *Spirulina*.	68
Multigenerational	Rats	*Spirulina* given over three generations did not affect fertility, gestation, size of litters, or fetus viability. F_{3b} generation animals were kept for 13 weeks at the same diet levels as their parents. These animals did not show adverse effects on subchronic toxicity parameters either.	76

* Unless otherwise specified, *Spirulina* was added to the diet at 10, 20, and 30% concentrations, using the corresponding controls.

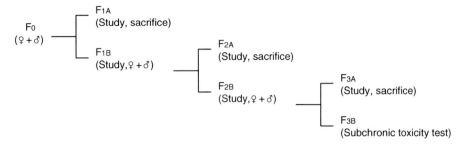

FIGURE 2.1 Three-generation reproductive assay of Spirulina in rats. $♀ + ♂ =$ mating; in the Study, animals were weighed, observed and weaned. On F_{3B} generation a subchronic toxicity test was carried out.

the pre- and postimplantation losses were calculated *Spirulina*, even at a 30% dietary concentration is not toxic to reproduction (Table 2.3). Therefore we would not expect *Spirulina* to be a reproductive hazard.[67,68]

MULTIGENERATION TESTS

Information pertaining to developmental toxicity can also be obtained from studies where animals are continuously exposed to the test substance over one or more generations.[75]

In our study, *Spirulina* was given to three generations over a period of approximately 2 years, following the schedule shown in Figure 2.1. Fertility, gestation, viability and lactation indices were recorded. A test of subchronic toxicity was carried out on the F_{3B} generation.

Analyses of reproduction and lactation results showed no adverse effects from *Spirulina* on fertility or gestation or any other parameters usually considered in this kind of study[76] (Table 2.3).

GENETIC TOXICITY

The primary objective of genetic toxicity testing is to determine the effects of chemical and physical agents on inheritance material (DNA) and the genetic processes of living cells.[77] There are nonmammalian and mammalian mutagenicity tests available to determine this kind of effects. Among the latter, the dominant-lethal assay is known to determine genetic changes in mammals. In this test males are treated with the test substance and mated with untreated females. The dominant-lethal mutation will arise in the sperm and can kill the zygote at any time during development. Females are dissected near the end of gestation and the numbers of fetal deaths and various other reproductive abnormalities are recorded.[69] This test has become the standard and a large number of compounds have been screened by using it.[78]

Spirulina genotoxicity has been studied in rats and mice after a short- and long-term use of dosage as well as in bacteria (Table 2.4). Models have been developed that allow for the detection of potential damage induced in germ cells at a specific stage

TABLE 2.4
Spirulina **Genotoxic Studies**

Study	Model	Methods and results summary	Reference
Lethal dominant	Mice	Short-term (5 days) and long-term (5 days/week, for 10 weeks) feeding of *Spirulina*, was followed by mating with untreated adult virgin females. Examination of uteri and ovaries of pregnant females at 12–14 days of gestation tp count preimplantation losses and nonliving implants failed and reveal dominant lethal effects.	80
	Rats	*Spirulina* given to males 5 days/week for 10 weeks, followed by mating with untreated virgin females during two weeks, failed to reveal germinal mutations of the dominant-lethal type.	81
	Rats	*Spirulina* incorporated into the experimental diet did not show germinal mutations, as shown by a dominant lethal test on males and females. No significant alterations were observed in semen counts, motility, and shape of sperm. Sex organ weights failed to reveal any alteration.	82
Ames	Bacteria	Negative results were reported in mutagenicity test with five strains of *Salmonella typhimurium* and *Schizosaccharomyces pombe* performed on urines of animals fed *Spirulina* for 4 months.	64

* Unless otherwise specified, *Spirulina* was added to the diet at 10, 20, and 30% concentrations, using the corresponding controls.

of development, to be expressed through weekly mating, or of the potential damage induced in germ cells at various stages of development, to be expressed during the first week of mating, respectively. However, this test does not allow for the detection of the most sensitive stage.[79] In both cases, *Spirulina* showed no damage in germ cells.[80–82]

Human Studies

Since extrapolating data from animals to humans poses some problems because of the differences between the animal and human species, not to mention the individual variations in the same strain, human studies are also conducted to determine the toxicities of different chemicals.[55]

So far, no systematic studies on clinical toxicology with *Spirulina* in humans have been found in the literature. There are only some isolated reports stating that people have lived solely on other forms algae for long periods of time, developing no negative symptoms whatsoever. Other studies report discomfort, vomiting, nausea, and poor digestibility of even small amounts of algae.[54] Some of these reports include studies conducted with *Chlorella, Scenedesmus acutus*[83] and *Scenedesmus obliquus*. It should be noted that for centuries *Spirulina* has been consumed and no significant adverse effect has ever been reported. This, of course, is not a scientific evidence for ruling out toxic effects, although it is an important consideration in relation to *Spirulina*, as it has been with the milenial use, of some plants and products occurring naturally.

However, toxicity studies have been indirectly conducted on humans with *Spirulina* such as in the study by Sautier and Tremolieres[85] in which this alga was given to undernourished humans as 50% of protein, leading to the conclusion that small doses, even for long periods of time, should be tolerable to normal subjects.

On the other hand, Becker[86] studied the effects of *Spirulina* on obesity by giving the alga at 2.8 g doses, three times a day for 4 weeks, resulting in statistically significant body weight loss in obese patients. No adverse effects were observed from clinical or biochemical parameters and no side effects were seen.

ANTITOXIC EFFECTS

Far from producing deleterious effects, *Spirulina* has instead showed itself to have antitoxic effects in tests conducted on cells, laboratory animals, and human beings. These properties have been expressed as a protective effect against toxic damage, such as cardiotoxicity, hepatotoxicity, nephrotoxicity, neurotoxicity, eye toxicity, testis toxicity, ovary toxicity, and other effects.

Table 2.5 shows some antitoxic properties reported for *Spirulina* and phycocyanin against deleterious effects of metals, pharmaceuticals and radiation. Both these antitoxic properties as well as some pharmacological effects can be attributed to the antioxidant capacity of this alga. For example, the hepatoprotection by phycocyanin from CCl_4 and R-(+)-pulegone toxicity is attributed to the inhibition of reactions involved in the production of reactive metabolites and possibly to its radical scavenging activity.[87] In the same way, Torres-Durán et al.[88] explain the potential hepatoprotective role of *Spirulina* against fatty liver induced by CCl_4 in rats. Moreover, Shastri et al.[89] found that *Spirulina* acts as an antagonist to testis toxicity from lead though its antioxidant activity.

DISCUSSION

Some authors have broadly shown the nutritional and therapeutic properties of *Spirulina* in several experimental models, which has led to the use of the alga in different countries at relatively high quantities. This alga produced by two companies in the United States was recently rated GRAS (Generally Recognized as Safe) for use in nutritional bars, drink mixes and snacks, as well a salad condiment and a pasta.[90]

Spirulina has probably been subject to more toxicology safety studies than any other algae, resulting in a high degree of confidence in its use by humans and animals without running any risk of deleterious effects on health.

Biogenic and nonbiogenic contamination determinations demonstrate that it complies with the greater part of the specifications about permissible limits, either those recommended by international agencies or implied in food legislation.

TABLE 2.5
Spirulina **Antitoxic Effects**

Effects against	Animals	Methods and results summary	Reference
Cardiotoxicity	Mice	Oral pretreatment with *Spirulina* (250 mg/kg) protected against doxorubicin-induced cardiotoxic effects as evidenced by lower mortality rates, less ascites, lower peroxidation levels, antioxidant enzyme normalization, and minimal damage to the heart (shown by ultrastructural studies). This effect could be due to the presence of antioxidant components.	99
	Rats	C-phycocyanin (10 μM) and *Spirulina* (50 μg/mL) attenuated the doxorubicin-induced reactive species formation, Bax expression, and cytochrome C release, while increasing caspase-3 activity, improving oxidative stress, and apoptosis in cardiomyocytes.	100
Hepatotoxicity	Rat	A preventive effect of *Spirulina* (5% in the diet) on the fructose-induced increase of liver triglyceride levels was seen together with an elevation of phospholipid concentrations in this tissue and a decreased plasma cholesterol level. It was concluded that *Spirulina* contain one or several factors affecting triglyceride accumulation.	101
	Rats	A 5% *Spirulina* diet prevented the fatty liver induced by $CHCl_4$. Liver triacylglycerols and cholesterol levels were lower that those in control rats. Hepatoprotective effects were related to its antioxidant activity.	102
	Rats	Intraperitoneal pretreatment with phycocyanin from *Spirulina* (200 mg/kg) resulted in reduced hepatotoxicity caused by $CHCl_4$ and R-(+)-pulegone. The mechanism may involve some cytochrome P450 reactions, in producing reactive metabolites.	87
	Mice	When *Spirulina* (10%) was added to the diet and given two weeks prior to simvastatin, it induced onset of fatty liver; a hypercholesterolemic diet and 20% ethanol decreased total liver lipids, mainly triacylglycerols, and increased serum lactate deshidrogenase (LDH) levels.	103
	Rats	After being treated with $CHCl_4$, total liver lipids and triacylglycerols decreased in rats fed on a diet with defatted *Spirulina* or oil fractions (5%). In addition, rats receiving whole *Spirulina* in their diet showed an increased HDL rate, while the levels in liver microsomal thiobarbituric acid-reactive substances decreased.	88

TABLE 2.5
Continued

Effects against	Animals	Methods and results summary	Reference
	Rat	Carotenoids extracted from *Spirulina* were given orally (100 mg/kg) to $CHCl_4$ treated animals. Carotenoids had a stronger antihepatotoxic effect as shown by biochemical parameters, compared to synthetic beta-carotene and beta-carotene only from a natural source. Carotenoids from *Dunaliella* showed better biological activity.	104
Genotoxicity	Mice	The micronucleus test showed *Spirulina* extract (1–5 mg/kg), given orally, protects mouse bone marrow polychromatic erythrocytes against gamma-radiation injury.	105
	Mice	Using the micronucleus test, pretreatment with *Spirulina* (250, 500, and 100 mg/kg) reduced chromosomal damage and lipid peroxidation induced by cyclophosphamide and mitomycin-C. Changes in antioxidant and detoxification systems were seen suggesting antioxidant effects.	106
	Mice and dogs	Polysaccharide of *Spirulina* 30 and 60 mg/kg increased the level of the white cells in blood and nucleated cells, as well as DNA in bone marrow in mice. At 12 mg/kg increased the level of the red cells, white cells, and hemoglobins in blood as well as nucleated cells in bone marrow in dogs.	107
	Cells	The hydrazide induced micronuclei frequency in a *Tradescantia* bioassay was decreased by the aqueous and dimethyl extracts of *Spirulina*. These data indicate that the alga is an anticlastogenic agent.	108
	Mice	The micronucleus test showed that pretreatment with *Spirulina* (250, 500, and 1000 mg/kg) inhibited genotoxicity and reduced lipid peroxidation induced by cisplatin and urethane. A concomitant increase in liver enzymatic and non-enzymatic antioxidants was seen.	109
	Mice	*Spirulina* given orally (200, 400, or 800 mg/kg) to male or female mice showed an antimutagenic effect against cyclophosphamide, evaluated by the dominant-lethal test. The results illustrate the alga's protective role in genetic-related damage to germ cells.	110
Nephrotoxicity	Rats	Phycocyanin (100 mg/kg) given orally controlled renal tubular damage and oxalate induced histopathological lesions. Biliprotein was suggested to have protected antioxidant defense systems in renal tissues and improve the thiol content in renal tissue and red blood cell lysate.	32, 33, 111

Continued

TABLE 2.5
Continued

Effects against	Animals	Methods and results summary	Reference
	Rats	Pretreatment with *Spirulina* (500 mg/kg) protected against cyclosporine-induced nephrotoxicity and prevented MDA rise in plasma and kidney tissues, isometric vacuolization and interstitial widening. These results suggested a crucial role played by *Spirulina*, given its antioxidant properties.	112
	Rats	*Spirulina* (500, 1000, 1500 mg/kg) restored renal functions, decreased lipid peroxidation, and increased previously reduced glutathione levels, superoxide dismutase, and catalase activities in gentamycin induced renal dysfunction.	113
	Rats	Oral *Spirulina* (1000 mg/kg) pretreatment buffered increased plasma urea, creatinine, urinary beta-*N*-acetyl-(D-glucose-aminidase), and plasma and kidney MDA as well as histomorphological changes in cisplatin-induced nephrotoxicity. This effect was attributed to its antioxidant properties.	114
Neurotoxicity	Rats	Oral pretreatment with phycocyanin (100 mg/kg) protected against kainic acid-induced hippocampus neuronal damage. Equivalent results were found in peripheral benzodiazepine receptors and heat shock protein 27 kD expression. Antioxidant effects of this protein were suggested.	115
Ocular toxicity	Rats	Lens glutathione, soluble protein and water content profiles showed a preventive effect of *Spirulina* at 1500 mg/kg doses in a naphthalene induced cataract model.	21
Ovary toxicity	Rats	*Spirulina* (300 mg/kg) showed a protective effect against lead-induced alterations in the number of mast cells in the cortex and medulla of rat ovaries during the oestrus cycle.	116
Testicular toxicity	Mice	*Spirulina* (800 mg/kg) given to males treated with lead for 30 days showed a significant recovery and less damage on histology, testes weight, tubular diameter, cell types, primary and secondary spermatocytes, and spermatids. The effect may be attributed to the presence of beta-carotene and superovide dismutase (SOD) enzymes.	89
	Mice	*Spirulina* given before or after mercury induced toxicity in testis protected the animals by increasing acid and alkaline phosphatase activity levels. The effect was attributed to the high β-carotene content and its antioxidant activity.	117

TABLE 2.5
Continued

Effects against	Animals	Methods and results summary	Reference
Other effects	Rats	Alterations in serum and liver enzymes such as glutamate oxaloacetate transaminase, glutamate pyruvate transaminase and alkaline phosphatase of rats fed on diets with hexachlorocyclohexane were improved by diets with 0.0628 and 3.18% *Spirulina*, added as a retinol supplement.	118
	Rats	*Spirulina* (1500 mg/kg) decreased the liver, lung, and kidney malondialdehyde, conjugated diene and hydroperoxide levels, in lead treated animals showing antioxidant activity.	119
	Rats	*Spirulina* (1500 mg/kg) included in the diet prevented lipid peroxidation and restored endogenous antioxidant contents to normal levels in the liver, lungs, heart, and kidneys of animals exposed to lead. The alga prevented lead deposition in the brain.	120
	Mice	*Spirulina* intake by a 6-month old mice for 28 days decreased hematological damage induced by ultraviólet (UVC)-irradiation.	121
	Rats	*Spirulina* (500 mg/kg) in combination with Liv-52 showed protective effects against biochemical parameters and histopathological changes caused by cadmium in the liver and kidneys.	122
	Fish	*Spirulina* feed improved tolerance of *Poecilia reticulate* to an azo dye methyl red expressed by a substantial decrease in the cytotoxic effects of red blood cells and a lower mortality rate at higher dye concentrations.	123
	Mice	*Spirulina* (800 mg/kg) given pre- and post-treatment with $HgCl_2$ significantly modified mercury induced biochemical alterations such as increased alkaline and acid phosphatase activity, serum iron and calcium levels, lipid peroxidation and blood glutathione levels. The alga relieved deleterious reactive oxygen species or lipid peroxides responsible for Hg-induced toxicity.	124
	Humans	*Spirulina* extract (250 mg) plus zinc (2 mg), twice daily for 16 weeks may be useful in the treatment of chronic arsenic poisoning with melanosis and keratosis. The treatment resulted in strongly increased urinary arsenic excretion and removal of hair.	125

Toxicity evaluation through short- and long-term studies on animals has shown that toxicity is absent in *Spirulina*. However, mention must be made once again of the problem of extrapolation from the animal model to human beings, especially the possibility that toxicity in animals and humans is not necessarily the same. Another problematic factor is the extrapolation of high doses, given to small populations of test animals in contrast to low exposures for large human populations.[91]

Administration of *Spirulina* in the mentioned animal studies have sometimes been at doses or concentrations (30% or more of alga in diets) much higher than the expected consumption by humans. On the other hand, the consumption of *Spirulina* by humans may extend for a major portion of their lives with therapeutic or nutritional purposes. Since the safety of *Spirulina* has been virtually shown for human and animal use, further research on other pharmacological and nutritional aspects with the alga can be carried out on humans without any risk of harm.

ACKNOWLEDGMENTS

The authors extend their gratitude to María Angélica Mojica Villegas for her assistance in the preparation of this chapter.

REFERENCES

1. Ramírez-Moreno, L. and Olvera-Ramírez, R., Uso tradicional y actual de *Spirulina* sp. (*Arthrospira* sp.), *Interciencia*, 31, 657, 2006.
2. Sánchez, M. et al., *Spirulina* (*Arthrospira*): an edible microorganism. A review. *Univer. Scient.*, 8, 7, 2003.
3. Khan, A., Bhadouria, P., and Bise, P.S., Nutritional and therapeutic potential of *Spirulina*, *Curr. Pharm. Biotech.*, 6, 373, 2005.
4. Belay, A., Current knowledge on potential health benefits of *Spirulina*, *J. Appl. Phycol.*, 5, 235, 1993.
5. Belay, A., Kato, T., and Ota, Y., *Spirulina* (*Arthrosrpira*): potential application as an animal feed supplement, *J. Appl. Phycol.*, 8, 303, 1996.
6. Fox, D.R., *Spirulina*, production and potential, *Aix-en Provence*, France, Edisud, 1996.
7. Mendes, R.L. et al., Supercritical carbon dioxide extraction of compounds with pharmaceutical importance from microalgae, *Inorg. Chim. Acta.*, 356, 328, 2003.
8. Campanella, L., Crescentini, G., and Avino, P., Chemical composition and nutritional evaluation of some natural and commercial food products based on *Spirulina*, *Analusis*, 27, 533, 1999.
9. Remirez, D., Ledon, N., and Gonzalez, R., Role of histamine in the inhibitory effects of phycocyanin in experimental models of allergic inflammatory response, *Mediat. Inflamm.*, 11, 81, 2002.
10. Belay, A., The potential application of *Spirulina* (*Arthrospira*) as a nutrition and therapeutic supplement in health management, *J. Am. Nutr. Ass.*, 5, 27, 2002.
11. Becker, E.W., Comparative toxicological studies with algae in India, Thailand, and Peru, In *Algae biomass*, Shelef, G. and Soeder, C.J., Eds., Elsevier/North-Holland Biomedical Press, Tübingen, West Germany, 1980, 767.
12. Dillon, J.C., Phuc, A.P., and Dubacq, J.P., Nutritional value of the alga *Spirulin*, *World Rev. Nutr. Diet.*, 77, 32, 1995.
13. Chamorro, G. et al., Farmacología y Toxicología del alga *Spirulina*, *Rev. Invest. Clín.*, 48, 389, 1996.
14. Chamorro, G. et al., Actualización en la farmacología de *Spirulina* (*Arthrospira*), un alimento no convencional, *Arch. Latinoam. Nutr.*, 52, 232, 2002.
15. Hernández-Corona, A. et al., Antiviral activity of *Spirulina maxima* against herpes simples virus type II, *Antivir. Res.*, 56, 279, 2002.

16. Ozdemir, G. et al., Antibacterial activity of volatile component and various extracts of *Spirulina platensis*, *Phytother. Res.*, 18, 754, 2004.

17. Hsiao, G. et al., C-Phycocyanin, a very potent and novel platelet aggregation inhibitor from *Spirulina platensis*, *J. Agric. Food Chem.*, 53, 7734, 2005.

18. Nagaoka, S. et al., A novel protein C-phycocyanin plays a crucial role in the hypocholesterolemic action of *Spirulina platensis* concentrate in rats, *J. Nutr.*, 135, 2425, 2005.

19. Rasool, M., Sabina, E.P., and Lavanya, B., Anti-inflammatory effect of *Spirulina fusiformis* on adjuvant-induced arthritis in mice, *Biol. Pharm. Bull.*, 29, 2483, 2006.

20. Chamorro, G. et al., *Spirulina maxima* pretreatment partially protects against 1-methyl-4-phenyl-1,2,3,6-tetrahydropyridine neurotoxicity, *Nutr. Neurosc.*, 9, 207, 2006.

21. Haque, S.E. and Gilani, K.M., Effect of ambroxol, *Spirulina* and vitamin-E in naphthalene induced cataract in female rats, *Indian J. Physiol. Pharmacol.*, 49, 57, 2005.

22. Khan, M. et al., C-phycocyanin protects against ischemia-reperfusion injury of heart through involvement of p38 and ERK signaling, *Am. J. Physiol Heart Cire Physiol.*, 290, H2136, 2005.

23. Wang, Y. et al., Dietary supplementation with blueberries, spinach, or *Spirulina* reduces ischemic brain damage, *Exp. Neur.*, 193, 75, 2005.

24. Mao, T.K., Vann der Water, J., and Gershwin, M.E., Effects of *Spirulina*-based dietary supplement cytokine production from allergic rhinitis patients, *J. Med. Food*, 8, 27, 2005.

25. Mascher, D. et al., Ethanolic extract of *Spirulina maxima* alters the vasomotor reactivity of aortic rings form obese rats, *Arch. Med. Res.*, 37, 50, 2005.

26. Miranda, M.S. et al., Antioxidant activity of the microalga *Spirulina maxima*, *Braz. J. Med. Biol. Res.*, 31, 1075, 1998.

27. Piñero-Estrada, J.E., Bermejo-Bescós, P., and Villar del Fresno, A.M., Antioxidant activity of different fractions of *Spirulina Platensis* protean extract, *Il farmaco*, 56, 497, 2001.

28. Wu, L.C. et al., Antioxidant and antiproliferative activities of *Spirulina* and chlorella water extracts, *J. Agric. Food Chem.*, 53, 4207, 2005.

29. Romay, C., Ledón, N., and González, R., Further studies on anti-inflammatory activity of phycocyanin in some models of inflammation, *Inflamm. Res.*, 47, 334, 1998.

30. Romay, C. et al., Antioxidant and anti-inflammatory properties of C-phycocyanin from blue-green algae, *Inflamm. Res.*, 47, 36, 1998.

31. Romay, C. et al., C-phycocyanin; a biliprotein with antioxidant, anti-inflammatory and neuroprotective effects, *Curr. Protein Sci.*, 4, 207, 2003.

32. Farooq, S.M. et al., Prophylactic role of phycocyanin: a study of oxalate mediated renal cell injury, *Chem. Bio. Interact.*, 149, 1, 2004.

33. Farooq, S.M. et al., Oxalate-mediated nephronal impairment and its inhibition by c-Phycocyanin: a study on urolithic rats, *Mol. Cell. Biochem.*, 284, 95, 2006.

34. Kotsonis, F.N., Burdock, G.A., and Famm, W.G., Food toxicology, In *Cassarett and Doull's essentials of toxicology*, Klaassen, C.D. and Watkins III J.B., Eds., McGraw-Hill, New York, 2003, 431.

35. Becker, E.W., *Microalgae. Biotechnology and microbiology*, Cambridge University Press, 1995.

36. Eaton, D.L. and Klaassen C.D., *Principles of toxicology*, In Klaassen C.D. and Watkins III J.B., Eds., McGraw-Hill, New York, 2003, 6.

37. Omaye, S.T., *Food and nutritional toxicology*, CRC Press, Boca Ratón, 2004.

38. Carmichael, W.W., The toxin of cyanobacteria, *Sci. Am.* 270, 78, 1994.
39. Aldridge, W.N., *Mechanisms and concepts in toxicology*, Taylor and Francis, London, 1996.
40. Becker, E.W. and Venkataraman, L.V., Production and utilization of the blue-green alga *Spirulina* in India, *Biomass*, 4, 105, 1984.
41. Ciferri, O., *Spirulina*, the edible microorganism, *Microbiol. Rev.*, 47, 551, 1983.
42. Corrado, A. et al., Pathogenesis, clinical findings and management of acute and chronic gout, *Minerva Med.*, 97, 495, 2006.
43. Mathews, C.K., Van Holde, K.E., and Ahern, K.G., *Bioquímica*, Tercera Edición, Pearson Addisson Wesley, Madrid, 2005.
44. Curtis M.J. et al., *Pharmacologie Intégrée*, DeBoeck Université, Paris, 1999.
45. Kim, S.K. et al., Selective cadmium accumulation using recombinant *Escherichia coli*, *J. Biosci. Bioeng.*, 99, 109, 2005.
46. Lu, F.C. and Kacew, S., *Lu's basic toxicology*, 4th ed., Taylor and Francis, London, 2002.
47. Hughes, W.W., *Essentials of environmental toxicology*, Taylor and Francis, London, 1996.
48. Goyer, R.A. and Clarkson, T.W., Toxic effects of metals, In *Casarett and Doull's essentials of toxicology*, Klaassen, C.D. and Watkins III J.B., Eds., McGraw-Hill, New York, 2003, 348.
49. Perales-Vela, H.V., Peña-Castro, J.M., and Cañizares-Villanueva, R.O., Heavy-metal detoxification in eukaryotic microalgae, *Chemosphere*, 64, 1, 2006.
50. Chen, H. and Pan, S., Bioremediation potential of *Spirulina*: toxicity and biosorption of lead, *J. Zhejiang Univ. Sci. B.*, 6, 171, 2005.
51. Gong, R. et al., Lead biosorption and desorption by intact and pretreated *Spirulina maxima* biomass, *Chemosphere*, 58, 125, 2005.
52. Rangsayator, N. et al., Phytoremediation potential of *Spirulina* (*Arthrospira*) *platensis*: biosorption and toxicity studies of cadmium, *Environ. Pollut.*, 119, 45, 2002.
53. Jagiello, M. et al., Mode of biosorption of chromium (III) by *Spirulina* species cells from aqueous solutions, *Water Environ. Res.*, 78, 740, 2006.
54. Becker, W., Microalgae in human and animal nutrition, In *Handbook of microalgal culture: biotechnology and applied phycology*, Amos Richmond, Ed., Blackwell Science, Oxford, 312, 2004.
55. Altug, T., *Introduction to toxicology and food*, CRC Press, Boca Raton, 2003.
56. Dirección General de Sanidad Vegetal, Secretaría de Agricultura y Recursos Hidráulicos, *Reporte, 238*, 46, México.
57. Alimentos esenciales para la humanidad. (AEH), *Report*, México.
58. Chamorro, G., Etude toxicologique de l' alga *Spirulina* plante pilote productrice de proteines (*Spirulina* de Sosa Texcoco S.A.), *Report, UNIDO* 10, 387, 1980.
59. Woolley, A., *A guide to practical toxicology. Evaluation, prediction and risk*, Taylor and Francis, London, 2003.
60. Bello Gutiérrez, J., Fundamentos de ciencia toxicológica, Díaz de Santos, Madrid, 2001.
61. Ecobichon, D.J., The basis of toxicity testing, 2nd ed., CRC Press, Boca Ratón, 1997.
62. Elias, P.S. and Chem, C., *Subchronica toxicity studies: methodology, interpretation and problems*, Galli, C.L. and Paoletti, R., Eds., Elsevier/North-Holland Biomedical Press, Amsterdam, 1980, 169.
63. Till, H.P. and Williams, M., *Sub-chronic (90 day)toxicity study with dried algae (M₂)in albino rats*, Rapport Nr. R 3352, Central Institute for nutrition and food research.

64. Bizzi, A. et al., Trattamenti prolungati nel ratto con diete conntenenti proteine di *Spirulina*. Aspetti biochimici, morfologici e tossicologici, In *Prospettive della coltura di Spirulina in Italia*. Consiglio Nazionale delle Ricerche and Materassi, R., Eds., Accademia dei Geo rgofili, Firence, 205, 1980.

65. Chamorro, G.A. et al., Etude de la toxicité chronique de la Spiruline chez le rat, *Med. Nutr.*, 24, 104, 1988.

66. Christian, M.S. and Hoberman, A.M., Current *in vivo* reproductive toxicity and development toxicity (Teratology) test methods, In *A guide to general toxicology*, Judith K. Marquis, Ed., Karger, Basel, 1983, 91–10.

67. Salazar, M. et al., Effect of *Spirulina maxima* consumption on reproduction and peri- and post-natal development in rats, *Food Chem. Toxicol.*, 34, 353, 1996.

68. Chamorro, G. et al., Reproductive and peri- and post-natal evaluation of *Spirulina maxima* in mice, *J. Appl. Phycol.*, 9, 107, 1997.

69. Shibamoto, T. and Bjeldanes L.F., *Introduction to food toxicology*, Academic Press, Inc., Harcout Brace and Company, San Diego, 1993.

70. Timbrell, J.A., *Principles of biochemical toxicology*, 2nd ed., Taylor and Francis, London, 1994.

71. Chamorro, G. et al., Evaluation teratologique de la *Spiruline* chez le hamster, *Belg. J. Food Chem. Biotechnol.*, 42, 189, 1988.

72. Chamorro, G., Salazar, M., and Salazar, S., Estudio teratogénico de *Spirulina* en rata, *Arch. Lationamer. Nutr.*, 29, 641, 1989.

73. Chamorro, G. and Salazar, M., Estudio teratogénico de *Spirulina* en ratón, *Arch. Latinoamer. Nutr.*, 40, 86, 1990.

74. Tuchmann-Duplessis, H., *Drug effects on the fetus*, ADIS Press, New York, 1975.

75. Rogers, J.M. and Kavlock, R.J., Developmental toxicology, In *Casarett and Doull's essentials of toxicology*, Klaassen, C.D. and Watkins, J.B III., Eds., McGraw-Hill, New York, 2003, 146–160.

76. Chamorro, G. et al., Multi-generation study on reproduction and lactation in rats fed *Spirulina*, *Arch. Hydrobiol. Beih. Ergerbn. Limnol.*, 20, 165, 1985.

77. Preston, R.J. and Hoffmann, G.R., Genetic toxicology, In *Casarett and Doull's essentials of toxicology*, Curtis, D. Klaassen and John, B. Watkins III, Eds., McGraw-Hill, New York, 2003, 131–145.

78. Teaf, C.M. and Middendorf, P.J., Mutagenesis and genetic toxicology, In *Principles of toxicology*, Williams, P.L., James, R.C., and Roberts, S.M., Eds., 2nd ed., A Wiley-Interscience Publication, New York, 2000, 239.

79. Green, S. et al., Current status of bioassays in genetic toxicology-dominant lethal assay, *Mut. Res.*, 154, 4967, 1987.

80. Chamorro, G.A. and Salazar, M., Dominant-lethal assay of *Spirulina maxima* in male CD-1 mice after short-term and prolonged-term feeding, *J. Food Protect.*, 52, 127, 1989.

81. Salazar, M. and Chamorro, G., Study of lethal dominant of *Spirulina maxima* in male rats, *Sci. Alim.*, 10, 713, 1990.

82. Chamorro, G. and Salazar, M., Dominant-lethal study of *Spirulina maxima* in male and female rats after short-term feeding, *Phytother. Res.*, 10, 28, 1995.

83. Powell, R.C., Nevel, E.M., and McDowell, M.E., Algae feedings in humans, *J. Nutr.*, 75, 7, 1961.

84. Gross, R. et al., The nutritional quality of *Scenedesmus acutus* produced in a semi industrial plant in Peru, *Ber. Dtsch. Bot. Ges.*, 95, 323, 1982.

85. Sautier, C. and Trémolieres, Valeur alimentaire des algues spirulines chez l'homme, *Ann. Nutr. Alim.*, 30, 517, 1976.

86. Becker, E.W. et al., Clinical and biochemical evaluations of the alga *Spirulina* with regard to its application in the treatment of obesity: a double-blind cross-over study, *Nutr. Rep. Int.*, 33, 565, 1986.

87. Vadiraja, B.B., Gaikwad, N.W., and Madyastha, K.M., Hepatoprotective effect of C-phycocyanin: protection for carbon tetrachloride and R-(+)-pulgeone-mediated hepatotoxicity in rats, *Biochem. Biophys. Res. Commun.*, 249, 428, 1998.

88. Torres-Durán, P.V. et al., Studies on the preventive effect of *Spirulina maxima* on fatty liver development induce by carbon tetrachloride, in the rat, *J. Ethnopharm.*, 64, 141, 1999.

89. Shastri, D., Kumar, M., and Kumar, A., Modulation of lead toxicity by *Spirulina fusiformis, Phytother. Res.*, 13, 258, 1999.

90. Belay, A., Algae and health: *Spirulina* (Arthospira) as a case in point, presented at Biotecnología algal. Nuevas perspectivas para Latinoamérica, 1er. Congreso latinoamericano sobre biotecnología algal, Buenos Aires-Argentina, October 25–29, 2004, 69.

91. Shank, R.C., General toxicology, In *Toxicogenomics. Principles and applications*, Hamadeh, H.K. and Afshari, C.T., Eds., Hoboken, New Jersey, Wiley-Liss, 2004, 1.

92. IUPAC, Proposed guidelines for testing of single cell protein destined as major protein source for animal feed, Information Bulletin, International Union of Pure and Applied Chemistry. Technical Reports, No. 12, Oxford, IUPAC Secretariat, 1974.

93. Becker, E.W. and Venkataraman, L.V., *Biotechnology and explotation of algae. The Indian approach*, German Agency for Technical Cooperation, Eschborn, 1982.

94. Boudene, C., Collas, E., and Jenkins, C., Recherche et dosage de divers toxiques mineraux dans les algues spirulines de différents origins et evaluation de la toxicité a long terme chez le rat d'un lot d'algues spirulines de provenance mexicaine, *Ann. Nutr. Alim.*, 29, 577, 1975.

95. Krishnakumari, M.K., Ramesh, H.P., and Venkataraman, L.V., Food Safety Evaluation: acute oral and dermal effects of the algae *Scenedesmus acutus* and *Spirulina platensis* on albino rats, *J. Food Protect.*, 44, 934, 1981.

96. Naidu, K.A., Toxicity assessment of phycocyanin-a blue colorant from blue-green alga *Spirulina platensis, Food Biotechnol.*, 13, 51, 1999.

97. Chamorro, G.A. et al., Subchronic toxicity in rats fed *Spirulina, J. Pharm. Belg.*, 43, 29, 1988.

98. Salazar, M. et al., Subchronic toxicity study in mice fed *Spirulina maxima, J. Ethnopharmacol.*, 62, 235, 1998.

99. Bourges, H. et al., Utilization of the alga *Spirulina* as a protein source, *Nutr. Rep. Intern.*, 4, 31, 1971.

100. Khan, M., C-Phycocyanin ameliorates doxorubicin-induced oxidative stress and apoptosis in adult rat cardiomycetes, *J. Cardiovas. Pharmacol.*, 47, 9, 2006.

101. González de Rivera, et al., Preventive effect of *Spirulina maxima* on the fatty liver induced by a fructosa-rich diet in the rat, a preliminary report, *Life Sciences*, 53, 57, 1993.

102. Torres-Durán, P.V. et al., *Spirulina maxima* prevents induction of fatty liver by carbon tetrachloride in the rat, *Biochem. Mol. Biol. Int.*, 44, 787, 1998.

103. Ble-Castillo, J.L. et al., *Arthrospira maxima* prevents the acute fatty liver induced by administration of simvastatin, ethanol and a hypercholesterolemic diet in mice, *Life Sci.*, 70, 2665, 2002.

104. Murthy, K.N. et al., Comparative evaluation of hepatotoxicity activity of carotenoids of microgoalgae, *J. Med. Food*, 8, 523, 2005.

105. Qishen, P., Baojiang, G., and Kolman, A., Radio-protective effect of extract from *Spirulina platensis* in mouse bone marrow cell studied by using the micronucleous test, *Tox. Lett.*, 48, 165, 1989.

106. Prekumar, K. et al., Effect of *Spirulina fusiformis* on cyclophosphamide and mitomycin-C induced genotocicity and oxidative stress in mice, *Fitoterapia*, 77, 906, 2001.

107. Zhang, H. et al., Chemo- and radio-protective effects of polysaccharide of *Spirulina platensis* on hemopoietic system of mice and dogs, *Acta Pharmacol. Sin.*, 22, 1121, 2001.

108. Ruiz-Flores, E. et al., Anticlastogeanic effect of *Spirulina maxima* on the micronuclei induced by maleic hydrazide in *Tradescantia*, *Life Sci.*, 72, 1345, 2003.

109. Prekumar, K. et al., Protective effect of *Spirulina fusiformis* on chemical-induced genotoxicity in mice, *Fitoterapia*, 75, 24, 2004.

110. Chamorro, G. et al., Antimutagenic effect of *Arthrospira* (*Spirulina*) *maxima* evaluated by the dominant-lethal test in mice, presented at Toxicologie de la pharmacodependance aux medicaments, Congres annuel de la Societé de Toxicologie. Paris-France, October, 23–24, 2006, 51.

111. Farooq, S.M. et al., Salubrious effect of C-phycocyanin against oxalate-mediated renal cell injury, *Clin. Chim. Acta.*, 348, 199, 2004.

112. Khan, M. et al., *Spirulina* attenuates cyclosporine-induced nephrotoxicity in rats, *J. Appl. Toxicol.*, 26, 444, 2006.

113. Kuhad, A. et al., Renoprotective effect of *Spirulina fusiformis* on cisplatin-induced oxidative stress and renal dysfunction in rats, *Ren. Fail.*, 28, 247, 2006.

114. Mohan, I.K. et al., Protection against cisplatin-induced nephrotoxicity by *Spirulina* in rats, *Cancer Chemother. Pharmacol.*, 58, 802, 2006.

115. Rimbau, R. et al., Protective effects of C-phycocyanin against kainic acid-induced neuronal damage in rat hippocampus, *Neuros. Lett.*, 276, 75, 1999.

116. Karaca, T. and Simsek, N., Effects of *Spirulina* on the number of ovary mast cells in lead-induced toxicity in rats, *Phytother. Res.*, 21, 44, 2007.

117. Saxena, P.S. and Kumar, N., Modulatory potential of *Spirulina fusiformis* on testicular phosphatases in Swiss albino mice against mercury intoxication, *Indian J. Exp. Biol.*, 42, 998, 2004.

118. Venkataraman, L.V. et al., *Spirulina platensis* as retinol supplement for protection against hexachlorocyclohexane toxicity in rats, *J. Food Sci. Tech.*, 31, 430, 1994.

119. Upasani, C.D., Khera, A., and Balaraman, R., Effect of lead with vitamin E, C, or *Spirulina* on malondialdehyde, conjugated dienes and hydroperoxides in rats, *Indian J. Exp. Biol.*, 39, 70, 2001.

120. Upasani, C.D. and Balaraman, R., Protective effect of *Spirulina* on lead-induced deleterious changes in the lipid peroxidation and endogenous antioxidants in rats, *Phytother. Res.*, 17, 330, 2003.

121. Zaccaro, M. et al., Efecto de la ingesta de *Spirulina platensis* en ratones expuestos a estrés ambiental, presented at *Biotecnología algal*, Nuevas perspectivas para Latinoamérica, 1er. Congreso latinoamericano sobre biotecnología algal, Buenos Aires-Argentina, October, 25–29, 2004, 81.

122. Jeyaprash, K. and Chinnaswamy, P., Effect of *Spirulina* and Liv-52 on cadmium induced toxicity in albino rats, *Indian J. Exp. Biol.*, 43, 773, 2005.

123. Sharma, S., Sharma, S., and Sharma, K.P., Protective role of *Spirulina* feed in freshwater fish (*Poecilia reticulate* Peters) exposed to an azo dye-methyl red, *Indian J Exp. Biol.*, 43, 1165, 2005.

124. Sharma, M.R. et al., Modification of mercury-induced biochemical alterations in blood of Swiss albino mice by *Spirulina fusiformis*, *Environ. Tox. Pharm.*, 20, 289, 2005.
125. Misbahuddin, M. et al., Efficacy of *Spirulina* extract plus zinc in patients of chronic arsenic poisoning: a randomized placebo-controlled study, *Clin. Toxicol.*, 44, 135, 2006.

3 *Spirulina* and Its Therapeutic Implications as a Food Product

Uma M. Iyer, Swati A. Dhruv, and Indirani U. Mani

CONTENTS

INTRODUCTION

Good nutrition is vital to good health, optimal growth, and development, and for the prevention of diseases. The recognition that nutrients have the ability to interact and modulate molecular mechanisms underlying human physiological functions has resulted in the neutraceutical revolution in the field of nutrition. The human body is perfectly capable of healing itself if its needs are satisfied with the necessary vitamins, minerals, enzymes, and other nutrients. There are many foods that have healing and preventative health qualities, but one such powerful, wide-ranging, and diverse group of nutrients is *Spirulina*. Since *Spirulina* contains an array of bioactive chemicals, considerable potential exists for *Spirulina* to be used in various recipes where its incorporation and supplementation can help in enhancing the nutritional qualities of the food as well as in therapeutic management of various disorders. Some of the diet-related disorders that are gaining importance are the noncommunicable diseases such as diabetes, hypertension, and heart disease. A primary influence on the onset of these diseases is due to changes in lifestyle, that is, an abundance of food coupled with low levels of physical activity. It has been reported that in 2001, chronic diseases contributed approximately 60% of the 56.5 million total reported deaths in the world and 46% of the global burden of the disease. The proportion of the burden of NCDs is expected to rise to 57% by 2020. The prevalence of these diet-related noncommunicable disorders is increasing globally at an unprecedented rate, whereby the management of the same from the nutritional point of view is of utmost importance. Hence, several recipes incorporating spray-dried *Spirulina*—the wonder food was tested and the sensory qualities of the same were evaluated so as to be able to incorporate them into the dietary management of these disorders.

SENSORY EVALUATION OF *SPIRULINA* INCORPORATED RECIPES

The study was planned to develop various recipes supplemented with spray-dried *Spirulina* at three different levels and to rank the recipes according to the degree of acceptance.

India is a country with heterogenic population having diverse food habits. Some of the commonly consumed foods across the country were identified for practical feasibility. In all, there were 22 recipes, which can be broadly classified into four categories:

1. Different types of parathas with curd
2. Different types of vegetables with chapati
3. Different types of rice with curd
4. Snacks

All the recipes had the following characteristics:

1. All the recipes were made of equicarbohydrate containing 50 g carbohydrates.

2. For each recipe spray-dried *Spirulina* was added at three different levels, namely, 1 g, 2.5 g, and 5 g level.

Sensory evaluation of the recipes was performed by a selected trained panel consisting of 10 members using the scientific method of "Hedonic scale" to evaluate the recipe. The sensory attributes evaluated were color and appearance, texture, flavor and taste, and overall acceptability. In all there were four samples for each recipe, that is, three samples with *Spirulina* incorporated at different levels and a control (without spray-dried *Spirulina*). The recipes were scored on a 5-point scale on the basis of highly desirable, desirable, moderately desirable, slightly undesirable, and undesirable. On this basis, the scores for each characteristic were calculated.

DIFFERENT TYPES OF PARATHAS WITH CURD

Sensory evaluation of seven different types of parathas was performed, and the results of which have been discussed below.

Seven different types of parathas were prepared, namely, plain paratha, potato paratha, methi paratha, spinach paratha, mint and cabbage paratha, peas paratha, and coriander paratha, respectively. No significant difference in the sensory qualities between the control and *Spirulina* incorporated (1 g/2.5 g/5 g) parathas were seen. The overall acceptability scores of *Spirulina* incorporated parathas with curd ranged from 3.15 to 4.23 and was comparable to the control score of 3.63–4.15 (Table 3.1). The overall acceptability decreased with increase in *Spirulina* supplementation but was not statistically significant. The attributes, such as taste, color, and texture, were comparable within the groups but was best acceptable up to 2.5 g level.

DIFFERENT TYPES OF RICE WITH CURD

Rice is another cereal, which is widely consumed in India. In view of this, it was thought worthwhile to see if *Spirulina* could be incorporated in various rice preparations. There were four different types of rice that were prepared, for example, coriander rice, fenugreek rice, spinach rice, and vegetable pulao. All the different types of rice were served with 50 g of curd. As evident from Table 3.2, no significant difference was observed in the scores between the control and *Spirulina*-supplemented recipes in all rice preparations. It was heartening to know that spinach rice with raita supplemented with *Spirulina* at 1 g and 2.5 g levels was more acceptable than the control sample. With regard to coriander rice, fenugreek rice, and vegetable pulao, the overall acceptability though nonsignificant showed a decreasing trend with increasing level of *Spirulina* supplementation (Table 3.2). In addition to this, it was observed that the color and appearance of *Spirulina*-supplemented rice at 1 g and 2.5 g levels was more acceptable than the control sample. These observations highlight that the green color of *Spirulina* did not affect the overall sensory attributes of rice up to 2.5 g level.

VEGETABLE WITH CHAPATI

The sensory evaluation of *Spirulina*-supplemented vegetables showed that out of four vegetables prepared (kofta curry, potato spinach, spinach paneer, and potato

TABLE 3.1

Effect of *Spirulina* Supplementation on the Sensory Qualities of Various Types of Parathas (Mean ± SD)

Group	Color/appearance	Texture	Taste/flavor	Overall acceptability
Plain paratha				
Control	4.10 ± 1.34	3.88 ± 1.17	4.53 ± 0.63	3.63 ± 1.29
Level 1 (1.0 g)	3.58 ± 1.32	3.53 ± 1.33	4.08 ± 0.75	3.25 ± 1.16
Level 2 (2.5 g)	3.91 ± 0.95	3.71 ± 1.38	3.58 ± 0.95	3.69 ± 1.38
Level 3 (5.0 g)	3.33 ± 1.31	3.38 ± 1.21	3.36 ± 1.21	3.15 ± 1.09
Potato paratha				
Control	4.46 ± 0.74	3.50 ± 1.32	3.81 ± 1.33	3.84 ± 1.29
Level 1 (1.0 g)	4.28 ± 0.28	3.28 ± 1.43	3.91 ± 1.38	3.76 ± 1.30
Level 2 (2.5 g)	4.10 ± 0.98	3.91 ± 1.44	3.58 ± 1.49	3.41 ± 1.44
Level 3 (5.0 g)	3.21 ± 1.45	3.75 ± 1.58	3.46 ± 1.54	3.07 ± 1.38
Peas paratha				
Control	3.66 ± 1.69	4.27 ± 1.42	4.00 ± 1.47	4.00 ± 1.38
Level 1 (1.0 g)	3.84 ± 1.34	3.91 ± 1.49	4.00 ± 1.47	3.92 ± 0.70
Level 2 (2.5 g)	4.00 ± 1.35	4.00 ± 1.52	4.09 ± 0.79	4.07 ± 0.88
Level 3 (5.0 g)	3.71 ± 1.27	3.92 ± 1.33	3.45 ± 1.30	3.80 ± 0.83
Methi paratha				
Control	3.64 ± 1.17	4.04 ± 1.39	3.91 ± 1.32	3.69 ± 1.38
Level 1 (1.0 g)	3.92 ± 1.32	4.09 ± 0.79	4.00 ± 1.34	3.84 ± 1.45
Level 2 (2.5 g)	3.77 ± 1.58	3.85 ± 1.35	3.64 ± 1.28	3.57 ± 1.34
Level 3 (5.0 g)	2.91 ± 1.18	2.84 ± 1.16	3.14 ± 1.55	3.41 ± 1.11
Coriander paratha				
Control	4.16 ± 0.68	4.00 ± 0.72	4.08 ± 0.86	4.15 ± 0.86
Level 1 (1.0 g)	4.40 ± 0.66	3.78 ± 1.26	3.60 ± 1.50	4.23 ± 0.69
Level 2 (2.5 g)	4.00 ± 0.35	3.75 ± 1.29	3.61 ± 1.27	4.07 ± 0.72
Level 3 (5.0 g)	3.27 ± 1.48	3.53 ± 1.49	3.54 ± 1.15	3.53 ± 1.21
Mint and cabbage paratha				
Control	4.00 ± 0.61	3.66 ± 1.17	4.06 ± 0.77	3.75 ± 1.23
Level 1 (1.0 g)	3.90 ± 1.32	3.84 ± 1.29	4.08 ± 0.75	3.84 ± 1.23
Level 2 (2.5 g)	3.30 ± 0.60	3.25 ± 1.23	3.93 ± 0.70	3.18 ± 1.11
Level 3 (5.0 g)	2.60 ± 0.66	3.08 ± 1.18	3.25 ± 0.82	2.84 ± 1.02
Spinach and cauliflower paratha				
Control	3.75 ± 1.53	3.71 ± 1.38	4.16 ± 0.79	3.84 ± 1.34
Level 1 (1.0 g)	3.46 ± 1.27	3.66 ± 1.39	3.63 ± 0.88	3.56 ± 1.16
Level 2 (2.5 g)	3.08 ± 1.25	3.76 ± 1.52	3.41 ± 0.95	3.64 ± 0.97
Level 3 (5.0 g)	2.53 ± 0.74	3.69 ± 1.32	3.33 ± 1.10	3.53 ± 0.84

fenugreek) palak paneer and potato methi vegetables were found to be more acceptable with regard to all sensory qualities at all the three levels, 1 g, 2.5 g, and 5 g (Table 3.3). And even in the other two vegetables, that is, kofta curry and potato palak vegetable, though the mean scores were lower than the control sample, the scores for almost

TABLE 3.2
Effect of *Spirulina* Supplementation on the Sensory Qualities of Various Types of Rice (Mean ± SD)

Group	Color/appearance	Texture	Taste/flavor	Overall acceptability
Coriander rice				
Control	3.71 ± 1.22	4.27 ± 0.61	3.91 ± 1.98	4.00 ± 0.66
Level 1 (1.0 g)	4.00 ± 0.94	4.00 ± 0.89	3.61 ± 1.94	3.45 ± 0.89
Level 2 (2.5 g)	3.90 ± 0.86	4.20 ± 0.74	3.80 ± 0.74	3.16 ± 1.28
Level 3 (5.0 g)	3.40 ± 1.00	4.10 ± 0.83	3.00 ± 1.41	3.40 ± 0.91
Fenugreek rice				
Control	4.18 ± 1.40	4.36 ± 1.43	4.27 ± 1.48	4.36 ± 1.43
Level 1 (1.0 g)	4.18 ± 1.40	4.18 ± 1.40	4.27 ± 1.48	4.33 ± 1.37
Level 2 (2.5 g)	33.81 ± 1.40	4.18 ± 1.46	4.00 ± 1.47	3.90 ± 1.44
Level 3 (5.0 g)	3.71 ± 1.38	4.00 ± 1.35	4.00 ± 1.52	3.58 ± 1.49
Spinach rice				
Control	4.00 ± 1.41	4.00 ± 1.38	4.00 ± 1.41	4.09 ± 1.37
Level 1 (1.0 g)	3.90 ± 1.37	4.00 ± 1.38	4.18 ± 1.46	4.16 ± 1.40
Level 2 (2.5 g)	3.72 ± 1.48	3.90 ± 1.44	4.09 ± 1.50	4.16 ± 1.40
Level 3 (5.0 g)	3.63 ± 1.55	3.92 ± 1.38	3.90 ± 1.40	3.30 ± 1.43
Vegetable pulao (rice)				
Control	4.27 ± 1.42	4.27 ± 1.42	4.36 ± 1.43	4.33 ± 1.37
Level 1 (1.0 g)	3.81 ± 1.40	3.81 ± 1.40	3.75 ± 1.78	3.91 ± 1.38
Level 2 (2.5 g)	3.91 ± 1.49	4.09 ± 1.44	4.00 ± 1.41	3.91 ± 1.38
Level 3 (5.0 g)	3.00 ± 1.41	4.10 ± 0.70	3.72 ± 1.28	3.58 ± 1.25

all the qualities were found to be higher at 5 g *Spirulina*-supplemented vegetable in comparison to 1 g and 2.5 g level. Thus, spray-dried *Spirulina* can be incorporated in various vegetables without affecting the sensory attributes.

DIFFERENT TYPES OF SNACKS

There were seven types of snacks prepared for sensory evaluation of different levels of *Spirulina* supplementation. Out of the seven snack preparations two were shallow fried (i.e., dhebra and muthia), one was baked (i.e., biscuit), and the rest four were deep fried (i.e., samosa, matar chop, methi vada, and cutlets). Out of the seven different types of snacks prepared, the overall acceptability of four snacks (i.e., dhebra, matar chop, methi vada, and cutlets) at 1 g/2.5 g *Spirulina* supplementation was more acceptable in comparison to the control samples (Table 3.4). In the case of muthia, the mean scores for color was lower than the control sample. The mean scores for texture were comparable with the mean score of the control sample. In case of biscuits, the mean scores for all the sensory attributes showed a decreasing trend in comparison to the control samples except for texture wherein 1 g *Spirulina*-supplemented biscuits showed higher acceptability in comparison to control. Similar trend was also seen for samosas.

TABLE 3.3

Effect of *Spirulina* Supplementation on the Sensory Qualities of Various Types of Vegetables (Mean ± SD)

Group	Color/appearance	Texture	Taste/flavor	Overall acceptability
Kofta curry				
Control	4.04 ± 1.37	4.25 ± 1.42	4.27 ± 1.48	4.18 ± 1.40
Level 1 (1.0 g)	3.84 ± 1.29	3.53 ± 1.54	3.72 ± 1.48	3.66 ± 1.37
Level 2 (2.5 g)	3.83 ± 1.40	3.76 ± 1.47	3.35 ± 1.62	3.57 ± 1.23
Level 3 (5.0 g)	3.90 ± 1.31	3.91 ± 1.32	4.08 ± 1.32	3.83 ± 1.28
Potato spinach				
Control	4.00 ± 1.34	3.91 ± 1.32	4.36 ± 0.64	4.00 ± 1.41
Level 1 (1.0 g)	3.69 ± 1.32	3.92 ± 1.26	3.84 ± 1.29	3.69 ± 1.32
Level 2 (2.5 g)	3.90 ± 1.37	3.50 ± 1.19	3.76 ± 1.42	3.50 ± 1.54
Level 3 (5.0 g)	3.66 ± 1.37	4.00 ± 1.34	3.91 ± 1.49	3.84 ± 1.34
Palak (spinach) paneer				
Control	3.53 ± 1.21	3.41 ± 1.25	2.61 ± 1.00	2.58 ± 0.95
Level 1 (1.0 g)	3.69 ± 1.43	3.76 ± 1.42	3.61 ± 1.38	3.23 ± 1.30
Level 2 (2.5 g)	3.75 ± 1.29	3.53 ± 1.21	2.84 ± 1.16	2.92 ± 1.20
Level 3 (5.0 g)	4.09 ± 0.60	3.61 ± 1.21	2.84 ± 1.16	3.16 ± 0.68
Potato fenugreek				
Control	4.00 ± 1.34	3.53 ± 1.21	2.58 ± 0.98	3.69 ± 1.32
Level 1 (1.0 g)	3.75 ± 1.29	3.50 ± 1.19	3.76 ± 1.42	2.58 ± 0.95
Level 2 (2.5 g)	4.09 ± 0.60	4.00 ± 1.34	3.91 ± 1.49	3.84 ± 1.34
Level 3 (5.0 g)	3.69 ± 1.43	3.91 ± 1.49	2.84 ± 1.16	3.76 ± 1.42

Conclusions

Thus, all the 22 Indian recipes incorporated with *Spirulina* were acceptable with regard to appearance/color, texture, taste/flavor, and overall acceptability at 1 g and 2.5 g levels.

From the sensory evaluation of *Spirulina*-based recipes, the following conclusions can be made:

1. Spray-dried *Spirulina* can be effectively incorporated into various Indian recipes, which would help in the dietary management of diabetes as well as hyperlipidemia as it is low in carbohydrate, has gamma linolenic acid, high in protein, and high in antioxidant content.
2. Owing to its multinutrient property, various recipes that can be supplied in the supplementary feeding programs can be tried out for combating various nutritional disorders such as vitamin A and iron-deficiency anemia.

After the standardization of various *Spirulina*-supplemented recipes, the glycemic index (GI) of foods supplemented with *Spirulina* was carried out, so as to

TABLE 3.4
Effect of *Spirulina* Supplementation on the Sensory Qualities of Various Types of Snacks (Mean ± SD)

Group	Color/appearance	Texture	Taste/flavor	Overall acceptability
Dhebra				
Control	4.08 ± 1.44	4.09 ± 1.37	4.16 ± 1.40	3.90 ± 1.37
Level 1 (1.0 g)	4.09 ± 1.44	4.09 ± 1.37	4.27 ± 1.42	4.09 ± 1.37
Level 2 (2.5 g)	3.75 ± 1.53	3.00 ± 1.17	3.71 ± 1.48	3.80 ± 0.97
Level 3 (5.0 g)	3.25 ± 1.47	3.10 ± 1.13	3.36 ± 1.66	3.30 ± 1.26
Muthia				
Control	4.00 ± 1.41	3.90 ± 1.31	3.66 ± 1.31	3.90 ± 1.37
Level 1 (1.0 g)	3.80 ± 1.46	4.10 ± 0.70	3.61 ± 1.38	3.76 ± 1.30
Level 2 (2.5 g)	3.40 ± 1.25	3.58 ± 0.86	3.72 ± 0.96	3.18 ± 1.19
Level 3 (5.0 g)	3.00 ± 1.30	3.30 ± 1.26	3.20 ± 1.24	3.07 ± 1.22
Biscuits				
Control	3.58 ± 1.32	3.20 ± 1.07	4.40 ± 1.35	3.54 ± 1.37
Level 1 (1.0 g)	3.38 ± 0.73	3.50 ± 0.80	3.33 ± 1.24	3.00 ± 1.17
Level 2 (2.5 g)	2.54 ± 1.07	3.00 ± 0.95	3.27 ± 0.96	2.66 ± 1.02
Level 3 (5.0 g)	2.60 ± 0.91	3.10 ± 0.83	2.70 ± 0.90	2.41 ± 1.03
Samosa				
Control	4.40 ± 0.48	3.89 ± 0.78	3.98 ± 0.87	4.03 ± 0.85
Level 1 (1.0 g)	4.40 ± 0.48	3.88 ± 0.87	3.89 ± 0.86	3.90 ± 0.85
Level 2 (2.5 g)	4.10 ± 0.70	5.71 ± 0.57	3.78 ± 0.86	3.84 ± 0.87
Level 3 (5.0 g)	3.33 ± 0.94	4.09 ± 0.81	3.83 ± 0.88	3.86 ± 0.91
Matar chop				
Control	4.16 ± 1.46	4.00 ± 1.47	4.00 ± 1.41	4.00 ± 1.41
Level 1 (1.0 g)	4.45 ± 1.43	4.36 ± 1.43	4.45 ± 1.43	4.40 ± 1.38
Level 2 (2.5 g)	4.45 ± 1.43	4.45 ± 1.43	4.45 ± 1.43	4.45 ± 1.43
Level 3 (5.0 g)	4.36 ± 1.49	4.45 ± 1.43	4.45 ± 1.43	4.36 ± 1.49
Methi vada				
Control	4.06 ± 0.94	4.10 ± 0.70	3.80 ± 1.07	3.72 ± 1.05
Level 1 (1.0 g)	3.90 ± 0.94	4.10 ± 0.70	3.90 ± 1.22	3.80 ± 0.79
Level 2 (2.5 g)	3.81 ± 0.94	3.99 ± 0.87	3.70 ± 1.26	3.70 ± 0.64
Level 3 (5.0 g)	3.75 ± 0.99	4.00 ± 0.86	3.23 ± 1.40	3.70 ± 0.95
Cutlets				
Control	4.60 ± 0.88	4.30 ± 0.64	4.27 ± 1.05	4.50 ± 0.80
Level 1 (1.0 g)	4.60 ± 0.88	4.30 ± 0.64	4.80 ± 0.40	4.70 ± 0.45
Level 2 (2.5 g)	3.60 ± 0.80	4.18 ± 0.57	4.30 ± 0.78	4.20 ± 0.74
Level 3 (5.0 g)	2.70 ± 0.64	3.70 ± 0.61	3.90 ± 0.83	3.80 ± 0.74

enable the diabetics to judiciously choose the foods that they consume to delay the postprandial excursion in glucose levels. A brief description regarding the GI has been discussed below before presenting the GI of various *Spirulina* incorporated recipes.

GLYCEMIC INDEX

Diet plays a central role in the management of type 2 diabetes mellitus (T2DM). Diet contains a multitude of nutritional and chemical molecules each capable of regulating a number of biological processes. One of the nutrients, which is of prime importance, is the quantity and quality of carbohydrates (CHO). The diabetics are advised to select carbohydrate foods that minimize the postprandial blood glucose excursions, which on a long run would help to prevent the development of secondary complications. This has led to the introduction of GI where the effects of various CHO-containing foods on postprandial plasma glucose concentrations are classified in relation to the response elicited by an index glucose challenge. The concept of GI of foods was first introduced by Jenkins et al.[2] and is defined as the ratio between area under the 2 h postprandial glycemic curve on ingestion of carbohydrate (test food) and on ingestion of glucose.

$$GI = \frac{\text{Area under 2-h blood glucose curve on ingestion of test food}}{\text{Area under 2-h blood glucose curve on ingestion of standard glucose}} \times 100$$

Factors Affecting Glycemic Index

The way the gastrointestinal tract handles the CHO is modulated by a number of food factors present in the food, as a result different equicarbohydrate foods produce different glycemic responses. There are several factors affecting the GI of a food. These include:

- Nature of starch and its digestibility
- Method of cooking and processing
- Physical characteristics of food/starches
- Protein and fat content
- Fiber content of food
- Antinutrients

The factors affecting GI along with their postulated mechanisms are summarized below:

Factors affecting GI	Postulated mechanism
Starch digestibility	Amylopectin—larger surface area per molecule than amylose, therefore, easy enzymatic attack
Nutrient-starch interaction	Starch protein complex: unavailable for enzymatic attack
Antinutrients	Binds with nutrients or enzymes and delays digestion process
Method of cooking and processing	Starch becomes more soluble, therefore, easy enzymatic digestion
Protein and fat content	Protein stimulates insulin secretion, fat delays gastric emptying
Fiber	Delays gastric emptying and gel formation

THERAPEUTIC IMPLICATIONS OF GLYCEMIC INDEX

The clinical utility of GI lies in classifying foods into low-, moderate-, and high-GI foods, which would help in developing appropriate exchange lists for diabetics. Apart from this, the therapeutic implications of low-GI foods have been documented in literature and are as follows:

- Helps to control established diabetes
- Helps to lose weight
- Improves the insulin sensitivity
- Reduces appetite for quick sugars and carbohydrates, thus avoiding blood sugar spikes
- Can help to minimize the hypoglycemic effect of sudden intensive exercise

STUDIES ON GLYCEMIC INDEX

Over the years, several researchers across the globe have carried out research pertaining to GI and its implications in health and disease.[2–7] Similarly, in the Indian context, research related to low-GI foods and their therapeutic importance has also been studied extensively. The GI of traditional Indian CHO foods, conventional CHO meals, cereal pulse mix, combination of cereals and green leafy vegetables, and regional Indian meals have been carried out.[8–12] In this context, *Spirulina*, which has bioactive compounds that enhance health, was incorporated into various recipes and tested for their glycemic and lipemic responses, the results of which are discussed below.

Glycemic and Lipemic Responses of *Spirulina*-Supplemented Rice-Based Preparations

Recipes tested: Rice alone, Rice with green gram dal, Rice with red gram dal, Rice with peas, Vegetable pulao with curd
Subjects: Normal subjects
Carbohydrate load: 50 g
Level of Spirulina supplementation: 2.5 g spray-dried powder
Number of subjects: Six for each recipe

The nutritive value of rice-based recipes incorporated with *Spirulina* is depicted in Table 3.5.

The GI of the various recipes ranged from 38% to 50%. Rice alone elicited a higher GI in comparison to rice preparations with a combination of pulses and vegetables. Similarly, on comparing the glycemic response of the *Spirulina*-supplemented recipes with that of unsupplemented recipes carried out on T2DM, a marked reduction in GI was noticed. A similar trend was observed with respect to the lipemic response (Table 3.5).

TABLE 3.5
Nutrient Composition, Glycemic and Lipemic Responses of *Spirulina*-Supplemented Rice-Based Recipes

Recipes	Protein (g)	Fat (g)	Fiber (g)	% GI[a] (mean ± SD)	% GI[b] (mean ± SD)	% TG rise/fall	% TG rise
Rice	6.2	5.5	0.2	59.0 ± 4.0	80.0 ± 14.0	−9	40
Rice + green gram dal	11.0	5.7	0.3	51.0 ± 8.0	62.0 ± 8.0	−5	86
Rice + red gram dal	10.7	5.8	0.5	38.0 ± 11.7	64.0 ± 6.0	−4	39
Rice + peas	10.1	5.7	1.3	48.0 ± 11.0	74.0 ± 8.0	−8	20
Vegetable pulao	8.7	6.4	1.8	46.0 ± 8.4	—	2	—

[a] GI (*Spirulina* supplemented) in normal subjects.
[b] GI (*Spirulina* unsupplemented) in diabetic subjects.

TABLE 3.6
Nutrient Composition, Glycemic and Lipemic Responses of *Spirulina*-Supplemented Wheat-Based Recipes

Recipes	Protein (g)	Fat (g)	Fiber (g)	% GI[a] (mean ± SD)	% GI[b] (mean ± SD)	% TG[a] rise	% TG[a] rise
Plain paratha	12.3	14.0	2.2	74.0 ± 7.9	82.0 ± 9.9	5.52	22.8
Methi paratha	14.3	14.2	2.2	37.0 ± 16.4	52.0 ± 20.5	11.5	51.3
Spinach paratha	13.9	14.3	2.4	64.0 ± 8.9	72.0 ± 12.7	4.2	13.9

[a] *Spirulina* supplemented.
[b] *Spirulina* unsupplemented.

Glycemic and Lipemic Responses of *Spirulina*-Supplemented Wheat-Based Preparations

Recipes tested: Plain paratha, Fenugreek paratha, and Spinach paratha
Subjects: Type 2 diabetics
Carbohydrate load: 50 g
Level of Spirulina supplementation: 2.5 g spray-dried powder
Number of subjects: Six for each recipe

The glycemic and lipemic responses of wheat-based recipes with and without *Spirulina* incorporation have been depicted in Table 3.6. The addition of *Spirulina* resulted in a reduction in the GI values of plain paratha (GI reduction from 81% to 74%), methi paratha (GI reduction from 52% to 37%), and spinach paratha (GI reduction from 72% to 64%). Similarly, a reduction in the triglyceride (TG) response was seen with *Spirulina*-supplemented recipes as compared with the unsupplemented ones (Table 3.6).

TABLE 3.7
Nutrient Composition, Glycemic and Lipemic Responses of Regional Meals with and without *Spirulina* Supplementation

Recipes	Protein (g)	Fat (g)	Fiber (g)	% GI[a] (mean ± SD)	% GI[b] (mean ± SD)	% TG[a] rise	% TG[a] rise/fall
Punjabi meal	18.9	20.6	3.1	34.0 ± 16.64	68.0 ± 19.21	3.3	10.24
South Indian meal	15.5	15.1	3.2	53.0 ± 21.18	63.0 ± 4.26	6.9	−6.34
Gujarati meal	17.1	17.3	2.1	61.0 ± 21.89	83.0 ± 11.41	46	18.05
West Bengal meal	26.8	24.8	1.3	58.0 ± 8.87	70.0 ± 16.5	18.2	16

[a] *Spirulina* supplemented.
[b] *Spirulina* unsupplemented.

Glycemic and Lipemic Responses of *Spirulina*-Supplemented Regional Meals

Recipes tested: Punjabi meal, South Indian meal, Gujarati meal, and West Bengali meal
Subjects: Normal subjects
Carbohydrate load: 75 g
Level of Spirulina supplementation: 2.5 g spray-dried powder
Number of subjects: Six for each recipe

The Indian cuisine in various parts of India is different and has its own speciality; hence, composite meals from various parts of India were tested for their GI. The nutrient composition and glycemic and lipemic responses of various regional meals are depicted in Table 3.7. A favorable reduction in the glycemic response was observed with 2.5 g of *Spirulina* supplementation. Highest reduction in the GI was seen in Punjabi meal (68 vs. 34), followed by Gujarati meal, West Bengali meal, and South Indian meal. The least rise in % TG was seen for Punjabi meal supplemented with *Spirulina* (3.3%). The remaining three regional meals showed a rise in the range of 6.9–46%.

Glycemic and Lipemic Responses of *Spirulina*-Supplemented Snacks

Recipes tested: Matar chops, Samosa, Biscuits, Dhebra with curd, Methi wada, and Vegetable cutlets
Subjects: Type 2 diabetics
Carbohydrate load: 50 g
Level of Spirulina supplementation: 2.5 g spray-dried powder
Number of subjects: Six for each recipe

TABLE 3.8
Nutrient Composition, Glycemic and Lipemic Responses of *Spirulina*-Supplemented Snacks

Recipes	Protein (g)	Fat (g)	Fiber (g)	% GI mean ± SD	% TG rise mean
Matar chops	13.0	28	4.6	37.0 ± 18.5	27.5
Vegetable cutlets	10.5	21.3	2.4	44.0 ± 21.5	29.4
Samosa	8.2	21.2	1.8	40.0 ± 18.4	14.4
Dhebra with curd	15.0	16.5	1.3	54.0 ± 10.3	29.4
Biscuits	7.0	17.0	0.5	43.0 ± 23.1	27.1
Methi vada	20.6	25.7	1.9	33.0 ± 17.9	12.8

The nutritive value and glycemic and lipemic responses of *Spirulina*-supplemented snacks are given in Table 3.8. Results indicated that among the test snacks Methi wada was most suitable in terms of glycemic (38%) and lipemic (12%) responses, followed by Matar chops (37%) and Samosa (39%). Biscuits and vegetable cutlets also produced a low-glycemic response but were higher than the previous three snacks. Dhebra produced the highest GI with curd (53%). The lower value for vegetable cutlets could be due to the frying process.

Discussion

Spirulina, the blue-green algae, has some potent probiotic compounds that enhance health with more than 60% good quality proteins, vitamins, β-carotene, and γ-linolenic acid, and has become a favored material of health care. Therefore, spray-dried *Spirulina* was incorporated in various recipes to exploit its nutritional properties and to see its efficacy in terms of glycemic and lipemic responses. *Spirulina*, which contains single cell protein of high biological value, was added to the recipes at 2.5 g level. From the results of the present study, it is clear that the multiple components present in *Spirulina* could have played a role in eliciting relatively lower glycemic and lipemic responses as compared to the corresponding recipes without *Spirulina*. It has been well established that amino acids affect the postprandial glucose concentration.[13] It could be speculated that the addition of 2.5 g of *Spirulina*, which is rich in protein, may bring in the insulin peak earlier in the recipes with *Spirulina* compared to recipes without *Spirulina*. This could be one of the possible mechanisms by which a lowered glycemic response was seen in recipes supplemented with *Spirulina* than in recipes without *Spirulina*. Further *Spirulina* contains γ-linolenic acid and antioxidants, which may modulate the lipid metabolism favorably. It has been reported that low-GI diets bring about a 20% reduction in the TG levels in patients with hypertriglyceridemia.[14,15] The positive shifts in the glycemic and lipemic responses have been substantiated by clinical trials with long-term *Spirulina* supplementation (2 g/day) for a period of 2 months in diabetics.[16] All these observations confirm the efficacy of *Spirulina* as a hypoglycemic and hypolipidemic agent.

Conclusions

Hence, on the basis of sensory evaluation of data and looking at the glycemic and lipemic responses of the *Spirulina*-supplemented recipes it can be concluded that spray-dried *Spirulina* can be effectively used as an supportive therapy in the management of hyperglycemia and hyperlipidemia.

METHOD OF PREPARATION AND COMPOSITION OF RECIPES

The details of the recipes used for standardization as well as GI are given below. Please make a note that wherever the incorporation of *Spirulina* is mentioned, it is indicative that in case of standardization, *Spirulina* was supplemented at three levels in the recipes, namely, 1 g, 2.5 g, and 5 g levels; whereas, for finding the GI, *Spirulina* was incorporated at the level of 2.5 g.

Plain Paratha with Tomato–Onion Raita: Wheat flour (60 g) was sieved. *Spirulina* powder was added. Stiff dough was made and was divided into equal balls. These balls were rolled into triangular shapes and fried on both the sides with little oil (10 g used for all parathas) until they turn golden brown in color. This was served with tomato–onion Raita. Raita was prepared by beating the curd (50 g) to a smooth consistency and then adding tomato (30 g), onion (30 g), and 5 g of cumin seeds powder to it.

Methi (Fenugreek) Paratha with Curd: Wheat flour (20 g) and suji (35 g) were sieved together. To this, chopped fenugreek leaves (100 g), green chilli (2.5 g), ginger (2.5 g), cumin seeds powder (2.5 g), salt, and *Spirulina* powder were added. Mixture was made into soft dough. The dough was divided into small balls and rolled into triangular-shaped chapatis. The chapatis were placed on a hot tava and after a minute, they were turned on to the other side. Little oil (10 g used for all parathas) was applied, and it was fried on both the sides until they turn golden brown in color and served with 50 g curd.

Potato Paratha with Curd: Potatoes (50 g) were boiled, peeled, and mashed. To this, chopped chillies (2.5 g), coriander leaves (2.5 g), dry green mango powder (2.5 g), cumin seeds powder (2.5 g), salt (as per taste), and *Spirulina* powder were added and mixed well. Wheat flour (50 g) was made into dough. The dough was made into small balls and each small ball was then rolled into small round flat shaped chapati. A spoonful of potato mixture was placed on each chapati and enclosed with another. The ball so formed was dusted with dry flour and rolled out again into medium thick chapati. The chapati was then placed on a hot tava and after a minute, it was turned on to the other side. Little oil (10 g used for all parathas) was applied, and it was shallow fried on both sides until it turn golden brown in color and served with 50 g curd.

Spinach Paratha with Curd: Cauliflower (100 g), ginger (5 g), and green chillies (2.5 g) were grated. All these were added together with salt, dry green mango powder (2.5 g), and cumin seeds powder (2.5 g). This mixture was mixed well and kept aside.

Spinach leaves (50 g) paste was prepared and *Spirulina* powder was added to it. This was then incorporated into wheat flour and soft dough was made. Dough was divided into small balls and were rolled into small round chapatis. A spoonful of mixture was placed on each chapati and enclosed with another. The chapati was placed on a hot tava and after a minute, it was turned on to the other side. Little oil (10 g used for all parathas) was applied, and it was fried on both sides until it turn golden brown in color and served with 50 g curd.

Mint and Cabbage Stuffed Paratha with Curd: Cabbage (100 g), onion (30 g), and green chillies (2.5 g) were chopped. To this, dry green mango powder (2.5 g), salt, and cumin seeds (2.5 g) were added, mixed well, and kept aside. Mint leaves (50 g) paste was made and *Spirulina* powder was added to it. Soft wheat flour (25 g) dough was made by adding mint paste and *Spirulina* powder. Dough was divided into small balls and they were rolled into small chapatis. A spoonful of mixture was placed on each chapati and was enclosed with another. This was placed on a hot tava and after a minute, it was turned on to the other side. Little oil (10 g used for all parathas) was applied, and it was fried on both sides until it turn golden brown in color and served with 50 g curd.

Peas Paratha with Curd: Potatoes (15 g) and peas (50 g) were boiled and mashed. Onion (20 g), green chillies (2.5 g), and coriander leaves (5 g) were chopped, and added to peas and potato mixture. To this, gingelly seeds (5 g), dry green mango powder (2.5 g), and *Spirulina* powder were added and mixed well. Wheat flour (45 g) was made into a dough. Dough was divided into small balls and were rolled out into small chapatis. A spoonful of mixture was placed on each chapati and enclosed with another. The chapati was placed on a hot tava and after a minute it was turned on to the other side. Little oil (10 g used for all parathas) was applied, and it was fried on both the sides until it turn golden brown in color and served with 50 g curd.

Coriander Paratha with Curd: Coriander leaves (50 g) were chopped. Soft wheat flour (65 g) was made adding coriander leaves, cumin seeds (2.5 g), salt, and *Spirulina* powder. The dough was divided into small balls and were rolled into triangular-shaped rotis. Each roti was placed on a hot tava and after a minute it was turned on to the other side. Little oil (10 g used for all parathas) was applied, and each roti was fried on both sides until it turn golden brown in color and served with 50 g curd.

Potato Palak with Chapati: Spinach (150 g), garlic (5 g), ginger (5 g), and tomato (20 g) were chopped separately. Potato (50 g) was cut and peeled into equal pieces. Oil (5 g) was heated in a pan and the garlic and ginger were fried until they turn golden brown in color. Potato and palak (spinach) were added along with salt and red chilli. When it was half cooked, tomato and *Spirulina* powders were added and cooked for sometime. This vegetable was served with rotis/chapatis, which were made using 45 g of whole wheat flour. "Roti" or "Chapati" is an Indian flat bread much like the Mexican Tortilla. Roti is rolled out of unleavened whole wheat dough. The small balls of dough (approximately 15 g each) are rolled out with the help of a rolling pin and then partially cooked on a hot tava or griddle and then finished directly over high heat. The high heat makes the rotis puff up into a ball.

Potato Methi with Chapati: Methi (fenugreek leaves, 100 g) was chopped finely. Onion (30 g) was cut into slices. Potato (20 g) was peeled and cut into equal pieces. Oil (5 g) was heated; onion and cumin seeds (2.5 g) were added and fried until they turn light brown in color. Potato, methi, salt, and red chilli were added. When half cooked, dried green mango powder (2.5 g) and *Spirulina* powder were added and cooked for some more time. This vegetable was served with rotis/chapatis, which were made using 50 g of whole wheat flour. "Roti" or "Chapati" is an Indian flat bread much like the Mexican Tortilla. Roti is rolled out of unleavened whole wheat dough. The small balls of dough (approximately 15 g each) are rolled out with the help of a rolling pin and then partially cooked on a hot tava or griddle and then finished directly over high heat. The high heat makes the rotis puff up into a ball.

Palak Paneer with Chapati: Palak (Spinach, 100 g) was chopped and the paste was made in a mixer with *Spirulina* powder. Tomato (30 g), garlic (10 g), and ginger (10 g) were chopped separately. Oil (5 g) was heated in a pan. Cumin seeds (2.5 g), ginger, and garlic were added and fried until they turn dark brown in color. Tomato, salt, and red chillies were added and fried until the oil left the sides of the pan. Spinach and *Spirulina* powders along with paneer pieces (25 g) were cooked for 10 min. This vegetable was served with rotis/chapatis, which were made using 60 g of whole wheat flour. "Roti" or "Chapati" is an Indian flat bread much like the Mexican Tortilla. Roti is rolled out of unleavened whole wheat dough. The small balls of dough (approximately 15 g each) are rolled out with the help of a rolling pin and then partially cooked on a hot tava or griddle and then finished directly over high heat. The high heat makes the rotis puff up into a ball.

Dudhi Kofta with Chapati: Dudhi (bottlegourd, 100 g) was grated and water was squeezed out. Ginger (2.5 g), coriander leaves (5 g), onion (30 g), and tomato (30 g) were finely chopped and added separately. Grated dudhi, Bengal gram flour (22 g), *Spirulina* powder, salt, dry green mango powder (2.5 g), and ginger were mixed well and made into a stiff dough. Equal balls were made out of this and deep fried in oil until they turn dark brown in color. Oil (20 g) was heated, cumin seeds (2.5 g) were added, and onions were fried until they turn dark brown in color. Tomato, salt, and red chillies were added and fried till the oil left the sides of the pan. Some water was added and the koftas were added and cooked for 2–3 min. This vegetable was served with rotis/chapatis, which were made using 40 g of whole wheat flour. "Roti" or "Chapati" is an Indian flat bread much like the Mexican Tortilla. Roti is rolled out of unleavened whole wheat dough. The small balls of dough (approximately 15 g each) are rolled out with the help of a rolling pin and then partially cooked on a hot tava or griddle and then finished directly over high heat. The high heat makes the rotis puff up into a ball.

Methi Rice with Curd: Oil (10 g) was heated in a pan. Onion (20 g), ginger (5 g), and green chillies (2.5 g) were chopped. They were fried until they turn light brown in color. Chopped methi (fenugreek leaves, 100 g) and washed rice (50 g) were added with equal amount of water. *Spirulina* powder was added and mixed well. This mixture was cooked in pressure cooker till done and it was garnished with chopped tomatoes (20 g) and served with curd (50 g).

Coriander Rice with Potato Raita: Coriander leaves paste (50 g) was prepared. Oil (5 g) was heated in a pan and chopped green chill (2.5 g) and ginger (2.5 g) were added and fried until they turn brown in color. Washed rice (50 g) was added with equal amount of water. *Spirulina* powder was added and cooked till done.

Potato Raita: Potatoes (25 g) were boiled and mashed properly. Curd (50 g) was whipped and mashed potatoes along with salt and cumin seed powder (2.5 g) were added.

Vegetable Pulao with Curd: Vegetables (10 g potato, 20 g peas, 20 g carrot, and 20 g cauliflower) were cut into small pieces. When oil (5 g) was hot two cloves were added. Sliced onions (20 g) were added and fried until they turn dark brown in color. All the vegetables were added and were fried with rice (50 g) for 1 min. *Spirulina* powder was added with equal amount of water and cooked in pressure cooker till done, garnished with chopped tomato (20 g), and served with curd (50 g).

Spinach Raita with Onion Rice: Potatoes (10 g) were sliced and fried in half teaspoon oil and taken out when they turn light brown in color. Some more oil (2.5 g) was taken and sliced onions (20 g) and ginger (2.5 g) were fried until they turn light brown in color. Washed rice (50 g) was added with equal amount of water and cooked in pressure cooker till done.

Spinach Raita: Spinach paste (100 g) was made and *Spirulina* powder was added to this paste. Curd (50 g) was whipped and the paste was added along with salt and cumin seed powder (2.5 g).

Muthia: Rice (35 g), Bengal gram dal (15 g), and red gram dal (15 g) were coarsely powdered. To this, chopped fenugreek leaves (30 g), sugar (1.5 g), salt, and *Spirulina* powder were added. Stiff dough was made with the help of curd. Dough was divided into equal oblong rolls. They were steamed for 30 min till done. The rolls were then cut into small equal pieces. Oil was heated in a pan and gingelly seeds (2 g) were added and the pieces were shallow fried for 2 min.

Dhebra: Methi leaves (25 g) were chopped. Bajra flour (40 g) and wheat flour (25 g) were sieved. Chopped methi, curd (15 g), sugar (2.5 g), salt, gingelly seeds (2.5 g), and *Spirulina* powder were added. Mixture was made into a soft dough. Dough was divided into small balls and rolled into chapatis. Each chapati was shallow fried in a pan until it turn golden brown in color.

Samosa: Potatoes (50 g) were boiled, peeled, and mashed. Carrot (15 g) was grated, and onion (15 g), green chillies (2.5 g), and coriander leaves (5 g) were chopped. Chopped onion was fried in 3 ml oil. Green chillies, cumin seeds (2.5 g), mango powder (2.5 g), mashed potatoes, carrot, and peas (20 g) were added and cooked for 2 min. *Spirulina* powder was then added and mixed well. Wheat flour refined (40 g) was mixed with a pinch of salt and made into soft dough. The dough was divided into small balls and were rolled into thin chapatis, each chapati cut into two halves and twisted into a cone. A spoonful of mixture was filled into each cone and enclosed with the help of water. The cones were deep fried in hot oil (20 g oil for consumed while frying) until the cones turn brown in color uniformly on all the sides.

Matar Chop: Potatoes (90 g) and peas (100 g) were boiled and mixed well. To this, arrowroot flour (5 g), dry green mango powder (2.5 g), sugar (5 g), green chilli (2.5 g), coriander leaves (5 g), and chopped ginger (2.5 g) were added. *Spirulina* powder was added and mixed well. Half teaspoon oil was heated in a pan and gingelly seeds (2 g) and dry coconut (10 g) was added. To this, potato and peas mixture was added and fried for 1 min. From this, equal balls were made. Oil (20 g oil for consumed while frying) was heated in a pan. Balls were deep fried.

Vegetable Cutlets: Potatoes (50 g) were boiled, peeled, and mashed. Carrot (20 g) was grated and coriander leaves (5 g), onion (20 g), ginger (2.5 g), and green chillies (2.5 g) were chopped finely. All this was mixed with cumin seeds (2.5 g), dry green mango powder (2.5 g), salt, and *Spirulina* powder well. Bread was soaked in water for 1 min and squeezed out. Bread (50 g) was mixed well with the above mixture. Mixture was divided into equal parts and made into oval shape. Bread crumb powder was sprinkled on each piece and deep fried in hot oil (20 g oil for consumed while frying) until they turn brown in color.

Methi Wada: Methi (50 g), green chillies (2.5 g), and ginger (2.5 g) were chopped. These were added to Bengal gram flour (75 g) along with gingelly seeds (2 g), salt, dry green mango powder (2.5 g), and *Spirulina* powder. All these were mixed with enough water and made into stiff dough. Small balls of this mixture were then deep fried in oil (20 g oil for consumed while frying) until they turn brown in color.

Biscuits: Sugar (15 g) was powdered and sieved along with whole wheat flour (22.5 g), refined wheat flour (22.5 g), baking powder, and *Spirulina* powder. Butter (20 g) was added and the mixture was made into medium stiff dough, then vanilla essence was added. The dough was divided into five balls and flattened slightly, and baked in an oven for around 40 min at 150°C.

Rice: *Spirulina* powder (2.5 g) was added to rice (64 g). Oil (5 g), salt (as per taste), and green chillies (as per taste) were added to improve the palatability. It was then pressure cooked with equal amount of water till done.

Rice with Green Gram Dal: *Spirulina* powder (2.5 g) was added to rice (45 g) and green gram dal (25 g). Oil (5 g), salt (as per taste), and green chillies (as per taste) were added to improve the palatability. It was then pressure cooked with equal amount of water till done.

Rice with Red Gram Dal: *Spirulina* powder (2.5 g) was added to rice (45 g) and red gram dal (26 g). Oil (5 g), salt (as per taste), and green chillies (as per taste) were added to improve the palatability. It was then pressure cooked with equal amount of water till done.

Rice with Peas: *Spirulina* powder (2.5 g) and peas green (27 g) were added to rice (45 g). Oil (5 g), salt (as per taste), and green chillies (as per taste) were added to improve the palatability. It was then pressure cooked with equal amount of water till done.

REGIONAL MEALS

Punjab Meal

1. *Dal Makhani:* Rajmah (15 g) and whole black gram (10 g) were soaked together for about 8 h in 200 ml of water and then pressure cooked for 12 min. Onions (25 g), tomatoes (30 g), ginger (2 g), and garlic (2 g) were chopped finely. In hot oil (5 g), chopped onions were fried until they turn golden brown in color. Chopped tomatoes, ginger, and garlic were added to make smooth gravy. Cooked legumes were added along with turmeric powder (one-fourth tsp), chilli powder (one-fourth tsp), and some garam masala (one-fourth tsp), and cooked for another 15 min on slow fire. Before removing from the fire, ghee (5 g) was added.

2. *Brinjal Bhurta:* Brinjal (80 g) was roasted on direct flame until the outer skin blackened. The skin was removed and the brinjal mashed. Onions (30 g), tomatoes (20 g), ginger (2 g), garlic (2 g), and one green chilli were chopped finely. In hot oil (10 g), the ingredients were fried. Turmeric (one-fourth tsp) and salt (according taste) were added and fried. Mashed brinjal (80 g) was added, mixed well, and cooked for 5 min. After removing from the fire, chopped coriander (5 g) was added.

3. *Phulka:* "Phulka", "Roti" or "Chapati" is an Indian flat bread much like the Mexican tortilla. Roti is rolled out of unleavened whole wheat dough. The small balls of dough (approximately 15 g each) are rolled out with the help of a rolling pin and then partially cooked on a hot tava or griddle and then finished directly over high heat. The high heat makes the phulka puff up into a ball.

Gujarati Whole Meal

1. *Kichadi:* Red gram rice (20 g) was soaked for 8 h. In hot oil (5 g), one broken red chilli and a few mustard seeds were added. After the seeds crackled, rice (50 g) and red gram dal (20 g) were added and fried. Salt (according to taste), turmeric (one-fourth tsp), and about 140 ml of water were added and pressure cooked for 8 min. Ghee (2.5 g) was added before serving.

2. *Kadhi:* Curd (65 g) was beaten well after adding water. A paste of ginger (2 g) and chilli (2 g) was made and added to the curd (65 g) along with Bengal gram flour (5 g) and mixed well to make a smooth paste. In hot oil (2.5 g), cumin seeds (1), one cinnamon, one clove, and one pepper were tempered and poured in the Kadhi. Kadhi was allowed to cook for 10 min after the addition of 5 g of jaggery with constant stirring.

3. *Potato Bhaji:* Potatoes (65 g) were boiled in their jackets and the skin was peeled off on cooling. They were diced and kept aside. In hot oil (7.5 g), mustard seeds (1 g) were added. On crackling, green chilli, salt, and turmeric as per taste were added and fried. Diced potatoes were added and cooked for 5 min.

Bengali Meal

1. *Fried Fish:* Fish (80 g) was cleaned and washed thoroughly. After adding salt as per taste and turmeric (one-fourth tsp) to the fish, it was kept aside for 20 min. Mustard oil (5 g) was heated and the fish (80 g) was fried until it was golden brown on both sides. It was served with some lemon slices.
2. *Dal:* Green gram dal (25 g) was roasted to a light brown color and then pressure cooked with salt as per taste. Mustard oil (2.5 g) and ghee (2.5 g) were heated and cumin seeds (1 g), one bay leaf, one red chilli, and grated ginger (2 g) were tempered. Cooked dal (25 g) was added with turmeric (one-fourth tsp) and sugar (2 g), and simmered for 5 min. Grated coconut (5 g) was added and then removed from the fire.
3. *Charchari:* Peeled potato (20 g) and sweet potato (20 g) were cut into cubes. Brinjal (40 g) was cut into even sized pieces. In hot mustard oil (10 g), one broken red chilli, one slit green chilli, and 2 g mixture of mustard seeds, onion seeds, and cumin seeds were tempered. Vegetables were added and sauted. Salt (as per taste), sugar (1 g), turmeric (one-fourth tsp), and 100 ml of water were added to cook the vegetables. It was covered with a lid and allowed to cook, until the vegetables were tender and water was absorbed.
4. *Rice:* Rice (55 g) was washed and pressure cooked in double quantity of water with salt for 5–7 min.

South Indian Meal

1. *Rice:* Rice (55 g) was washed and pressure cooked in double quantity of water with salt for 5–7 min.
2. *Sambhar:* Red gram dal (20 g) was pressure cooked in 100 ml of water for 5–7 min. Tamarind (10 g) was soaked in about 25–30 ml water for 30 min and the juice was extracted. Brinjal (10 g) and tomato (10 g) were cubed and onion was finely chopped. In hot oil (5 g), mustard seeds (30 g), one red chilli, two curry leaves, and a pinch of asafetida were added and after it spluttered, vegetables were added and sauteed for a few minutes. The tamarind juice was added and brought to a boil. Cooked dal with water, salt (as per taste), and sambhar powder (5 g) were added and brought to a boil.
3. *Cabbage Curry:* Cabbage (100 g) was finely chopped and fresh coconut (20 g) was grated. To hot oil (10 g), mustard seeds (3 g), black gram dal (2.5 g), and cabbage were added and allowed to cook on a low flame. Water was sprinkled and the vegetables were stirred from time to time. After cabbage was cooked, salt (as per taste) and chilli powder (2 g) were added, and the vegetable was garnished with fresh coconut.

ACKNOWLEDGMENTS

The authors wish to acknowledge the financial assistance received by the University Grants Commission (New Delhi, India) and Parry Agro Industries Ltd. (Chennai,

India) for the work that has been reported in this communication. The authors would also like to thank the research scholars, Ms. Shweta Sachdeva, Ms. Namita Bhakar, Ms. Shirali Parikh, Ms. Sophia Ahmedi, and Ms. Shilpa Deshmukh, for their contributions in carrying out the work.

REFERENCES

1. World Health Organization (WHO) Report. Diet, Nutrition and the prevention of chronic diseases. WHO Technical Report Series 916, Report of a Joint WHO/FAO Expert Consultation, 2003.
2. Jenkins, D.J.A. et al., Glycemic index of foods: A physiological basis for carbohydrate exchange. *Am. J. Clin. Nut.*, 34, 362, 1981.
3. Jenkins, D.J.A., Wolever, T.M., and Colier, G.R., Metabolic effects of low glycemic index diet. *Am. J. Clin. Nutr.*, 46, 968, 1987.
4. Jenkins, D. J.A. et al., Glycemic index: Overview of implications in health and disease. *Am. J. Clin. Nutr.*, 76 (Suppl.), 266S, 2002.
5. Miller, J.B., Glycemic index/glycemic load. *Am. J. Clin. Nutr.*, 76, 5, 2001.
6. Miller, J.B. et al., Low glycemic index diets in the management of diabetes: A meta analysis of randomized controlled trials. *Diabetes Care*, 26, 2261, 2003.
7. Ludwig, D. et al., High glycemic index foods, overeating and obesity. *Pediatrics*, 103, e26, 1999.
8. Mani, U.V. et al., Glycemic index of traditional Indian carbohydrate foods. *J. Am. Coll. Nutr.*, 9, 573, 1990.
9. Mani, U.V. et al., Glycemic index of some commonly consumed foods in Western India. *Asia Pacific J. Clin. Nutr.*, 2, 111, 1993.
10. Mani, U.V. et al., Glycemic index of cereal–pulse mix (diabetic mix) in NIDDM subjects. *Int. J. Fd. Sci. Nutr.*, 45, 141, 1994.
11. Mani, U.V. et al., Study on the glycemic index of selected cereal–green leafy vegetables combination in NIDDM patients. *J. Nutr. Med.*, 4, 321, 1994.
12. Mani, U.V. et al., Long-term effect of cereal pulse mix supplementation on serum lipid profile in NIDDM subjects. *J. Nutr. Environ. Med.*, 7, 3, 1997.
13. Westphal, S.A., Gannon, M.C., and Nuttall, F.Q., Metabolic response to glucose ingested with various amounts of protein. *Am. J. Clin. Nutr.*, 52, 267, 1990.
14. Wolever, T.M.S. et al., The glycemic index: Methodology and clinical implications. *Am. J. Clin. Nutr.*, 54, 846, 1991.
15. Mani, U.V. et al., Glycemic index of conventional carbohydrate meals. *Br. J. Nutr.*, 68, 445, 1992.
16. Parikh, P., Mani, U., and Iyer, U., Role of *Spirulina* in the control of glycemia and lipidemia in type 2 diabetes mellitus. *J. Med. Fds.*, 4, 193, 2001.

4 Therapeutic Utility of *Spirulina*

Uliyar V. Mani, Uma M. Iyer, Swati A. Dhruv, Indirani U. Mani, and Kavita S. Sharma

CONTENTS

INTRODUCTION

Spirulina, the blue-green algae, has today emerged as a great nutraceutical phenomenon. Worldwide medical research has discovered that *Spirulina* with its unique blend of nutrients (good-quality proteins, balanced fatty acid profile, antioxidant vitamins, and minerals) has helped to combat many health problems like diabetes, arthritis, anemia, cancer, and so forth.

Over the past decade, studies have been carried out in the department on *Spirulina* supplementation in the management of various disorders. Initial studies were conducted by supplementing *Spirulina* in T2DM (Type 2 diabetes mellitus) and hyperlipidemic subjects for a period of 2 months. The results of these studies showed that *Spirulina* supplementation in T2DM patients at a level of 2 g/day for a period of 2 months resulted in a significant reduction in fasting and postprandial blood glucose.[1] Similarly, *Spirulina* supplementation (2 g/day) for a period of 2 months also had a favorable impact on lipid metabolism of hyperlipidemic subjects.[2]

These initial observations encouraged us to carry out long-term *Spirulina* supplementation studies in various disorders, namely, diabetes, asthma, nephrotic syndrome, and anemia, which have been discussed at length in this chapter.

THERAPEUTIC UTILITY OF *SPIRULINA* IN DIABETES MELLITUS

INTRODUCTION

Noncommunicable diseases are increasing to alarming proportions and gaining their hold over the developing countries. One of the noncommunicable diseases that has gained importance is diabetes mellitus because of its rising prevalence. Worldwide, the number of cases of diabetes is currently estimated to be around 150 million. This number is predicted to double by 2025, with the greatest number of cases being expected in China and India.[3] The rising prevalence of diabetes and its associated complications place a high burden on the health care systems. The major therapeutic goal in diabetic patients therefore, is to optimize blood glucose control in order to improve the well-being of the patients and reduce the risk of diabetes-induced complications. The recent years have witnessed a renewed interest in identifying probiotics, antioxidants, neutraceuticals, and designer foods that can be used as alternative therapies for sustaining and managing health. This prompted us to assess the efficacy of *Spirulina* in the management of diabetes mellitus.

METHODOLOGY

The study was designed as a clinical intervention trial. Patients with T2DM were recruited from the Diabetes Clinics of Vadodara with the consent of the consulting physician and patients. The patients were kept under an observation for a period of 4 months. After the observation period, the patients ($n = 30$, females: $n = 13$, males: $n = 17$) were supplemented with 2 g/day *Spirulina* tablets for 4 months. The patients were asked to take two tablets (500 g each) along with lunch and two tablets (500 g each) with dinner. Patients were asked to maintain their habitual diet, medication regimen and level of physical activity throughout the study period. Follow-up evaluations were carried out at intervals of 2 and 4 months.

TABLE 4.1

Patient Characteristics at Baseline and after Observation Period

Variables	At baseline	After observation period
Anthropometric indices		
Body mass index (kg/m^2)	25.9 ± 4.0	26.0 ± 4.9
WC (cm)	96.2 ± 11.4	98.9 ± 17.1
Waist hip ratio	0.95 ± 0.1	0.95 ± 0.1
General habits, n (%)		
Nonsedentary	18 (60.0)	19 (63.3)
Tobacco consumers	1 (3.3)	2 (6.7)
Smokers	5 (16.7)	3 (10.0)
Alcohol takers	8 (26.7)	8 (26.7)
Biochemical indices, mg%		
HbA$_{1c}$ (%)	8.4 ± 1.2	8.8 ± 1.8
Triglycerides	155.8 ± 41.6	160.8 ± 62.4
TC	202.4 ± 28.5	198.5 ± 37.2
HDL-C	45.0 ± 9.3	43.6 ± 13.0
LDL-C	125.0 ± 23.4	123.9 ± 28.4

RESULTS AND DISCUSSION

The results of the study are as follows:

There was no significant difference in the characteristics of the patients at enrolment and after 4 months of observation (Table 4.1). This indicates that any change obtained after intervention may be attributed to the inclusion of *Spirulina*.

Data from the current study clearly shows a steady and substantial improvement in the glycemic status of patients supplemented with *Spirulina* at 2 g/day level for a period of 4 months. Significant reductions not only in the fasting but also in the 2-h postprandial blood glucose levels were noticed after 2 months as well as after 4 months of intervention (Table 4.2).

Concomitant to the decrease in fasting and postprandial hyperglycemia, *Spirulina* supplementation resulted in a significant decrease in the HbA$_{1c}$ (glycated hemoglobin) levels, which is an integrated index of blood sugar levels over past 2–3 months (Table 4.2). And it may also be indicative of a reduced risk for the development of coronary heart disease (CHD), which has been demonstrated in the Kumamoto Study and the United Kingdom prospective diabetes study (UKPDS).[4,5]

Improvement in the glycemic control as observed in this study is in accordance with the earlier observations on supplementation with *Spirulina* in patients with diabetes.[1,6,7] Various theories validating this hypoglycemic potential of *Spirulina* have been proposed. One such theory attributes this effect to its fiber content. Well-executed clinical intervention trials have established a strong association between intake of fiber and blood glucose lowering.[8–20] Viscosity of fiber has been proposed

TABLE 4.2

Effect of *Spirulina* Supplementation on Blood Glucose, HbA$_{1c}$, Glucosamine, and Uronic Acid Levels of Diabetic Patients (Mean ± SD)

Variables	0 months	2 months	4 months	F value
FBG				
Total patients ($n = 30$)	168.0 ± 52.2	150.2 ± 39.3*	137.7 ± 44.0***	8.20***
Males ($n = 17$)	168.7 ± 57.1	149.6 ± 35.5	138.6 ± 39.2*	3.05
Females ($n = 13$)	167.2 ± 47.3	150.9 ± 45.2	136.5 ± 51.4**#	9.23**
PP$_2$BG				
Total patients ($n = 30$)	262.0 ± 57.6	245.5 ± 66.4**	209.6 ± 50.3***	10.43***
Males ($n = 17$)	269.4 ± 60.6	251.1 ± 64.3	212.2 ± 43.1**#	7.10**
Females ($n = 13$)	252.3 ± 45.4	238.1 ± 70.9	206.2 ± 60.0*	3.23
HbA$_{1c}$				
Total patients ($n = 30$)	8.8 ± 1.8	8.2 ± 1.3*	8.1 ± 1.5*	
Males ($n = 17$)	8.5 ± 1.2	8.2 ± 0.9	8.1 ± 0.8*	
Females ($n = 13$)	8.4 ± 1.2	7.8 ± 1.3*	7.4 ± 1.3*	
Glucosamine				
Total patients ($n = 30$)	4.3 ± 1.3	3.9 ± 1.3**	3.8 ± 1.4**	5.65**
Males ($n = 17$)	4.5 ± 1.4	4.2 ± 1.3*	4.1 ± 1.2*	3.58*
Females ($n = 13$)	3.9 ± 1.3	3.6 ± 1.3*	3.5 ± 1.7*	2.07
Uronic acid				
Total patients ($n = 30$)	50.7 ± 10.3	44.8 ± 10.3***	43.2 ± 11.2***	15.46***
Males ($n = 17$)	53.4 ± 11.3	47.5 ± 10.3***	46.9 ± 9.9**	10.70***
Females ($n = 13$)	47.2 ± 8.0	41.3 ± 9.1*	38.4 ± 11.4*	5.84**

ANOVA: **$p < .01$, ***$p < .001$.
*$p < .05$, **$p < .01$, ***$p < .001$ vs. 0 months.
#$p < .05$, ##$p < .01$, ###$p < .001$ vs. 2 months.

as the principal mechanism. Evidence suggests that gel forming capacity of fiber slows the rate of glucose absorption, consequently improving the glycemic status.[1,21,22]

Another theory suggests the role of *Spirulina* proteins. Dietary proteins by themselves are known to stimulate insulin secretion and when coingested with a carbohydrate source, they markedly potentiate insulin response.[23,24] Thus it is possible that the ingestion of *Spirulina* proteins along with the meals, as was done in the present study, may have an insulin secretagogue effect resulting in a reduction in the 2-h postprandial glycemia.[1,21] This improvement in the postprandial glycemia in turn may be responsible for the decrease observed in HbA$_{1c}$ concentrations.

Several investigations have established an association between the presence of hyperglycemia and the end products of Hexoseamine Biosynthesis Pathway (HBP) flux.[25–27] Results of the present study also highlight the strong correlation between HbA$_{1c}$ and the levels of glucosamine and uronic acid. With the significant improvements observed in hyperglycemia, the reaction in the glucosamine and uronic acid levels of the patients given *Spirulina* did not come as a surprise.

Results of the present analysis clearly highlight the efficacy of *Spirulina* as a lipid as well as cholesterol lowering agent. Significant reductions in the triglycerides, total lipids, total cholesterol, and its fractions except high density lipoprotein cholestrol (HDL-C) were observed after supplementation of *Spirulina* (Table 4.3). These observations are in line with the results reported by Mani[1] and Nayaka.[28] Various hypotheses have been proposed in an attempt to identify direct mechanisms responsible for the hypolipidemic and hypocholesterolemic potency of *Spirulina*. Focus has been laid on the high gamma linolenic acid (GLA) content. *Spirulina* is the only natural whole food source of GLA in the plant kingdom.[22] GLA is a precursor for the body's prostaglandins (PG). The prostaglandin PGE1 is essential for regulating a variety of basic biochemical functions in the body including the regulation of blood pressure, cholesterol synthesis, inflammation, and cell proliferation.[22,29,30] Under normal conditions, the human body can convert GLA from linoleic acid through activity of the enzyme delta-6-desaturase. Diabetes, however, is associated with inhibition of the delta-6-desaturase enzyme.[30] An external food source of GLA such as *Spirulina* therefore, plays a crucial role in regulating the cholesterol levels in diabetic patients.

In recent years, emphasis has also been laid on the favorable effects of the amino acid compositions of "good-quality" plant proteins on serum lipoproteins. Studies have highlighted the associations of high arginine intake with decreases in serum cholesterol levels and low methionine intake with lower incidence of CHD.[14,31-33] Interestingly, nutritional analysis of *Spirulina* proteins revealed this desirable amino acid composition.[22,29] It is, however, plausible that the hypocholesterolemic properties of *Spirulina* may in fact be due to the integrated effect of amino acids and the nonprotein components, namely, fiber, phytonutrients, and antioxidants.[13,14,22,31,34]

The hypocholesterolemic and hypolipidemic property of *Spirulina* can also be attributed to its plausible insulin secretagogue effect. As mentioned earlier, the additive effect of *Spirulina* proteins and fiber may result in improved insulin secretion. Howard[35] has reported decreased very low density lipoprotein (VLDL) triglyceride production as well as decreased Fractional Clearance Rate (FCR) coupled with an improvement in the peripheral VLDL clearance in the presence of insulin. This is reflected by the significant reductions seen in VLDL and triglyceride levels (Table 4.3). Furthermore, under the sustaining influence of insulin an increase in the turnover of VLDL-apoB and LDL receptor activity is seen. The hypocholesterolemic effect can also be attributed to this mechanism.[31,34]

The favorable shift in the lipid and lipoprotein profile in response to *Spirulina* supplementation was further supported by a significant increase in the HDL-C levels, may be a result of the additive effects of various proteins and nonprotein components of *Spirulina*.

Apart from the standard lipid parameters, efforts are being made to identify other risk factors of CHD.[36] Since apo A1 and B are the major protein components of HDL-C and LDL-C respectively, these have been most frequently investigated as the quantitative risk factors of CHD. Apo A1 and B are used independently and as a ratio to assess the risk of CHD. Studies have demonstrated that the changes as observed in this study with *Spirulina* supplementation, that is, a highly significant reduction in apo B causing a marked increment in the A1:B ratio (Table 4.4) is well correlated with less incidence of CHD.[34] Furthermore, because apo B is independently associated with

TABLE 4.3

Effect of *Spirulina* Supplementation on Lipids and Lipoprotein Levels of Diabetic Patients (Mean ± SD)

Variables	0 months	2 months	4 months	F value
Triglycerides				
Total patients ($n = 30$)	160.8 ± 62.4	149.5 ± 78.8	$132.7 \pm 53.0^{**\#}$	5.18^{**}
Males ($n = 17$)	155.9 ± 79.8	150.1 ± 81.8	137.8 ± 53.5	1.56
Females ($n = 13$)	151.3 ± 52.8	132.5 ± 50.7	$116.8 \pm 39.6^{*\#}$	6.85^{**}
Total lipids				
Total patients ($n = 30$)	648.9 ± 166.4	618.6 ± 157.1	$582.9 \pm 145.4^{**\#}$	5.86^{**}
Males ($n = 17$)	652.1 ± 179.5	640.8 ± 162.8	604.2 ± 153.4	1.46
Females ($n = 13$)	644.6 ± 154.8	589.6 ± 150.7	$555.1 \pm 135.1^{*\#}$	7.81^{**}
TC				
Total patients ($n = 30$)	198.5 ± 37.2	190.6 ± 31.7	$183.4 \pm 25.7^{***\#}$	6.62^{**}
Males ($n = 17$)	189.5 ± 38.6	186.4 ± 34.4	184.9 ± 29.2	0.47
Females ($n = 13$)	210.2 ± 33.0	196.2 ± 28.0	$181.4 \pm 21.2^{**\#\#\#}$	10.32^{***}
HDL-C				
Total patients ($n = 30$)	43.6 ± 13.0	44.4 ± 11.4	$48.4 \pm 12.2^{***\#\#}$	8.01^{***}
Males ($n = 17$)	39.8 ± 8.1	40.0 ± 7.5	$44.2 \pm 8.7^{**\#\#}$	1.46
Females ($n = 13$)	48.4 ± 17.0	50.4 ± 13.1	53.8 ± 14.4	2.28
LDL-C				
Total patients ($n = 30$)	123.9 ± 28.4	$116.4 \pm 23.9^{*}$	$108.3 \pm 21.0^{**\#\#}$	10.25^{***}
Males ($n = 17$)	118.0 ± 30.5	114.1 ± 25.7	111.6 ± 23.6	1.63
Females ($n = 13$)	131.6 ± 24.4	119.4 ± 22.0	$103.9 \pm 17.0^{**\#\#}$	11.60^{***}
VLDL-C				
Total patients ($n = 30$)	30.9 ± 13.4	29.9 ± 15.7	$27.1 \pm 10.5^{*}$	2.54
Males ($n = 17$)	32.5 ± 18.8	31.5 ± 15.5	29.0 ± 11.9	0.94
Females ($n = 13$)	30.2 ± 10.6	26.5 ± 10.0	$23.5 \pm 7.5^{*\#}$	6.42^{**}
Non HDL-C				
Total patients ($n = 30$)	154.8 ± 33.4	$146.4 \pm 29.2^{*}$	$135.0 \pm 25.8^{***\#\#\#}$	13.55^{***}
Males ($n = 17$)	149.5 ± 37.6	146.8 ± 34.2	140.6 ± 28.8	1.92
Females ($n = 13$)	161.8 ± 26.7	$145.8 \pm 22.4^{*}$	$127.6 \pm 16.6^{***\#\#\#}$	20.17^{***}
TC:HDL-C				
Total patients ($n = 30$)	4.8 ± 1.1	4.5 ± 1.1	$3.9 \pm 1.1^{***\#\#\#}$	16.51^{***}
Males ($n = 17$)	4.8 ± 1.2	4.7 ± 1.2	$4.3 \pm 1.0^{**\#}$	5.55^{**}
Females ($n = 13$)	4.7 ± 1.1	$4.1 \pm 0.9^{**}$	$3.6 \pm 0.8^{***\#\#}$	21.78^{***}
LDL-C:HDL-C				
Total patients ($n = 30$)	3.0 ± 0.9	$2.5 \pm 0.9^{**}$	$2.4 \pm 0.7^{***}$	11.61^{***}
Males ($n = 17$)	3.0 ± 0.9	2.8 ± 0.7	$2.6 \pm 0.8^{*}$	3.81^{*}
Females ($n = 13$)	3.0 ± 0.9	$2.5 \pm 0.6^{*}$	$2.0 \pm 0.6^{***\#\#\#}$	21.34^{***}

ANOVA: $^{*}p < .05$, $^{**}p < .01$, $^{***}p < .001$.
$^{*}p < .05$, $^{**}p < .01$, $^{***}p < .001$ vs. 0 months.
$^{\#}p < .05$, $^{\#\#}p < .01$, $^{\#\#\#}p < .001$ vs. 2 months.

TABLE 4.4
Effect of *Spirulina* Supplementation on Apolipoprotein Levels of Diabetic Patients (Mean ± SD)

Variables	0 months	2 months	4 months	F value
APO A1				
Total patients ($n = 30$)	135.3 ± 27.1	135.7 ± 32.6	137.0 ± 31.9	0.17
Males ($n = 17$)	120.7 ± 14.4	121.0 ± 21.1	124.0 ± 19.7	0.13
Females ($n = 13$)	157.6 ± 32.7	162.0 ± 32.8	161.8 ± 34.2	0.43
APO B				
Total patients ($n = 30$)	112.5 ± 35.9	102.5 ± 21.7**	100.2 ± 18.8***	9.79***
Males ($n = 17$)	112.1 ± 29.1	100.5 ± 24.7*	100.5 ± 22.1**	7.76**
Females ($n = 13$)	113.0 ± 22.3	105.1 ± 17.7	99.8 ± 14.1	3.18
APO A1:B				
Total patients ($n = 30$)	1.2 ± 0.4	1.3 ± 0.3*	1.4 ± 0.4*	5.40**
Males ($n = 17$)	1.1 ± 0.3	1.2 ± 0.3*	1.2 ± 0.4*	4.43*
Females ($n = 13$)	1.4 ± 0.4	1.5 ± 0.3	1.6 ± 0.4	1.25

ANOVA: *$p < .05$, **$p < .01$, ***$p < .001$.
*$p < .05$, **$p < .01$, ***$p < .001$ vs. 0 months.

cardiovascular disease and identifies high-risk phenotypes in normocholesterolemic diabetic patients, the 12.3 mg% reduction induced by *Spirulina* is noteworthy.[37]

Analysis clearly highlights the improvement in the assortment of CHD risk factors with *Spirulina* supplementation. In diabetes, these risk factors often co-occur. A linear increase in the risk for CHD has been observed with an increase in the number of risk factors.[19] Investigators now emphasize the measure of non-HDL-C since it serves as an index of combined risk of all the lipoprotein changes in diabetes.[38] Striking reductions in the non-HDL-C levels were noticed in patients supplemented with *Spirulina* (Table 4.3), indicating a reduction in all the atherogenic apo B containing lipoproteins and therefore plausibly a reduced risk for CHD. These results added credence to the earlier observations highlighting the beneficial attributes of *Spirulina*.

CONCLUSIONS

In conclusion, improved metabolic control resulted in the correction of several risk factors that figure prominently in the etiology of CHD. The results for the current study therefore, strongly favors the use of *Spirulina* as an adjunctive therapy for the optimal management of diabetes.

THERAPEUTIC UTILITY OF *SPIRULINA* IN ASTHMA

INTRODUCTION

Bronchial asthma is a disorder that affects lungs and the airways that deliver air to the lungs. It is the most common respiratory disorder characterized by episodic intrathoracic airway obstruction, airway hyperresponsiveness and airway inflammation. *Spirulina* with its galaxy of antioxidant nutrients can thus be an effective therapeutic mode for combating detrimental damage and inflammation in the respiratory lining. It could be an ideal choice in such a context for two reasons, first it is a rich source of GLA, which might play a crucial role as an anti-inflammatory agent, and second it has a good antioxidant profile that might help to counteract the detrimental exposure to oxidants.

A pilot trial carried out for a period of 2 months in the department revealed the beneficial role of *Spirulina* in the treatment of bronchial asthma.[39] Thus with this background, the present study was undertaken further in this direction to explore the long-term effect of *Spirulina* supplementation for a period of 4 months in patients suffering from mild to moderate degree of bronchial asthma. Thus, the present study focused on the objective "to study the effect of *Spirulina* supplementation on the protein status, pulmonary function and IgE status of the asthma patients."

METHODOLOGY

The enrolled asthma patients (from Shri Sayajirao General Hospital, Vadodara) suffering from mild to moderate degree of bronchial asthma were categorized into three groups— Group A: the control group was kept only on medication for a period of 4 months, Group B: the experimental group was administered medication and *Spirulina* (1 g/day) for a period of 2 months after which the *Spirulina* was withdrawn for the next 2 months and the medication was continued; and Group C: also the experimental group that was administered only *Spirulina* (1 g/day) for a period of 4 months. The patient's in-group A and B were on bronchodilators and anti-inflammatory drugs and their medication was not altered during the intervention trial. The serum total protein, albumin, and globulin and IgE were analyzed at baseline and at the end of 2- and 4-month period.

RESULTS AND DISCUSSION

The anthropometric measurement of the three groups of asthmatics is depicted in Table 4.5. The mean ages were 46, 40, and 33 years of Group A, Group B, and Group C asthmatics, respectively. The three groups were comparable with respect to height, weight, waist–hip ratio (WHR), and body mass index (BMI).

An overall good nutrition is very important in the prevention of asthma. The results from dietary analysis reveal that the patient's intake in all the three groups was inadequate with respect to proteins, fats, β-carotene and calories intake (Table 4.6).

This may play an additional triggering role in the ongoing asthma attacks by weakening body's immunity to fight infections and hence the recommended guideline is to satisfy the minimum daily requirements of all nutrients. A high P/S ratio suggests a high intake of polyunsaturated fatty acids (PUFA) from the diet, which can be detrimental, leading to high release of free radicals. The fatty acid composition of the diet in particular, the relative amounts of n-6 and n-3 PUFA may also be associated with the risk of asthma.[40] However, in the present study the dietary analysis revealed

TABLE 4.5

Anthropometric Measurements of the Three Groups of Asthmatics (Mean ± SD)

Variable	Group A	Group B	Group C
n	17	30	20
Age, years	46 ± 14.56	40 ± 12.55	33 ± 13.34
Height, meters	1.58 ± 0.09	1.55 ± 0.09	1.60 ± 0.08
Weight, kg	58.24 ± 14.39	52.97 ± 13.65	55.95 ± 10.32
Waist–hip ratio	0.87 ± 0.07	0.84 ± 0.07	0.83 ± 0.06
Body mass index, kg/m^2	23.07 ± 4.69	22.01 ± 5.39	22.04 ± 4.56

TABLE 4.6

Dietary Intake of the Three Groups of Asthmatics (Mean ± SD)

Nutrients	Group A	Group B	Group C
n	17	30	20
Energy (kcal)	1257 ± 261.76	1245 ± 363.43	1278 ± 307.48
Carbohydrate (g)	197.4 ± 48.23	185.6 ± 56.29	197.9 ± 52.31
Protein (g)	43.7 ± 31.23	36.5 ± 11.04	36.5 ± 9.97
Fat (g)	33.7 ± 10.67	34.9 ± 17.97	36.5 ± 11.75
β-Carotene (μg)	1527.1 ± 1455.92	1247.4 ± 888.84	1706.8 ± 1730.19
Vitamin C (mg)	58.1 ± 48.79	54.3 ± 50.48	54.6 ± 35.33
Linoleic acid (g)	10.1 ± 4.86	9.3 ± 5.57	9.7 ± 6.42
P/S ratio	1.9 ± 1.56	2.0 ± 1.33	1.5 ± 0.88

that the daily requirement of linoleic acid was adequately met and thus it cannot be the reason for the poor provision of GLA in the body.

With regard to the effect of *Spirulina* on protein status, the total protein value remained unaltered in Group A (only medication) and it showed a slight nonsignificant increase in Group B (medication + *Spirulina*) after a period of 4 months. However, in Group C, which was on exclusive *Spirulina* supplementation, a significant rise in total protein value was observed after a period of 4 months. This significant improvement in total protein value in Group C suggests the presence of high quality proteins in *Spirulina* (Table 4.7).

Also, when a comparison of protein status was made on a 2-monthly interval, it was observed that the mean serum total protein and albumin values remained unaltered in Group A (only medication), while they showed an increasing trend in Group B (medication + *Spirulina*) and Group C (only *Spirulina*) over a 4-month supplementation period. In Group C, which was on exclusive *Spirulina* supplementation a significant increase in serum total protein and albumin values was observed especially when the values were compared from baseline to 4 months and from 2 to

TABLE 4.7

Effect of *Spirulina* Supplementation on Protein Status in the Three Groups of Asthamatics (Mean ± SD)

	Baseline	2 months	4 months	F value
Total protein (g/dL)				
Group A (*n* = 17)	6.62 ± 0.56	6.53 ± 0.61	6.62 ± 0.60	0.12
Group B (*n* = 30)	6.54 ± 0.70	6.78 ± 0.67	6.77 ± 0.60	1.31
Group C (*n* = 20)	6.46 ± 0.72	6.63 ± 0.71	7.02 ± 0.70^{ba,b*,c***}	3.32*
F value	0.25	0.84	2.03	
Serum albumin (g/dL)				
Group A (*n* = 17)	4.01 ± 0.60	3.92 ± 0.62	4.03 ± 0.65	0.14
Group B (*n* = 30)	4.24 ± 0.53	4.37 ± 0.60	4.40 ± 0.49	0.81
Group C (*n* = 20)	3.94 ± 0.47	4.05 ± 0.52	4.29 ± 0.44^{bc,d**,c**}	2.72
F value	2.07	3.8*	2.88	
Serum globulin (g/dL)				
Group A (*n* = 17)	2.61 ± 0.65	2.61 ± 0.56	2.59 ± 0.62	0.13
Group B (*n* = 30)	2.30 ± 0.74	2.41 ± 0.65	2.37 ± 0.55	0.33
Group C (*n* = 20)	2.52 ± 0.60	2.58 ± 0.65	2.73 ± 0.58	0.73
F value	1.85	0.49	2.76	
Albumin/globulin (A/G) ratio				
Group A (*n* = 17)	1.67 ± 0.56	1.58 ± 0.48	1.66 ± 0.54	0.16
Group B (*n* = 30)	2.06 ± 0.86	2.01 ± 0.9	1.97 ± 0.61	0.08
Group C (*n* = 20)	1.65 ± 0.50	1.68 ± 0.59	1.61 ± 0.38	0.11
F value	2.67	2.31	3.49*	

Group A: medication only, Group B: medication + *Spirulina*, Group C: *Spirulina* only

ANOVA: * significant at $p < .05$.

[a] 2 months–4 months, significant at $p < .05$.

[b] Baseline—4 months, significant at $p < .001$.

[c] 2 months–4 months, significant at $p < .01$.

[d] Baseline—4 months, significant at $p < .01$.

4 months (Table 4.7). Thus these findings suggest the beneficial effect of good quality proteins in improving the protein status in the *Spirulina*-supplemented groups as against the medication group (Group A).

The pulmonary function tests (PFT) namely, forced vital capacity (FVC), forced expiratory volume in first second (FEV1), peak expiratory flow rate (PEFR), and FEV1/FVC revealed an overall improvement in pulmonary function efficacy in all the three groups. The patients in Group A (only medication) showed a significant improvement in % FEV1 and % FEV1/FVC values over a period of 4 months (Table 4.8).

Majority of the patients (65%) in Group A were on both bronchodilators (like salbutamol, salmeterol, deriphylline, aminophylline) and anti-inflammatory drugs (such as budesonide, prednisone). Thus this conjunction therapy with bronchodilators and

TABLE 4.8

Effect of *Spirulina* Supplementation on Pulmonary Function in the Three Groups of Asthmatics (Mean ± SD)

	Baseline	2 months	4 months	F value
FVC (% predicted)				
Group A ($n = 17$)	73 ± 22	76 ± 17^a	80 ± 18	0.61
Group B ($n = 30$)	72 ± 17	$83 \pm 17^{a**}$	$78 \pm 16^{b,c}$	3.28*
Group C ($n = 20$)	79 ± 20	82 ± 18	$89 \pm 18^{d,e}$	1.62
F value	0.69	0.92	2.47	
FEV 1 (% predicted)				
Group A ($n = 17$)	68 ± 12	70 ± 16	$79 \pm 11^{f,g}$	3.66*
Group B ($n = 30$)	61 ± 14	$74 \pm 19^{a**}$	$67 \pm 16^{b,c}$	5.14**
Group C ($n = 20$)	63 ± 14	$70 \pm 15^{a**}$	$80 \pm 14^{d,e}$	6.95***
F value	1.54	0.51	6.38**	
PEFR (% predicted)				
Group A ($n = 17$)	53 ± 26	53 ± 18	$60 \pm 22^{b,g}$	0.56
Group B ($n = 30$)	43 ± 18	$56 \pm 19^{a**}$	55 ± 18^e	4.69**
Group C ($n = 20$)	55 ± 20	60 ± 17^a	62 ± 17^c	0.85
F value	2.29	0.63	0.9	
FEV1/FVC (% predicted)				
Group A ($n = 17$)	77 ± 11	87 ± 13^h	$92 \pm 13^{b,e}$	6.61**
Group B ($n = 30$)	82 ± 19	88 ± 15^i	81 ± 16^b	1.43
Group C ($n = 20$)	82 ± 22	85 ± 14	92 ± 15	1.54
F value	0.49	0.23	4.12*	

Group A: medication only, Group B: medication+ *Spirulina*, Group C: *Spirulina* only.
ANOVA: significant at *$p < .05$, **$p < .01$, ***$p < .001$.
[a] Baseline—2 months ($p < .05$).
[b] 2–4 months ($p < .01$).
[c] Baseline—4 months ($p < .01$).
[d] 2–4 months ($p < .001$).
[e] Baseline—4 months ($p < .001$).
[f] 2–4 months ($p < .05$).
[g] Baseline—4 months ($p < .05$).
[h] Baseline—2 months ($p < .001$).
[i] Baseline—2 months ($p < .01$).

anti-inflammatory drugs has helped to improve the pulmonary function in Group A patients, as evidenced by significant improvement in % FEV1 and % FEV1/FVC over a period of 4 months. However, the patients in Group A reported to experiencing certain side effects such as palpitation, weakness, and tremors on use of these medications. Literature has cited a few to more increasing side effects of drugs on prolonged use.[41]

The Group B patients (medication+*Spirulina*) showed a significant improvement in % FVC (72 ± 17 to 78 ± 16), % FEV1 (61 ± 14 to 67 ± 16) and % PEFR values (43 ± 18 to 58 ± 18) over a period of 4 months (Table 4.8). It is interesting to note in this group that when the *Spirulina* supplements were withdrawn after a period of 2 months, the pulmonary function variables showed a decrease from 2 to 4 months. This indicates that *Spirulina* might be playing an important contributory role over and above the given medication. *Spirulina* could have probably contributed to improvement in pulmonary function owing to two reasons. First, it is a rich source of GLA, which might play a crucial role as an anti-inflammatory agent and second it has a good antioxidant profile that might help to counteract the detrimental exposure to oxidants.

Further, the role of *Spirulina* gets pronounced when a significant decrease in % FVC, % FEV1, and % FEV1/FVC was observed in the next 2 months when the *Spirulina* supplements were withdrawn while the medication was continued. Similar supplementation studies with GLA-rich agents or by altering the essential fatty acid content of the diet have been carried out, and these have shown a beneficial effect in patients with inflammatory diseases.[42–44] Also, a study by Hayashi et al.[45] reported that *Spirulina* may be beneficial in treating some forms of atopic bronchial asthma. Thus, the above-mentioned studies support our findings that supplementation with GLA rich agents (*Spirulina*) could possibly have helped to improve the pulmonary function in asthmatics.

The probable contributory factor in *Spirulina* is its rich antioxidant profile. Symptoms of ongoing asthma in adults appear to be increased by exposure to detrimental oxidants, which can be released endogenously in the lungs or can be exogenous in nature. It has been reported that inflammatory cells obtained from lungs of patients with asthma generate increased amounts of reactive oxygen species (ROS) and ROS can reproduce the key abnormalities of asthma.[46–49]

Thus, *Spirulina* with its good content of antioxidant nutrients such as β-carotene, vitamin E, selenium could possibly play a role in alleviating the pulmonary function abnormalities by scavenging endogenous and/or environmental oxidant sources. In the present study the intake of most nutrients (energy, protein, β-carotene) by the asthmatics was below the recommended dietary allowance (RDA). In particular, β-carotene contributed to only 52% of RDA in group B patients (Table 4.6). A marked fall in consumption of antioxidants and mineral cofactors in fresh fruit and vegetables, fish, and meat has produced a general reduction in the ability of lungs to counter inflammatory reactions due to inhalation of irritants or allergens.[50]

Spirulina, which contains antioxidant vitamins and minerals, could have possibly improved the overall antioxidant status of group B patients. This would have resulted in improving their pulmonary function efficacy as evidenced by significant improvement in all the pulmonary function variables in the first 2 months of supplementation followed by significant reduction observed in % FEV1, % FVC, and % FEV1/FVC in next 2 months on withdrawal of *Spirulina*. Also, *Spirulina* with its richest source of proteins of high biological value and a good content of phytonutrients might have helped to improve the immunocompetance in asthma patients.

In patients of Group C who were on continued *Spirulina* supplementation for a period of 4 months significant improvement was observed in % FEV1 values from 63 ± 14 to 80 ± 14 (Table 4.8). In addition to antioxidant vitamins and minerals, the

TABLE 4.9

Effect of *Spirulina* Supplementation on IgE Status in the Three Groups of Asthmatics (Geometric Mean ± SD)

	Baseline	2 months	4 months	F value
Group A (n = 17)	749.70 ± 1.55	776.38 ± 1.51	785.57 ± 1.51	0.03
Group B (n = 30)	277.58 ± 3.89	275.50 ± 3.24[a]	304.71 ± 2.88	0.10
Group C (n = 20)	443.51 ± 1.86	377.77 ± 1.86	378.59 ± 1.74[b]	0.49
F value	3.17*	5.41**	6.93***	

Group A: medication only, Group B: medication + *Spirulina*, Group C: *Spirulina* only.

ANOVA: *significant at $p < .05$, **$p < .01$, ***$p < .001$.

[a] Baseline: 2 months, significant at $p < .05$.

[b] Baseline: 4 months, significant at $p < .05$.

other contributory factor could be the GLA which might have played a crucial role as an anti-inflammatory.

Epidemiological studies have related the prevalence of asthma to total IgE levels.[51,52] Also studies have shown a relation between serum total IgE levels and impairment of lung function if symptoms suggesting asthma are present. There is also a relation reported between reduced baseline pulmonary function and likelihood that airway hyper responsiveness will be detected.[53–55] This relation provides an indirect link between increase serum IgE levels and airway hyper responsiveness through impaired lung function.

In the present study the mean IgE values at baseline were 749.70 ± 1.55 IU/mL, 277.58 ± 3.89 IU/mL, and 443.51 ± 1.86 IU/mL in Group A, Group B, and Group C, respectively (Table 4.9).

A significant difference was observed at baseline between these values in the three groups of asthmatics. The higher IgE levels in Group A patients as compared to the other two groups could possibly be attributed to the longer duration of disease in them (mean 7 years) as compared to 5 years in group B and 4 years in Group C. In addition, a significant difference was observed between the three groups after a 2-month and 4-month supplementation period. In Group A (only medication) an increase in serum IgE values was observed over the 4-month period; however, this increase was nonsignificant. In Group B (medication + *Spirulina*) the IgE value showed a significant decrease in 2 months of *Spirulina* supplementation. However, when the supplements were withdrawn in the next 2 months, it increased by 29 IU/mL, though this increase was nonsignificant. In Group C (only *Spirulina*) patients who were on continued *Spirulina* supplementation for a period of 4 months the IgE value showed a significant decrease from the baseline (443.51 ± 1.86 IU/mL) value over a period of 4 months (378.59 ± 1.74 IU/mL) (Table 4.9). Thus, these findings suggest the beneficial effect of *Spirulina* in improving the IgE status in the *Spirulina*-supplemented groups as against the medication group (Group A). The decrease in the IgE levels observed in the *Spirulina*-supplemented group can possibly be explained through the effect of GLA on prostaglandin E2 (PGE2) formation. GLA gets converted to dihommogammalinolenic acid (DGLA), which takes a preferential pathway to synthesize prostanoids of 1, 3 series, which are anti-inflammatory in nature. Further, increase in DGLA, allows it to act as a competitive inhibitor of the proinflammatory 2-series PGs (PG2) and 4-series LTs (LT4).

There is evidence that PGE2 can modulate the cytokines by T-lymphocytes. The formation of IgE by B-lymphocytes in turn is influenced by cytokines produced by T-helper (CD4$^+$) lymphocytes. Interleukin-4 (IL4) acts to commit B-cells to the synthesis of IgE, whereas interferon γ (IFN-γ) inhibits the formation of IgE.[56,57] A low concentration of PGE2 inhibits the formation of IFN-γ although it has no effect on production of IL4.[58,59] By inhibiting the formation of IFN-γ but not IL4, PGE2 will increase the formation of IgE. There is also evidence that PGE2 can directly act on β-cells to stimulate the formation of IgE. Roper and coworkers[60] have reported that PGE2 promotes the action of IL4 to increase the number of lymphocytes producing IgE.

Thus, it can be postulated that *Spirulina*, which is a rich source of GLA would have possibly led to decrease in the proinflammatory PGE2 production, which in turn would have led to a decrease of IgE in the *Spirulina*-supplemented groups. Further, withdrawal of supplements in Group B could possibly have led to an increase in PGE2 formation, which in turn could have led to an increase in the IgE levels.

CONCLUSIONS

Thus, from the positive results obtained in protein status, pulmonary function, and IgE status in supplemented groups it can be concluded that *Spirulina* can be introduced along with medicine as a therapeutic and dietary supplement in the treatment of asthmatics, and in the long run this may not only help to control asthma but also reduce the need of drugs in its treatment.

THERAPEUTIC UTILITY OF *SPIRULINA* IN NEPHROTIC SYNDROME

INTRODUCTION

Nephrotic syndrome is defined as a clinical condition in which >3.5 g/1.73 m^2/day of proteins are excreted in the urine. The defects in the change or size of selective barriers of the glomerular capillary wall that underline the excessive filtration of plasma proteins can arise as a consequence of a variety of diseases processes, including immunological disorders, toxic injuries, metabolic abnormalities, biochemical defects, and vascular disorders. Thus, nephrotic syndrome is a common end point of a variety of disease processes that alter the permeability of the glomerular basement membrane (GBM) or glomerular capillary wall. Proteinuria is the hallmark of the nephrotic state. The other important characteristics of nephrotic syndrome are hypoalbuminemia, hyperlipidemia, and edema.

Spirulina, which has a balanced amino acid profile, fatty acid profile, vitamins, trace elements, antioxidants, rich source of GLA, and hypocholesterolemic effect, prompted us to supplement it to patients suffering from nephrotic syndrome and to study its therapeutic effect and anti-inflammatory effect on these patients.

METHODOLOGY

The study was designed to see the efficacy of *Spirulina* supplementation for a period of 4 months in nephrotic patients. Patients suffering from nephrotic syndrome were enrolled from the Special Paediatric Nephrotic Clinic of Shri Sayajirao General Hospital, Vadodara, Gujarat, India with the consent of the consulting physician as well as parents of the patients. The enrolled patients were divided into two groups; experimental ($n = 30$) and control ($n = 30$). The nephrotic patients in the control and experimental group were matched for age, gender, and severity of disease to ascertain the improvements witnessed in these patients after *Spirulina* therapy in comparison to the patients in the control group. Patients in the control group were treated only with medication and were studied for a period of 4 months. Patients in the experimental group were supplemented with 1 g/day *Spirulina* tablets for 4 months. The patients were asked to take one tablet (500 g each) along with lunch and one tablet (500 g each) with dinner.

RESULTS AND DISCUSSION

The results of the study are as follows:

The clinical profile of all the nephrotic patients supplemented with *Spirulina* for 4 months is depicted in Table 4.10. There was no significant change registered in BMI, WC, and WHR after 4 months of supplementation.

Hypoproteinaemia is a clinical manifestation of nephrotic syndrome.[61] In the current study also the patients exhibited hypoproteinaemia at baseline. An improvement in the levels of total protein was seen after supplementation of *Spirulina*. This

TABLE 4.10
Clinical Profile of Nephrotic Patients at Baseline and 4 Months of *Spirulina* Supplementation (Mean ± SD)

Variables	Baseline	4 months
n	30	30
Boys/girls	25/5	25/5
Height (cm)	114.6 ± 21.6	117.0 ± 22.0
Weight (kg)	23.3 ± 12.5	23.1 ± 12.5
Body mass index (kg/m²)	16.6 ± 3.2	16.1 ± 3.1
Waist (cm)	58.3 ± 10.2	56.8 ± 9.7
Hip (cm)	59.9 ± 12.7	59.3 ± 12.5
Waist–hip ratio	0.98 ± 0.07	0.96 ± 0.05
Medication	Steroids	Steroids

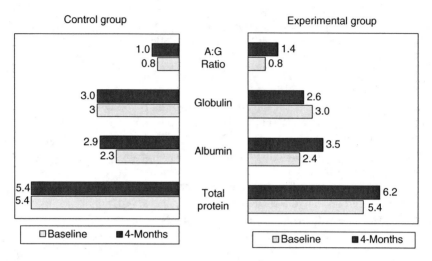

FIGURE 4.1   Protein status of nephrotic patients (g/dL).

significant improvement in total protein value suggests the presence of high quality proteins in *Spirulina*. In addition to this raised levels of albumin and A:G ratio was also seen after 4 months of *Spirulina* supplementation (Figure 4.1).

Thus, these findings suggest the beneficial effect of good quality proteins in improving the protein status in the *Spirulina*-supplemented group as against the control group. These results are in line with the trial carried out on asthmatics where *Spirulina* supplementation slowly improved the protein status.[62–64]

Hyperlipidemia is commonly seen in nephrotic syndrome patients. Characteristically TG and TC levels are elevated, as are VLDL-C and LDL-C and the concentration of HDL-C has been reported to be variable.[65–72] The mechanisms underlying these abnormalities are multifactorial, involving both increased rates of lipoproteins synthesis and defective clearance and catabolism of circulating particles.

In the present study, *Spirulina* was supplemented for a period of 4 months as it has been proved by many clinical studies[1,28,73–76] that it effectively reduces the elevated lipid levels. The results of the present study revealed significant reductions in the lipid levels in control and experimental groups (Table 4.11). But higher reduction in the lipid levels was observed in the experimental groups patients as compared to the control group patients (Table 4.11) after 2 and 4 months of supplementation.

This fall in the atherogenic lipid levels may be due to the supplementation of *Spirulina*. Various other trials[1,28,73–75] have proved that *Spirulina* effectively reduces the elevated cholesterol levels and similar results have been observed in the current study. The cholesterol reducing property of *Spirulina* may be due to its high content of GLA,[77] which has been discussed earlier in the chapter. The reduction observed in the TG and VLDL-C levels in nephrotic patients after *Spirulina* supplementation could be attributed to decreased VLDL triglyceride production and increased VLDL-C clearance in the periphery that might have been brought about by the high protein and fiber content of *Spirulina*. This in turn could have resulted in lowering LDL-C levels in these patients, due to the fact that most of the LDL-C is formed form VLDL-C. As

TABLE 4.11

Metabolic Profile of the Control and Experimental Group Patients after Matching for Age, Gender, and Severity of Disease at Two Monthly Intervals (mg/dL, Mean ± SD)

Parameters	Baseline	2 months	4 months
Triglyceride			
Control group	166.1 ± 53.2	131.8 ± 85.0*	142.6 ± 89.0
Experimental group	235.7 ± 142.0	116.6 ± 49.9*	115.3 ± 42.3**
Total cholesterol			
Control group	293.8 ± 147.5	215.3 ± 126.6***	210.6 ± 134.0*
Experimental group	367.5 ± 182.4	169.2 ± 40.6***	186.2 ± 82.1***
HDL-C			
Control group	56.8 ± 18.4	53.0 ± 15.1*	50.9 ± 18.4
Experimental group	65.5 ± 32.3	50.5 ± 11.6*	57.4 ± 19.6#
LDL-C			
Control group	203.9 ± 132.0	135.8 ± 102.8***	161.3 ± 97.0*
Experimental grp	254.9 ± 142.0	95.3 ± 31.6***	105.7 ± 59.0***
VLDL-C			
Control Group	33.2 ± 10.6	26.4 ± 17.0*	28.5 ± 17.8
Experimental group	47.1 ± 28.5	23.3 ± 10.0**	23.1 ± 8.5***
Non-HDL-C			
Control group	237.0 ± 139.2	162.3 ± 114.6***	159.7 ± 125.8*
Experimental group	302.0 ± 162.1	118.7 ± 32.5***	128.8 ± 65.1**
TC:HDL-C			
Control group	5.2 ± 2.0	3.9 ± 1.3***	4.1 ± 1.9
Experimental group	5.8 ± 1.8	3.4 ± 0.6***	3.2 ± 0.5***#
LDL-C:HDL-C			
Control group	3.6 ± 1.9	2.4 ± 1.1***	2.5 ± 1.7
Experimental group	4.0 ± 1.5	1.9 ± 0.6***	1.8 ± 0.5***
Apo A1			
Control group	156.3 ± 41.0	132.2 ± 28.0*	133.7 ± 45.4
Experimental group	157.4 ± 65.9	132.0 ± 34.4	145.1 ± 42.3#
Apo B			
Control group	160.9 ± 93.9	108.8 ± 79.6***	106.5 ± 79.7
Experimental group	230.5 ± 125.7	81.3 ± 24.0***	88.7 ± 43.7***
Apo A1:B			
Control group	1.3 ± 0.6	1.6 ± 0.7**	1.6 ± 0.6
Experimental group	0.8 ± 0.4	1.7 ± 0.4***	1.8 ± 0.5***#

*$p < .05$, **$p < .01$, ***$p < .001$ vs. baseline.
#$p < .05$ vs. 2 months.

Spirulina effectively lowered the lipids and lipoprotein fraction in these patients, a significant reduction in the atherogenic indices, that is, TC:HDL-C an LDL-C:HDL-C were also observed. Such changes in the lipid levels have also been associated with a lower incidence of CHD.[6]

The reduction in the elevated lipid levels led to an improvement in the apo A1:B ratio ($p < .001$) after 4 months of supplementation in the experimental group (Table 4.11). *Spirulina* supplementation also showed significant reduction in the apo B levels ($p < .001$) (Table 4.11) in the experimental group after 4 months of *Spirulina* supplementation. Thus, this beneficial effect of *Spirulina* suggests that it helped in decreasing the risk of developing cardiovascular disease in these patients and was also helpful in retarding the further progression of renal disease.

In addition, the supplementation of *Spirulina* in the experimental group also showed substantial reduction in the number of relapses. On the basis of this the clinician had brought down the level of drug to 54% of the initial requirements where as in the control group, the patients required 87% of the initial level for the treatment of nephrotic syndrome. These observations clearly demonstrate and substantiate that *Spirulina* had shown a remarkable improvement in the prognosis of nephrotic syndrome patients.

CONCLUSIONS

Hence, it can be said that *Spirulina* aided in improving the quality of the experimental group patients in a better way as compared to the patients in the control group.

THERAPEUTIC UTILITY OF *SPIRULINA* IN IRON DEFICIENCY ANEMIA

Two studies have been carried out in the department with regards to *Spirulina* supplementation in anemic subjects. One of the studies was carried out on adolescent girls and the other on pre school children, the details of the same are discussed below:

STUDY I: ADOLESCENT GIRLS

The present study was designed to investigate the effect of supplementation of spray-dried *Spirulina* powder on hemoglobin levels of anemic adolescent girls.

In all, 120 adolescent girls were screened for their anthropometric measurements and blood hemoglobin levels. All these girls belonged to high socioeconomic group. The age group of these girls was between 18–22 years with a mean age of 19 years. The mean blood hemoglobin levels and the prevalence of anemia in adolescent girls are displayed in Table 4.12. Out of 105 girls screened 29 were found to be anemic (28.2%), and out of these 20 gave their consent to participate in the study. The clinical profile of the adolescent anemic girls is depicted in Table 4.13. The mean height and weight of these adolescent girls was 158.8 cm and 49.4 kg. The mean BMI was found to be 19.56. Thus the overall growth profile of the girls seemed to be satisfactory. Mean nutrient intake of anemic adolescent girls based on 24-h dietary recall method

TABLE 4.12
Prevalence of Anemia and Mean Hemoglobin Levels of Adolescent Girls

Parameter	Mean ± SD
Total number of girls screened	105
Hemoglobin Levels of adolescent girls (g/dL)	12.46 ± 1.96
Number of girls found to be anemic	29 (28.2%)
Hemoglobin levels of anemic girls (g/dL)	11.35 ± 0.75

TABLE 4.13
Clinical Profile of Anemic Adolescent Girls (Mean ± SD)

Parameter	Mean ± SD
Number	20
Age (y)	20 ± 0.80
Height (cm)	158.78 ± 5.27
Weight (kg)	49.38 ± 7.28
Body mass index (kg/m^2)	19.56 ± 2.80
Waist–hip ratio	0.73 ± 0.06
Mid upper arm circumference (MUAC) (cm)	23.06 ± 2.36
Mean blood hemoglobin (g/dL)	11.35 ± 0.75

is given in Table 4.14. The mean intake of proximate nutrient, that is, carbohydrate, protein and fat was above 70% of RDA. With regard to micronutrients, the intake of iron was very low meeting only 41.5% of RDA. Vitamin A (150%) and β-carotene (250%) intake was much higher than the RDA.

A significant increase in blood hemoglobin levels was seen in the adolescent girls after 1 month of *Spirulina* supplementation (Table 4.15). On an average the hemoglobin levels increased by 1.17 g/dL, that is, 10.33%. This data indicates the beneficial effect of *Spirulina* in improving the hemoglobin levels in anemic girls. As two modes for supplementing *Spirulina* was used, the data on pre- and posthemoglobin levels were classified on the basis of the modes of supplementation. The hemoglobin levels of anemic girls supplemented *Spirulina* as syrup and incorporated in paratha is given in Table 4.15. A significant 11.65% rise in blood hemoglobin levels was noticed after supplementing *Spirulina* as syrup. Similarly, the hemoglobin levels were raised by 7.72% after supplementing *Spirulina* in the form of paratha. The increase in blood hemoglobin was more pronounced in girls supplemented *Spirulina* as syrup than in girls supplemented *Spirulina* as parathas (1.32 g/dL vs. 0.88 g/dL). This could possibly be due to inhibitors of iron absorption that are present in wheat flour, which are phytates and oxalates. About 119 mg of phytates and 4 mg of oxalates were present

TABLE 4.14
Nutrient Intake of Anemic Adolescent Girls (Mean ± SD)

Nutrient	Nutrient intake	Recommended dietary allowance*
Energy (kcal)	1636 ± 384	2225
Carbohydrate (g)	225.0	
Protein (g)	47.17 ± 13.82	50
Fat (g)	51.37 ± 18.60	20
Iron (mg)	12.45 ± 4.98	30
Vitamin A	1034.59 ± 446.32	600
β-Carotene (μg)	5987.23 ± 6390.96	2400
Vitamin C (mg)	72.24 ± 86.10	40
Vitamin B$_{12}$ (μg)	0.71 ± 0.74	1
Folic acid (μg)	169.49 ± 124.30	100
Oxalate (mg)	356.26 ± 283.37	—
Phytate (mg)	90.79 ± 83.10	—

* *Source:* Gopalan, C., Rama Sastri, B.V., and Balasubramanian, S.C.,
Nutritive Value of Indian Foods, 2nd ed., National Institute of Nutrition, Indian Council of Medical Research, Hyderabad, 1993.

TABLE 4.15
Effect of *Spirulina* Supplementation on Blood Hemoglobin Levels of Anemic Adolescent Girls (Mean ± SD)

Hemoglobin (g/dL)	Baseline	After 1 month of supplementation
Mean	11.35 ± 0.75	12.52 ± 0.68***
Spirulina incorporated in parathas	11.36 ± 0.54	12.23 ± 0.54***
Spirulina incorporated as a syrup	11.35 ± 0.84	12.66 ± 0.70***

*** Significant at $p < .001$.

in the *Spirulina*-supplemented parathas served to anemic adolescent girls, while in sugar syrup there was virtual absence of inhibitors.

The supplementation was carried out in between the meals, that is, between the breakfast and lunch. Therefore, this increase of hemoglobin levels can be attributed solely to iron content of *Spirulina*. Also care was taken to see that the dietary pattern of the girls did not change during the period of supplementation. Therefore, the supplementation of *Spirulina*, which contains a highly available form of iron, has led to the significant increase in hemoglobin levels in anemic adolescent girls. Although not many detailed studies are available regarding the effect of *Spirulina* supplementation on hemoglobin levels in anemic subjects, few pilot studies reported correlates the present findings. A study carried out in Japan on women having hypochromic anemia, were treated with 4 g *Spirulina* for 30 days. Their average blood hemoglobin content increased by 21% from 10.9 to 13.3 mg%.[78] In another study dietary supplementation of *Spirulina* fusiforms at 2 g/day over a period of 36 days showed 10% increase in hemoglobin content.[79]

Thus, it is clear from this study, that supplementation of 5 g of spray-dried *Spirulina* powder to anemic adolescent girls for a period of 30 days had a significant effect on iron metabolism, as is evident by the improved hemoglobin levels, and can be effectively used to combat iron-deficiency anemia, which is widely prevalent in the world.

STUDY II: PRESCHOOL CHILDREN

The major objective of the second study was to assess the effect of *Spirulina* supplementation on hemoglobin levels of preschool children (3–6 years) in urban slums of Vadodara.

The study was carried out in five anganwadis, two of which were selected as the experimental group and three as the control group. A total of 163 children (3–6 years) were selected, out of which 83 formed the experimental group and 80 formed the control group. Out of the total 163 subjects, 18 subjects from the experimental and 12 from the control group dropped out of the study. The subjects of the experimental group ($n = 65$) received daily 1 g spray-dried *Spirulina* supplementation for a period of 50 days and the control group received no supplementation.

Spirulina was supplemented for a period of 50 days to the subjects of the experimental group through door-to-door visits on a daily basis by an investigator. One gram spray dried *Spirulina* supplement was administered in 15-mL sugar syrup to the subjects by the investigator.

Table 4.16 shows the mean nutrient intake of the subjects by the control and experimental groups. There was no significant difference in the intake of any of the nutrients by the subjects in the two groups. In both the groups the subjects did not

TABLE 4.16
Mean Nutrient Intake of the Subjects

Nutrients	Experimental group ($n = 65$)	Control group ($n = 68$)	't' value
Energy (kcal)	824.87 ± 24.73	831.54 ± 22.51	0.20
Proteins (g)	24.74 ± 1.06	25.45 ± 1.22	0.43
Fats (g)	18.77 ± 1.09	16.30 ± 0.75	1.87
Calcium (mg)	267.15 ± 15.28	326.13 ± 24.78	2.004
Iron (mg)	8.74 ± 0.30	9.09 ± 0.23	0.924
β-Carotene (µg)	298.55 ± 30.48	319.65 ± 23.72	0.549
Vitamin C (mg)	25.98 ± 1.16	32.09 ± 3.61	1.57

TABLE 4.17

Impact of Supplementation on Mean Hemoglobin Levels of the Subjects

Groups	Hemoglobin levels (g/dL) (Mean ± SE) Experimental	Control	'*t*' values
All subjects	***n* = 65**	***n* = 68**	
Initial	10.20 ± 0.156	10.47 ± 0.185	1.11
Final	11.30 ± 0.11	10.15 ± 0.17	5.50
Difference	1.10 ± 0.15	−0.32 ± 0.096	8.07***
Paired 't'	7.09***	3.385**	
Anemic subjects	***n* = 46**	***n* = 46**	
Initial	9.58 ± 0.13	9.61 ± 0.13	0.145
Final	11.14 ± 0.16	9.40 ± 0.13	9.03***
Difference	1.55 ± 0.16	0.21 ± 0.09	9.52***
Paired 't'	9.27***	2.33*	
Non anemic subjects	***n* = 19**	***n* = 22**	
Initial	11.71 ± 0.12	12.28 ± 0.14	2.87***
Final	11.70 ± 0.16	11.72 ± 0.21	0.65
Difference	−0.005 ± 0.16	−0.56 ± 0.22	1.96*
Paired 't'	0.03	2.5*	

* Significant at $p < .05$.
** Significant at $p < .01$.
*** Significant at $p < .001$.

meet the daily requirements for any of the nutrients. Supplementation with *Spirulina* led to an increase in the intake of a few nutrients. The protein intakes increased by the 2.4% and the iron intake increased from a mean of 8.72 mg/day to 9.32 mg/day.

Effect of *Spirulina* supplementation on the mean hemoglobin levels is depicted in Table 4.17. While the initial hemoglobin level was similar in the two groups, at the end of the intervention period, the subjects in the experimental group had significant higher mean hemoglobin levels as compared to the control group, when the data were analyzed for two categories—all subjects and anemic subjects.

The *Spirulina*-supplemented group showed a significant increase in mean hemoglobin levels from an initial of 10.20 g/dL to a final of 11.30 g/dL. As against this, the control group showed a decrease from an initial 10.47 g/dL to 10.15 g/dL by the end of the study period. This change in hemoglobin levels from initial to final was statistically significant in both the groups. It can be seen that while the subjects who were anemic (<11 g/dL) initially and were supplemented showed an increase in mean hemoglobin levels form 9.58 g/dL to 11.14 g/dL, those who had normal hemoglobin levels to start with, maintained their hemoglobin levels. In contrast to this in the control group there was a significant decrease in hemoglobin levels in subjects with initially normal hemoglobin levels. The experimental group showed a rise in hemoglobin levels, which was significantly different from the drop seen in the control

TABLE 4.18
Percent Prevalence of Anemia among the Subjects:
Based on Hb Levels

Hemoglobin levels	Total $n = 133$	Experimental $n = 65$	Control $n = 68$
≥11 g/dL			
Before supplementation	30.83 (41)	29.23 (19)	32.35 (22)
After supplementation	43.61 (58)	58.5 (38)	29.4 (20)
10–10.99 g/dL			
Before supplementation	26.31 (35)	24.62 (16)	27.94 (19)
After supplementation	29.32 (39)	36.9 (24)	22.1 (15)
7–9.99 g/dL			
Before supplementation	42.11 (56)	46.15 (30)	38.24 (26)
After supplementation	27.07 (36)	4.6 (3)	48.5 (33)
≤7 g/dL			
Before supplementation	0.75 (1)	—	1.47 (1)
After supplementation	—	—	—

Values in parenthesis indicates number of subjects.

group. Of the subjects who received the *Spirulina* supplementation, the maximum rise in hemoglobin levels was seen in those who were anemic to begin with. The initially anemic in the control group, on the other hand, showed a significant drop in their mean hemoglobin levels by 0.21 g/dL.

It was interesting to note that the drop in hemoglobin levels seen in the initially anemic subjects was not as much as that seen in normal subjects of the control group, two compensatory processes, one of increased absorption and the other of accelerated erythropoiesis in deficiency may together have resulted in this finding.

Although many detailed studies are not available in literature regarding the effect of *Spirulina* supplementation on hemoglobin levels in humans, a few pilot studies done, corroborate the findings of the present study.[80] A study conducted in India using dietary supplementation of *Spirulina* fusiforms at 2 g/day on 20 subjects over a period of 36 days showed a 10% increase in hemoglobin concentration.[79] As stated earlier, a study conducted in Japan on 8 women having hypochromic anemia, assessed the effect of 4 g *Spirulina* supplementation for 30 days on hemoglobin levels. The average blood hemoglobin content increased by 21%, that is, from 10.9 to 13.3/dL.[78]

Supplementation of *Spirulina*, which brought about a rise in the hemoglobin levels of the experimental group, led to a drop in the percent prevalence of anemia in the subjects of experimental group (Table 4.18). While initially 70.8% of the subjects in experimental group were anemic, after the intervention period this had dropped to 41.5%. The percent prevalence of anemia in the control group increased from 67.7% to 70.6% by the end of the study. Initially, a larger proportion (46.2%) of the subjects in the experimental group was moderately anemic and 24.6% were mildly anemic.

TABLE 4.19

Percent Prevalence of Anemia among the Subjects: Before in Red Cell Morphology

Red cell morphology	Total n = 133	Experimental n = 65	Control n = 68
Normocytic normochromic			
Before supplementation	51.13 (68)	43.08 (28)	58.82 (40)
After supplementation	59.40 (79)	75.38 (49)	44.15 (30)
Microcytic hypochromic			
Before supplementation	42.10 (56)	49.23 (32)	35.29 (24)
After supplementation	39.10 (52)	24.62 (16)	52.94 (36)
Macrocytic hypochromic			
Before supplementation	6.77 (9)	7.69 (5)	5.88 (4)
After supplementation	1.50 (2)	0 (0)	2.94 (2)

Values in parenthesis indicates number of subjects.

After *Spirulina* supplementation, there was a shift from the moderate degree of anemia with only 4.6% of subjects being moderately anemic and 36.9% in mildly anemic.

In addition to bringing about a shift in the anemic status of the subjects the *Spirulina* supplementation also brought about changes in red cell morphology (Table 4.19). It was seen that initially there were 49.23% subjects having red cell morphology of microcytic hypochromia in experimental group. However, after supplementation the percent of subjects having microcytic hypochromia reduced to 24.6%. The reduction in the percent of microcytic hypochromia was reflected in the percent subjects with normocytic normochromic red cell at the end of the intervention period. The percent of normocytic normochromic category dramatically increased from an initial of 43 to 75.38%. The percent in the macrocytic hypochromic subjects also decreased after supplementation. The increase in normocytic normochromic subjects, indicates, that the low levels of hemoglobin seen initially in these two groups, were due to a deficiency of iron as supplementation of *Spirulina* brought about not only an improvement in hemoglobin but also in the red cell morphology.

Thus, supplementation with 1 g spray-dried *Spirulina* daily for 50 days, which contains a highly available form of iron brought about a significant increase in hemoglobin levels of the preschool children.

SUMMARY

From the various clinical studies with *Spirulina* supplementation in various disorders it can be concluded that:

- *Spirulina* supplementation in T2DM patients resulted in significant reduction in fasting and postprandial blood glucose, glycated Hb, and also helped in lowering the atherogenic lipid parameters.

- The positive results obtained in protein status, pulmonary function and IgE status in *Spirulina*-supplemented asthma patients strongly suggests that *Spirulina* can be introduced along with medicine as a therapeutic and dietary supplement in the treatment of asthmatics.
- Remarkable improvement in the prognosis of nephrotic syndrome patients with *Spirulina* supplementation substantiates the role of *Spirulina* as a health product in the management of nephrotic syndrome.
- Beneficial effect of *Spirulina* was also seen among preschool children and adolescent anemic girls whereby it helped in improving the blood hemoglobin levels thereby bringing about a reduction in the prevalence of anemia.

Thus to conclude it can be said that *Spirulina* with its potential therapeutic properties has been shown to be beneficial in the management of various disorders and may help to optimize health in the long run.

ACKNOWLEDGMENT

The authors wish to acknowledge the financial assistance received from The University Grants Commission, New Delhi, India, Parry Agro Industries Ltd, Chennai, India, and R. D. Birla Smarak Kosh, Mumbai, India, and Dr. Rhuta Labhe, Dr. Panam Parikh, Dr. Rohini Samuels, Ms. Alefia Sadliwala, and Ms. Ritika Taneja for their contributions in carrying out the work.

REFERENCES

1. Mani, U.V., Desai, S.A., and Iyer, U.M., Studies on the long-term effect of *spirulina* supplementation on serum lipid profile and glycated proteins in NIDDM patients, *J. Nutr. Functional, Med. Fds.*, 2, 25, 2000.
2. Shah, S., Role of *spirulina* in the management of hyperlipidemia, MSc Dissertation Thesis, Department of Foods & Nutrition, The M. S. University of Baroda, Vadodara, 1997.
3. World Health Organisation (WHO) Report. Diet, Nutrition and the prevention of chronic diseases. WHO Technical Report Series 916. Report of a Joint WHO/FAO Expert Consultation, 2003.
4. Bastyr, E.J. et al., Therapy focused on lowering postprandial glucose, not fasting glucose, may be superior for lowering HbA_{1c}, *Diabetes Care*, 23, 1236, 2000.
5. Stratton, I.M. et al., Association of glycaemia with macrovascular and microvascular complications of type 2 diabetes (UKPDS 35): prospective observational study, *BMJ*, 321, 405, 2000.
6. Parikh, P., Mani, U., and Iyer, U., Role of *Spirulina* in the control of glycemia and lipidemia in type 2 diabetes mellitus, *J. Med. Fds.*, 4, 193, 2001.
7. Parikh, P.M., Mani, U.V., and Iyer, U.M., Control of diabetes mellitus through the food supplement *spirulina*, *Ann. Nutr. Metab.*, 45, 1, 282, 2001.
8. Mani, I. and Mani, U.V., Effect of wheat bran supplementation on serum glycosylated protein and serum lipid profile in maturity onset diabetic patients, *Plant Fds. Hum. Nutr.*, 37, 184, 1987.

9. Mani, I., Patel, J.J., and Mani, U.V., Effect of wheat bran supplementation on serum lipids and urinary imino acids in maturity onset diabetics, *J. Clin. Biochem. Nutr.*, 3, 143, 1987.

10. Iyer, U.M., and Mani, U.V., Studies on the effect of curry leaves supplementation on lipid profile, glycated proteins and amino acids in NIDDM patients, *Plant Fd. Hum. Nutr.*, 40, 275, 1990.

11. Iyer, U.M. et al., Studies on the effect of sundakai (Solanum torvum) powder supplementation on lipid profile, glycated proteins and amino acids in NIDDM patients, *Plant Fd. Hum. Nutr.*, 42, 175, 1992.

12. Rai, V., Mani, U.V., and Iyer, U.M., Effect of Ocimum sanctum leaf powder supplementation on blood lipoproteins, glycated proteins and total amino acids in patients with NIDDM, *J. Nutr. Environ. Med.*, 7, 113, 1997.

13. Anderson, J.W. and Hanna, T.J., Impact of non-digestible carbohydrates on serum lipoproteins and risk for cardiovascular disease, *J. Nutr.*, 129, 1457S, 1999.

14. Anderson, J.W. et al., Effects of psyllium on glucose and serum lipid responses in men with type 2 diabetes and hypercholesterolemia, *Am. J. Clin. Nutr.*, 70, 466, 1999.

15. Bourdon, I. et al., Postprandial lipid, glucose, insulin, and cholecystokinin responses in men fed barley pasta enriched with β-glucan, *Am. J. Clin. Nutr.*, 69, 55, 1999.

16. Brown, L. et al., Cholesterol-lowering effects of dietary fiber: a meta-analysis, *Am. J. Clin. Nutr.*, 69, 30, 1999.

17. Anderson, J.W. et al., Cholesterol-lowering effects of psyllium intake adjunctive to diet therapy in men and women with hypercholesterolemia: meta-analysis of 8 controlled trials, *Am. J. Clin. Nutr.*, 71, 472, 2000.

18. Chandalia, M. et al., Beneficial effects of high dietary fibre intake in patients with type 2 diabetes mellitus, *N. Eng. J. Med.*, 342, 1392, 2000.

19. Vuksan, V. et al., Beneficial effects of viscous dietary fibre from Konjac–Mannan in subjects with insulin resistance syndrome, *Diabetes Care*, 23, 9, 2000.

20. Jenkins, D.J.A. et al., Effect of wheat bran on glycemic control and risk factors for cardiovascular disease in type 2 diabetes, *Diabetes Care*, 25, 1522, 2002.

21. Iyer, U., Deshmukh, S., and Mani, U., Glycemic indices of *spirulina*-supplemented meals, *Int. J. Diab. Dev. Countries*, 19, 108, 1999.

22. Henrikson, R., *Earth Food Spirulina*, 4th ed. Ronore Enterprises Inc., California, USA, 1999. <URL: http://www.spirulina.com>

23. Westphal, S.A., Gannon, M.C., and Nuttal, F.Q., Metabolic response to glucose ingested with various amounts of proteins, *Am. J. Clin. Nutr.*, 52, 262, 1990.

24. McCarty, M.F., The origins of Western obesity: a role for animal protein? *Med. Hypotheses*, 54, 488, 2000.

25. Hawkins, M. et al., Role of the glucosamine pathway in fat-induced insulin resistance, *J. Clin. Invest.*, 99, 2173, 1997.

26. Ciaraldi, T.P. et al., Glucosamine regulation of glucose metabolism in cultured human skeletal muscle cells: divergent effects on glucose transport/phosphorylation and glycogen synthase in non-diabetic and type 2 diabetic subjects, *Endocrinology*, 140, 3971, 1999.

27. Choi, C.S., Lee, F.N., and Youn, J.H., Free fatty acids induce peripheral insulin resistance without increasing muscle hexosamine pathway product levels in rats, *Diabetes*, 50, 418, 2001.

28. Nayaka, N., Homa, Y., and Goto, Y., Cholesterol lowering effect of *spirulina*, *Nutr. Rep. Int.*, 37, 1329, 1988.

29. Dillon, J.C. et al., Nutritional value of the alga *Spirulina*. In: *Plants in Human Nutrition. World Rev. Nutr. Diet.*, Simpoulos, A.P. (Ed.). Karger, Basel, 77, 32, 1995.

30. Cronin, J.R., Gamma linolenic acid: a building block for good health, *Alternative Complimentary Therapies*, 218, 2000.

31. Anderson, J.W., Johnstone, B.M., and Cook-Newell, M.E., Meta-analysis of the effects of soy protein intake on serum lipids, *N. Eng. J. Med.*, 333, 276, 1995.

32. Chambers, J.C. et al., Plasma homocysteine concentrations and risk of coronary heart disease in UK Indian Asian and European men, *Lancet*, 355, 523, 2000.

33. Teixeira, S.R. et al., Effects of feeding 4 levels of soy protein for 3 and 6 weeks on blood lipids and apolipoproteins in moderately hypercholesterolemic men, *Am. J. Clin. Nutr.*, 71, 1077, 2000.

34. Hermansen, K. et al., Beneficial effects of a soy-based dietary supplement on lipid levels and cardiovascular risk markers in type 2 diabetic subjects, *Diabetes Care*, 24, 228, 2001.

35. Howard, B.V., Lipoprotein metabolism in diabetes mellitus, *J. Lipid Res.*, 28, 613, 1987.

36. Niehauer, J. et al., Predictive value of lipid profile for salutary coronary angiographic changes in patients on a low fat diet and physical exercise programme, *Am. J. Cardiol.*, 78, 163, 1996.

37. Wagner, A.M. et al., Apolipoprotein (B) identifies dyslipidemic phenotypes associated with cardiovascular risk in normocholesterolemic type 2 diabetic patients, *Diabetes Care*, 22, 812, 1999.

38. Lu, W. et al., Non-HDL cholesterol as a predictor of cardiovascular disease in type 2 diabetes, *Diabetes Care*, 26, 16, 2002.

39. Mishra, M., The effect of *spirulina* in the treatment of bronchial asthma, MSc Dissertation Thesis, Department of Foods & Nutrition, The M. S. University of Baroda, Vadodara, 1998.

40. Troisi, R.J. et al., A prospective study of diet and adult-onset asthma, *Am. J. Respir. Crit. Care Med.*, 151, 1401, 1995.

41. Woolcock, A.J., Asthama. In: *Textbook of Respiratory Medicine*, 2nd ed., vol 2, Murray, J.F. and Nadel, J.A. (Eds). W B Saunders, Philadelphia, 1288, 1994.

42. Dayong, Wu. et al., Effect of dietary supplementation with black currant seed oil on the immune response of healthy elderly subjects, *Am. J. Clin. Nutr.*, 70, 536, 1999.

43. Ziboh, V.A. and Fletcher, M.P., Dose response effects of dietary gamma–linoleic acid enriched oils on human polymorphonuclear-neutrophil biosynthesis of leukotriene B4, *Am. J. Clin. Nutr.*, 55, 39, 1992.

44. Dry, J. and Vicent, D., Effect of fish oil diet on asthma: results of a one-year double-blind study, *Int. Arch. Allergy Appl. Immunol.*, 95, 156, 1991.

45. Hayashi, O., Katoh, T., and Okuwaki, Y., Enhancement of antibody production in mice by dietary *spirulina* platensis, *J. Nutr. Sci. Vitaminol.*, 40, 431, 1994.

46. Barnes, P.J., Reactive oxygen species and airway inflammation, *Free Radic. Biol. Med.*, 9, 235, 1990.

47. Chanez, P. et al., Generation of oxygen free radicals from blood eosinophils from asthma patients after stimulation with PAF or phorbol ester, *Eur. Respir. J.*, 3, 1002, 1990.

48. Schauer, U. et al., Enhanced superoxide generation by eosinophils from asthmatic children, *Int. Arch. Allergy Immunol.*, 96, 317, 1991.

49. Kumazawa, H. et al., The role free radicals in airway obstruction in asthmatic patients, *Chest,* 100, 1319, 1991.

50. Soutar, A., Seaton, A., and Brown, K., Bronchial reactivity and dietary antioxidants, *Thorax*, 52, 166, 1997.

51. Burrows, B. et al., Association of asthma with serum IgE levels and skin-test reactivity to allergens, *N. Engl. J. Med.*, 320, 271, 1989.

52. Sears, M.R. et al., Relation between airway responsiveness and serum IgE in children with asthma and in apparently normal children, *N. Engl. J. Med.*, 325, 1067, 1991.

53. Burrows, B. et al., Interactions of smoking and immnuologic factors in relation to airway obstruction, *Chest*, 84, 657, 1983.

54. Malo, J.L. et al., Reference values of the provocative concentrations of methacholine that cause 6% and 20% changes in forced expiratory volume in one second in a normal population, *Am. Rev. Respir. Dis.*, 128, 8, 1983.

55. Rijcken, B. et al., The relationship between airway responsiveness to histamine and pulmonary function level in a random population sample, *Am. Rev. Respir. Dis.*, 137, 826, 1988.

56. Gajeskwi, T.F., Joyce, J., and Fitch, F.W., Antiproliferative effect of IFN-γ in immune regulation III. Differential of Th1 and Th2 murine helper T-lymphocyte using recombinant IL-2 and recombinant IFN-γ, *J. Immunol.*, 143, 15, 1989.

57. Le Gros, G.S. et al., Generation of interleukin-4 producing cells *in vivo* and *in vitro*: IL-2 and IL-4 are required for *in vitro* production of IL-4 producing cells, *J. Exp. Med.*, 172, 921, 1990.

58. Snijdewint, F.G.M. et al., Prostaglandin E2 differentially regulates cytokine secretion profiles of human T-helper lymphocytes, *J. Immunol.*, 150, 5321, 1993.

59. Gold, K.N., Weyand, C.M., and Goronzy, J.J., Modulational helper T-cell function by prostaglandins, *Arthritis Res.*, 37, 925, 1994.

60. Roper, R.L., Brown, D.M., and Phipps, R.P., Prostaglandin E2 promotes B-lymphocyte Ig isotype switching to IgE, *J. Immunol.*, 154, 162, 1995.

61. Nayak, S.S. et al., Serum apolipoproteins A and B, lecithin: cholesterol acyl transferase activities and urinary cholesterol levels in nephrotic syndrome patients before and during steroid treatment, *Nephron*, 54, 234, 1990.

62. Labhe, R.U. et al., The effect of *spirulina* in the treatment of bronchial asthma, *J. Nutr. Functional and Med. Fds.*, 3, 53, 2001.

63. Labhe, R.U. et al., Management of bronchial asthma with *spirulina*. In: *Proc. Int. Symp. on Recent Advances in Mol. Biol., Allergy and Immunology*, Sept 3–5, 2000, 138.

64. Labhe, R.U., Mani, U.V., and Iyer, U.M., Effect of the functional food—*spirulina* in the management of bronchial asthma, *Ann. Nutr. Metab.*, 45, 1, 230, 2001.

65. Querfeld, U., Should hyperlipidemia in children with nephrotic syndrome be treated? *Pediatr. Nephrol.*, 13, 77, 1999.

66. Aguilar-Salinas, C.A. et al., Physiologic mechanisms of action of lovaststatin in nephrotic syndrome, *J. Lipid Res.*, 36, 18, 1995.

67. Wheeler, D.C. and Bernard, D.B., Lipid abnormalities in the nephrotic syndrome: cause, consequences and treatment, *Am. J. Kidney Dis.*, 23, 331, 1994.

68. D'Amico, G., Lipid changes in the nephrotic syndrome: new insights into pathomechanisms and treatment, *Clin. Wochenschr.*, 69, 618, 1991.

69. Olbricht, J., Pathophysiology and therapy of lipid metabolism disorders in kidney diseases, *Klin. Wochenschr.*, 69, 455, 1991.

70. Warwick, G.L. et al., Metabolism of apolipoprotein B-containing lipoproteins in subjects with nephrotic-range proteinuria, *Kidney Int.*, 40, 129, 1991.

71. de Sain-van Velden, M.G.M. et al., Increased VLDL in nephrotic patients results from a decreased catabolism while increased LDL resuls from increased synthesis, *Kidney Int.*, 53, 994, 1998.

72. Samuels, R. et al., Hypercholesterolemic effect of *spirulina* in patients with hyperlipidemic nephrotic syndrome, *J. Med. Fd.*, 5, 91, 2002.

73. Mani, U.V. et al., Glycemic and lipemic response to various regional meals and south Indian snacks, *Int. J. Diab.*, 17, 75, 1997.

74. Nayaka, N., Effect of *spirulina* on reduction of serum cholesterol, *Prog. Med.*, 36, 11, 1986.

75. Howard, B.V. et al., Plasma lipoprotein cholesterol and triglycerides in the Pima Indian population comparison of diabetic and non-diabetics, *Arteriosclerosis*, 4, 462, 1984.

76. Kato, T. and Takemoto, K., Effects of *spirulina* on hypercholesterolemia and fatty liver in rats, *Nutr. Foods Assoc. J.*, 37, 323, 1984.

77. Grattan Roughan, P., *Spirulina*: a source of dietary gamma-linolenic acid, *J. Sci. Food Agri.*, 47, 85, 1989.

78. Takeuchi, T., Clinical experiences of administration of *spirulina* to patients with hypochronic anaemia, Tokyo Medical and Dental University, Japan. C.F. National Symposium—*Spirulina* Ecology, Taxonomy, Technology and Application (ETTA) Shri AMM Murugappa Chettiar Research Centre (MCRC), Madras, India, 1978.

79. Seshadri, C.V. and Valliammai, V., The study of hemoglobin levels in humans fell on *spirulina* supplement, *Mono. Ser. Eng. Photo. Syn. Sys.*, vol 30, C.F. National Symposium—*Spirulina* Ecology, Taxonomy, Technology and Application (ETTA) Shri AMM Murugappa Chettiar Research Centre (MCRC), Madras, India, 1990.

80. Uliyar Mani, V. et al., Effect of *spirulina* supplementation on blood hemoglobin levels of anemic girls, *JFST*, 37, 6, 642, 2000.

5 Antioxidant Profile of *Spirulina*: A Blue-Green Microalga

Kanwaljit Chopra and Mahendra Bishnoi

CONTENTS

INTRODUCTION

Spirulina (*Arthrospira*), a filamentous, multicellular microalga, is a ubiquitous organism that was used as food in Mexico 400 years ago during the Aztec civilization. It is still being used as food by the Kanembu tribe in the Republic of Chad where it is sold as dried bread called "dihe."[1] Although it was first isolated by Turpin in 1827 from the freshwater stream, species of *Spirulina* (*Spirulina platensis*, *Spirulina maxima*, *Spirulina fusiformis*) have been found in variety of environments: soil,

101

sand, marshes, brackish water, sea water, and fresh water. This alga is a rich source of proteins, vitamins, amino acids, minerals, and other nutrients. It is considered as a valuable additional food source of some macro- and micronutrients including high quality protein, iron, gamma-linolenic fatty acid, carotenoids, vitamins B1, and B2. It is also used to derive additives in pharmaceuticals and foods. During *Spirulina* cultivation in open reservoirs and especially in closed photo bioreactors, its biomass may be additionally enriched with some trace elements such as iron, iodine, selenium, zinc, copper, manganese, and chromium in high bioavailable form.

In spite of the fact that the chemical composition of *Spirulina* varies widely when grown in open reservoirs, its efficiency in treatment and prophylaxis of different diseases is proved in a variety of experimental test systems and clinical trials. Over the past few years, however, it has been found to have many additional pharmacological properties. It has been experimentally proven, *in vivo* and *in vitro*, that it is effective to treat certain allergies, anemia, cancer, hepatotoxicity, viral and cardiovascular diseases, hyperglycemia, hyperlipidemia, immunodeficiency, and inflammatory processes, among others. Several of these activities are attributed to *Spirulina* itself or to some of its components including fatty acids omega-3 or omega-6, beta-carotene, alpha-tocopherol, phycocyanin, phenol compounds, and a recently isolated complex, Ca-Spirulan (Ca-SP).[2]

It is a well-known fact that reactive oxygen species (ROS) are involved in a diversity of important pathological processes in medicine including inflammation and neurodegenerative diseases, atherosclerosis, and cancer. There has been a global resurgence for alleviation of chronic diseases. The use of synthetic antioxidants has decreased because of their suspected activity as promoters of carcinogenesis as well as a general consumer rejection of synthetic food additives. The phenolic compounds in the plants are known to possess antioxidant activities in biological systems, however the antioxidant activities of algae are still being characterized. This chapter encompasses information on antioxidant effects of *Spirulina* and their implications in a multitude of oxidative pathologies.

MORPHOLOGY, BIOCHEMISTRY, AND CHEMICAL COMPOSITION OF *SPIRULINA*

Spirulina is a multicellular, filamentous cyanobacterium. Under the microscope, *Spirulina* appears as blue-green filaments composed of cylindrical cells arranged in unbranched, helicoidal trichomes (Figure 5.1). The filaments are motile, gliding along their axis, and heterocysts are absent. The helical shape of the trichome is characteristic of the genus but the helical parameters (i.e., pitch length and helix dimensions) vary with the species,[3,4] or may be induced by changing the environmental conditions.[5] Electron microscopy of ultra thin sections of *S. platensis* revealed that the cell wall is composed of possibly four layers. The most external or outer membrane layer (L-IV) is composed of material arranged linearly in parallel with the trichome axis and is considered analogous to that present in the cell wall of gram-negative bacteria. Layer III is possibly composed of protein fibrils wound helically around the trichomes, whereas the peptidoglycan-containing layer (L-II) folds

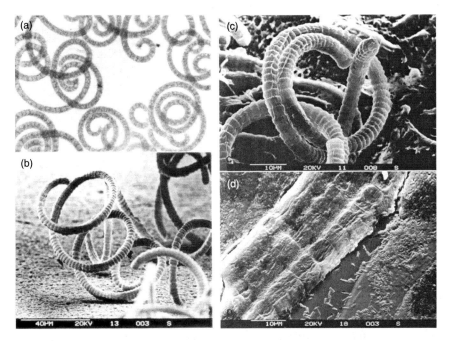

FIGURE 5.1   Morphology of *Spirulina*: (a) Optical microscopy of *S. platensis*. (b) Scanning electron micrograph of *S. platensis*. (c) Scanning electron micrograph of trichrome of *S. platensis*. (d) Scanning electron micrograph of nonaxenic of *S. platensis*. (Redrawn from Ciferri et al., 1983.)

towards the inside of the filament, giving rise, together with a putative fibrillar inner L-I, to the septum separating the cells. The most prominent cytoplasmic structure is the system of thylakoids originating from the plasmalemma but quite distinct from the well-evident mesosomes.[4,6]

LIFE CYCLE OF *SPIRULINA*

The life cycle of *Spirulina* (Figure 5.2) in laboratory culture is rather simple. A mature trichome is broken into several pieces through the formation of specialized cells, necridia, that undergo lysis, giving rise to biconcave separation disks. The fragmentation of the trichome at the necridia produces gliding, short (two to four cells) chains of cells, and the hormogonia, which move away from the parental filament to give rise to a new trichome. The cells in the hormogonium lose the attached portions of the necridial cells, becoming rounded at the distal ends with little or no thickening of the walls. During this process, the cytoplasm appears less granulated and the cells assume a pale blue-green color.[7]

Like most cyanobacteria, *Spirulina* is an obligate photoautotroph and cannot grow in the dark in media containing organic sources of carbon. The phycocyanin, biliproteins involved in the light-harvesting reactions, have been resolved by gel electrophoresis in *S. platensis* and *S. maxima* and isolated from the former. Both

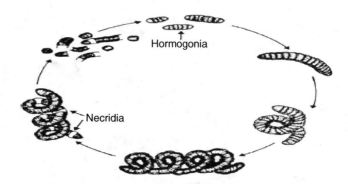

FIGURE 5.2   Life cycle of *Spirulina*. (Redrawn from Ciferri et al., 1983.)

c-phycocyanin and allophycocyanin appear to be oligomeric complexes composed of at least two different subunits that may be resolved by electrophoresis under denaturing conditions.[8,9] Cytochrome C_{554}, a cytochrome with high redox potential that links photosystems I and II, has been purified from *S. platensis* and *S. maxima*.[10] Ferredoxin, one of the electron carriers of photosynthesis, was purified from *S. maxima* and sequenced from *S. maxima* and *S. platensis*.[11]

Spirulina has high protein content 45% of the dry weight in the samples and 62% in laboratory-grown *S. platensis*. More recent analysis confirmed that protein represents more than 60% and, in certain samples, even 70% of the dry weight. The protein content of *Spirulina* appears to be high when compared with that of unicellular algae and other cyanobacteria.

ANTIOXIDANT EFFECTS OF *SPIRULINA*

IN VITRO AND IN VIVO ANTIOXIDANT EFFECTS OF VARIOUS EXTRACTS OF *SPIRULINA*

The antioxidant properties of *Spirulina* and its extracts have recently attracted the attention of researchers (Table 5.1). In one of the earliest studies, Manoj et al.[12] reported that the alcohol extract of *Spirulina* inhibited lipid peroxidation more significantly (65% inhibition) than the chemical antioxidants like α-tocopherol (35%), butylated hydroxyanisole, an antioxidant (BHA) (45%), and beta-carotene (48%). The water extract of *Spirulina* was also shown to have better antioxidant effect (76%) than gallic acid (54%) and chlorogenic acid (56%). An interesting aspect of their finding is that the water extract had a significant antioxidant effect even after the removal of polyphenols. In another study, by Zhi-gang et al.,[13] the antioxidant effects of two fractions of a hot water extract of *Spirulina* were studied using three systems that generate superoxide, lipid, and hydroxyl radicals. Both fractions showed significant capacity to scavenge hydroxyl radicals (the most highly reactive oxygen radical), but no effect on superoxide radicals. One fraction had significant activity in scavenging lipid radicals at low concentrations. Miranda et al.,[14] demonstrated the antioxidant

TABLE 5.1
Summary of Studies on Antioxidant Effects of *Spirulina*

Reference	Type of study	Summary of study
Manoj et al., 1992	*In vitro*	The alcohol extract of *Spirulina* inhibited lipid peroxidation more significantly than the chemical antioxidants like alpha-tocopherol, BHA, and beta-carotene. Water extract showed more antioxidant activity than gallic acid and chlorogenic acid.
Zhi gang et al., 1997	*In vitro*	Two fractions of hot water extracts showed marked scavenging of hydroxyl radical (the highly reactive oxygen radical); one of the fractions had significant activity in scavenging lipid radicals at low concentrations.
Miranda et al., 1998	*In vitro*	Peroxidation of rat brain homogenate was inhibited by almost 95% with 0.5 mg of the methanolic extract. The IC_{50} of the extract in this system was found to be 180 mcg.
Romay et al., 1998	*In vitro*	Phycocyanin was able to scavenge hydroxyl ($IC_{50} = 0.91$ mg/mL) and alkoxyl ($IC_{50} = 0.76$ μg/mL) radicals. It also inhibited liver microsomal lipid peroxidation ($IC_{50} = 12$ mg/mL).
Romay et al., 2000	*In vitro*	Phycocyanin inhibited 2,2′-azobis(2-amidinopropane) dihydrochloride (AAPH), a free radical generator induced human erythrocyte haemolysis in the same way as trolox and ascorbic acid, two well-known antioxidants. On the basis of the values of IC_{50} phycocyanin was found to be 16 times more efficient as antioxidant than trolox and about 20 times more efficient than ascorbic acid.
Hirata et al., 2000	*In vitro*	The antioxidant activity of phycocyanobilin (a component of phycocyanin) was greater than that of alpha-tocopherol, zeaxanthin, and caffeic acid on the molar basis.
Bhat and Madyastha, 2000	*In vitro*	Phycocyanin showed a potent peroxyl radical scavenger capacity with a rate constant ratio of 1.54 compared to 3.5 for uric acid (a known peroxyl radical scavenger).
Rimbau et al., 1999	Animal (Rats)	Oral administration of c-phycocyanin (100 mg/kg) in rats prevented kainic acid induced behavioral and glial reactivity in the rat hippocampus crossing the hematoencepphalic barrier. Authors postulate potential use of phycocyanin in the treatment of neurodegenerative disease such as Alzheimer's and Parkinson's disease induced by oxidative stress-induced neuronal injury.
Vadiraja et al., 1998	Animal (Rats)	Carbon tetrachloride (0.6 mL/kg) and R-(+)-pulegone (250 mg/kg) induced hepatotoxicity in rats was reduced significantly when phycocyanin was administered intraperitoneally to rats 1 or 3 h before the challenge.
Miranda et al., 1998	Animal (Rats)	Plasma antioxidant activity in brain homogenate incubated at 47°C showed that the antioxidant activity of plasma was 97% and 71% for the experimental group and 74% and 54% for the control group after 2 months and 7 months, respectively.
Bhat and Madyastha, 2000	Animal (Rats)	c-Phycocyanin from *Spirulina* effectively inhibited CCl_4–induced lipid peroxidation in rat liver *in vivo*.

activity of a methanolic extract of *Spirulina in vitro* and *in vivo*. The *in vitro* antioxidant assay involved a brain homogenate incubated with and without the extract at 37°C. Peroxidation of rat brain homogenate was inhibited by almost 95% with 0.5 mg of the methanolic extract. The IC_{50} of the extract in this system was found to be 180 mcg. The *in vivo* antioxidant capacity was evaluated in plasma and liver of animals receiving a daily dose of 5 mg for 2 and 7 weeks.[14] Plasma antioxidant activity in brain homogenate incubated at 47°C showed that the antioxidant capacity of plasma was 97% and 71% for the experimental group and 74% and 54% for the control group after 2 and 7 months of *Spirulina* treatment. The antioxidant effect was attributed to beta-carotene, tocopherol, and phenolic compounds working individually or in synergy.[14,15] Different extracts from the microalga *S. platensis* were obtained using pressurized liquid extraction (PLE) and four different solvents (hexane, light petroleum, ethanol, and water). All extracts demonstrated a significant antioxidant activity as tested using electro-chromatography with diode array detection (MEKC-DAD).[16]

Chlorella (*Chlorella vulgaris*), another microalga, has also been reported to show antioxidant activity[17] in exhibiting attenuating effects on oxidative stress and suppressing inflammatory mediators.[18] In one study, Wu et al.,[19] compared the antioxidant activity of *Spirulina* and chlorella extracts. Results of this study indicated that the total phenolic content of *Spirulina* was almost five times greater than that of chlorella (6.86 +/− 0.58 vs. 1.44 +/− 0.04 mg tannic acid equivalent/g of algae powder, respectively). The antioxidant activity of *Spirulina* determined by the ABTS*+ method was higher than chlorella (EC50: 72.44 +/− 0.24 μmol of trolox equivalent/g of *Spirulina* extract vs. 56.09 +/− 1.99 μmol of trolox equivalent/g of chlorella extract). Results of DPPH assay also showed a similar trend as the ABTS*+ assay (EC50: 19.39 +/− 0.65 μmol of ascorbic acid equivalent/g of *Spirulina* extract vs. 14.04 +/− 1.06 μmol of ascorbic acid equivalent/g of chlorella extract).[19]

PHYCOCYANIN, A MAJOR ANTIOXIDANT CONSTITUENT OF *SPIRULINA*

Phycobiliproteins are a small group of highly conserved chromo proteins that constitute the phycobilisome, a macromolecular protein complex whose main function is to serve as a light harvesting complex for the photosynthetic apparatus of cyanobacteria and eukaryotic groups. The most common classes of phycobiliproteins are allophycocyanin, phycocyanin (Pc), and phycoerythrin all of which are formed by a and b protein subunits and carry different isomeric linear tetrapyrrole prosthetic groups (bilin chromophore) that differ in the arrangement of their double bonds. The bilin groups are attached to the polypeptides through thioether linkages to specific cysteinyl residues.[20] Phycocyanin (Figure 5.3) is composed of two dissimilar a and b protein subunits of 17,000 and 19,500 Da, respectively, with one bilin chromophore attached to the subunit (a 84) and two to the b subunit (b 84, b 155).[21] Phycocyanin exists as a complex interacting mixture of trimer, hexamer, and decamer aggregates. It is obtained from the microalgae cellular biomass by a freeze thawing process or by using a French pressure cell, and is purified by successive steps of ammonium sulphate precipitation and further DEAE-cellulose chromatography. Phycocyanin is considered

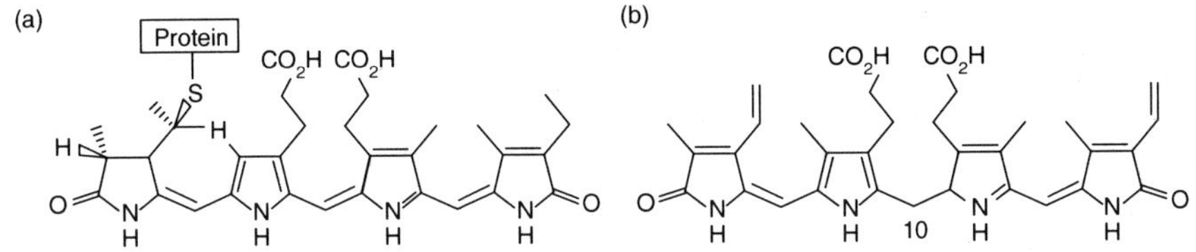

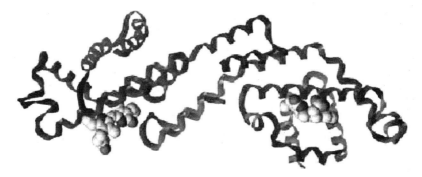

FIGURE 5.3   Chemical structure of phycocyanin bilin chromophore (a) and bilirubin (b).

FIGURE 5.4   Three dimensional structure of phycocyanin with alpha and beta dimers Pc is composed of two dissimilar a (red) and b (blue) protein subunits of 17 000 and 19 1500 Da, respectively, with one bilin chromophore attached to the a subunit (a 84) and two to the b subunit (b 84, b 155). (Redrawn from Romay et al., 2003.)

pure when the absorption ratio of visible maximum to 280 was greater than 4.[22,23] The chemical structure of the bilin chromophores (Figure 5.4) in phycocyanin is very similar to bilirubin, a heme degradative product. Bilirubin is considered to be a physiologically important antioxidant against reactive species.[24] It inhibits oxidative modification of plasma proteins and aromatic amino acid residues. Scavenging of oxygen radicals by bilirubin has been shown to protect serum albumin as well as other biological targets.[25,26] Similarly phycocyanin inhibits the reactive oxygen species generation as well as scavenges them in the variety of test systems and displays a powerful anti-oxidant activity (Table 5.2).

MECHANISMS OF ANTIOXIDANT ACTIVITY OF *SPIRULINA*

FREE RADICAL SCAVENGING

Harmful free radicals such as superoxide anion (an ROS) hydroxyl, alkoxyl, and peroxyl radicals are produced in various tissues because of the partial reduction of some oxygen molecules in the mitochondria. In various tissues (liver, lung, brain) an electron transport chain from NADPH to water occurs (with insertion of one oxygen atom into xenobiotic substrates) that use cytochrome P_{450} as the electron acceptor. Here futile recycling of electrons in the absence of substrates produces the superoxide

TABLE 5.2

Antioxidative Property of Phycocyanin (Major Constituent of *Spirulina*) in Different Test Systems (Redrawn from Romay et al., 2003)

Reaction system	Effect
Superoxide generated from hypoxanthine-xanthine oxidase	No effect
Alkoxyl radical generated from *t*-BOOH-ferrous sulfate	Scavenge
Hydroxyl radical generated from hydrogen peroxide-ferrous sulfate (Fenton reaction)	Scavenge
Peroxyl radical generated from AAPH thermolysis	Scavenge
Singlet oxygen	Quench
Lipid peroxidation induced by Fe^{+2}-ascorbic acid and AAPH thermolysis	Inhibit
Peroxynitrite generated from nitrite acidified hydrogen peroxide	Scavenge
Hypochlorite	Removed
Reactive oxygen production from neutrophils stimulated with opsonized zymosan	Inhibit

anion and all other different deleterious free radicals. Administration of hepatotoxic, nephrotoxic, and neurotoxic chemicals resulted into generation of free radicals and *Spirulina*, as an extract and its important constituent, phycocyanin, scavenge these free radicals.

Scavenging of alkoxyl and hydroxyl radicals by phycocyanin was demonstrated using a chemiluminescence (CL) assay.[27] Determination of alkoxyl radical scavenging activity of phycocyanin was performed by measuring the inhibition of the CL produced by the reaction of *tert*-butyl hydroperoxide with ferrous ions in the presence of luminol. Exposure of phycocyanin to peroxyl radicals generated by thermolysis of AAPH leads to a progressive loss of the chromatography. Phycocyanin is considered pure when the absorption ratio of visible maximum to 280 was greater than 4.[23] The inhibition of CL produced by the Fenton reaction with luminol was used to evaluate the phycocyanin scavenging capacity against hydroxyl radicals. In this system the CL signal was inhibited in a dose-dependent fashion by increasing phycocyanin concentrations. It was reported that 24.7 mM of phycocyanin caused the same inhibition (50%) as 1.6 mM of dimethyl sulfoxide, a specific hydroxyl radical scavenger used as control. Hydroxyl radical scavenging capacity of phycocyanin has also been assayed by the inhibition of damage to 2-deoxyribose. In this system, phycocyanin inhibited deoxyribose damage in a concentration-dependent fashion. The IC_{50} values reported for phycocyanin using this method were 19 mM and 28 mM.[27] Bhat and Madyastha,[28] also demonstrated the involvement of the bilin chromophore in the radical scavenging activity of phycocyanin by studying the reactivity of the protein with peroxyl radicals derived from AAPH thermolysis. It was also shown that both native phycocyanin and the reducing form (using $NaBH_4$) are able to scavenge peroxyl radicals.[29] This was supported by the fact that when reduced phycocyanin was incubated with AAPH (10 mM) at 37°C, there was a rapid decrease in the absorption at 418 nm with a concomitant appearance of peaks at 618 and 360 nm in the UV-visible spectrum indicating the oxidation of phycocyanorubin to phycocyanobilin (PCB) by peroxyl radical.[26,29] These authors, using the competition kinetics of crocin bleaching by peroxyl radicals, also analyzed the interaction of peroxyl radical with phycocyanin and its ability to scavenge this radical. These studies demonstrated that phycocyanin is a potent peroxyl radical scavenger with an IC_{50} of 5.0 mM. Under these experimental conditions, uric acid, a known peroxyl radical scavenger had an IC_{50} of 1.9 mM. The rate of constant ratios obtained for phycocyanin and uric acid were of 1.54 and 3.5, respectively. It also has been reported that phycocyanin is able to protect human erythrocytes against lysis induced by peroxyl radicals. In this assay phycocyanin (12–75 mM) inhibited erythrocyte haemolysis in the same way as trolox and ascorbic acid, well-known antioxidants.[30] On the basis of IC_{50} values, phycocyanin proved to be almost 16 times more efficient as an antioxidant than trolox and about 20 times more efficient than ascorbic acid. The scavenging of ONOO(−) by phycocyanin and its bilin chromophore was also evaluated using competitive kinetics of pyrogallol red bleaching assays. Pyrogallol red is one of the more efficient dyes that can be used to evaluate the ONOO(−) scavenging activity of any compound in aqueous solution.[31]

INHIBITION OF LIPID PEROXIDATION

Lipid peroxidation mediated by ROS is believed to be an important cause of destruction and damage to cell membranes, because a simple initiating event can result in the conversion of hundreds of fatty acids side chain into lipid peroxides, which alter the structural integrity and biochemical functions of membranes. It has been shown that phycocyanin, an important antioxidant constituent of *Spirulina*, significantly inhibits the increase in lipid peroxides of rat liver microsomes after treatment with Fe^{+2}-ascorbic acid [27] or the free radical initiator AAPH.[28] Addition of phycocyanin (200–540 mM) to isolated microsomes in the presence of Fe^{+2}-ascorbate resulted in a concentration dependent decrease in thiobarbituric acid reactive substances (TBARS) as an index of hepatic lipid peroxidation. The calculated IC_{50} was 327 mM. Thus, phycocyanin reduced both the rate and the final extent of lipid peroxidation. The phycocyanin effect on peroxyl radical-induced lipid peroxidation in rat liver microsomes also has been studied. It was demonstrated that phycocyanin inhibits the azo-initiated microsomal lipid peroxidation in a concentration-dependent fashion with an IC_{50} value of 11.35 mM. Phycocyanin at 200 mM concentration inhibited nearly 95% of peroxyl radical induced lipid peroxidation.[32] Reduced phycocyanin also efficiently inhibited this reaction with an IC_{50} value of 12.7 mM. In fact both native and reduced phycocyanin inhibited lipid peroxidation almost to the same extent. In correspondence with these results it was demonstrated that phycocyanin also reduced CCl_4-induced lipid peroxidation *in vivo*. Intraperitoneal administration of phycocyanin (50–200 mg/kg), 3 h prior to CCl_4 treatment resulted in significantly lower production of malondialdehyde (MDA) than was found in rats receiving only CCl_4. It is known that in CCl_4 intoxication, free radicals arising from its biotransformation induce lipid peroxidation. The trichloromethyl radical ($CCl_3^{\cdot}$) initially formed is relatively nonreactive and this carbon-centered radical readily reacts with O_2 to form a peroxyl radical that is a good initiator of lipid peroxidation. Since it was demonstrated that phycocyanin did not alter the liver function and the cytochrome P_{450} system, the protection by phycocyanin against CCl_4-induced lipid peroxidation may not be related to a reduced formation of reactive metabolites of CCl_4, but to the ability of phycocyanin to scavenge peroxyl radicals.[28]

MODULATION OF METABOLIZING AND DETOXIFICATION ENZYMES

Spirulina has modulatory effect on the various drug metabolizing and detoxifying enzymes as well as antioxidant enzymes. In one study, the effect of 250 and 500 mg/kg of *Spirulina* was examined on drug metabolizing phase I and phase II enzymes, antioxidant enzymes, glutathione content, lactate dehydrogenase (LDH) in the liver of 7-week-old Swiss albino mice.[33] Primary findings of the study reveal the "monofunctional" nature of *Spirulina* as deduced from its potential to induce only the phase II enzyme activities is associated mainly with carcinogen detoxification. The glutathione *S*-transferase and DT-diaphorase specific activities were induced in hepatic and all the extrahepatic organs examined (lung, kidney, and fore stomach) by *Spirulina* pretreatment.[33] With reference to antioxidant enzymes, namely, superoxide dismutase, catalase, glutathione reductase, glutathione peroxidase, and reduced glutathione were increased significantly by both the chosen doses of *Spirulina*.[27]

SPIRULINA AND OXIDATIVE DAMAGE

SPIRULINA AND DRUG-INDUCED OXIDATIVE DAMAGE

There are various drugs causing nephrotoxicity and cardiotoxicity through the free radical generation mechanism. Among them, cyclosporine (CsA)-induced nephrotoxicity, doxorubicin-induced cardiotoxicity, gentamicin-induced nephrotoxicity, and cisplatin-induced nephrotoxicity present considerable clinical challenge. CsA, gentamicin, and cisplatin cause a dose-related decrease in renal function in experimental animals and humans.[34] The generation of ROS has been implicated in nephrotoxicity induced by these drugs.[35] Pretreatment with *Spirulina* protected the rats from cisplatin-induced nephrotoxicity as evidenced by attenuation of decrease in creatinine clearance (Figure 5.5). The protection of renal function was coupled with prevention in the rise in kidney tissue malondialdehyde levels and enhancement of renal glutathione, superoxide dismutase (SOD) and catalase (Figure 5.6). The cardiotoxicity of doxorubicin is associated with oxidative stress and apoptosis.[36] In another study, the doxorubicin-induced enhancement of ROS in cells as measured by the 2′,7′-dichlorodihydrofluorescein diacetate and dihydroethidium fluorescence was markedly reduced by pretreatment of phycocyanin/*Spirulina*.[36,37]

SPIRULINA AND METAL-INDUCED OXIDATIVE DAMAGE

Systemic and oral administration of some metals leads to the initiation of oxidative damage. Lead (100 ppm) given in doubly deionized water for 30 days, oral administration of cadmium (6 mg/kg) as cadmium chloride ($CdCl_2$) for 30 days, intraperitoneal administration of $HgCl_2$ (50 mg/kg) resulted in a significant increase in thiobarbituric acid reactive substances (TBARS) levels, conjugated diene and hydroperoxide and a decrease in the levels of copper, zinc, iron, selenium, glutathione, superoxide dismutase, catalase, glutathione peroxidase when compared to normal control.[38,39] Administration of *Spirulina* produced a well-pronounced protective effect in respect

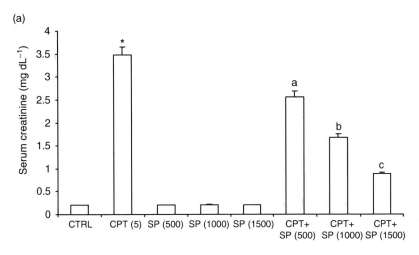

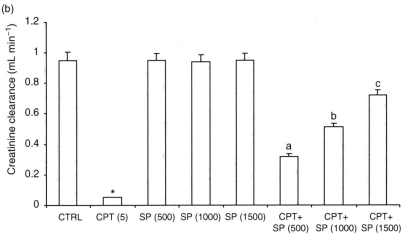

FIGURE 5.5 Effect of *Spirulina* (SP) (500, 1000, 1500 mg kg^{-1}, p.o.) on (a) serum creatinine and (b) creatinine clearance in cisplatin (100 mg kg^{-1}, p.o.) treated rats. $^*p < .05$ as compared to the control group (CTRL); [a,b,c]$p < .05$ as compared to the CPT group and with one another. (Kuhad et al., 2006.)

to these parameters in cadmium-intoxicated rats as well as lead-intoxicated animals by reducing various oxidative stress parameters such as malondialdehyde, conjugated diene and hydroperoxide.[38,39] Extract of *S. fusiformis* provided protection against oxidative damage induced by mercuric chloride.[40]

SPIRULINA AND EXERCISE-INDUCED OXIDATIVE DAMAGE

Spirulina supplementation prevents skeletal muscle damage in untrained human beings. Sixteen students were volunteered to take *S. platensis* in addition to their normal diet for 3 weeks. Blood samples were taken after finishing the Bruce incremental treadmill exercise before and after treatment. The results showed that plasma concentrations of malondialdehyde were significantly decreased after supplementation with *Spirulina*.[41] The activity of blood superoxide dismutase (SOD) was significantly raised after supplementation with *Spirulina*. Both the blood glutathione peroxide (GP(x)) and LDH levels were significantly different between *Spirulina* supplementation analysis[41] (Figure 5.6).

SPIRULINA AND NITROSATIVE STRESS

Peroxynitrite (ONOO(−)) is known to inactivate important cellular targets and also mediate oxidative damage in DNA. Phycocyanin, a biliprotein from *S. platensis*, and its chromophore, phycocyanobilin, efficiently scavenge ONOO(−), a potent physiological inorganic toxin. Scavenging of ONOO(−) by phycocyanin and PCB was established by studying their interaction with ONOO(−) and quantified by using competition kinetics of pyrogallol red bleaching assay. The relative antioxidant ratio and IC_{50} value clearly indicate that phycocyanin is a more efficient ONOO(−) scavenger than PCB. Increasing role of peroxynitrite species in different pathological conditions suggest that phycocyanin can be a potential therapeutic target for different disorders.[26]

The interaction of phycocyanin and its bilin chromophore with peroxynitrite (ONOO(−)) was studied spectroscopically by Bhat and Madyastha.[31] They demonstrated that the addition of increasing concentrations of ONOO(−) (0–200 mM) to phycocyanin (10 mM) significantly decreased its absorption at 618 nm, with no change in the absorption at 360 nm. Nearly, 50% of absorption at 618 nm was lost in the presence of 200 mM ONOO(−), although there was no shift in the absorption maxima. The spectra of bilin chromophores are characterized by absorption maxima at 610 and 365.5 nm. The addition of ONOO(−) (0–125 mM) to bilin chromophores (10 mM) decreased the absorbance peak at 610 nm and 365.5 nm, with a shift towards lower wavelength (563 and 329.5 nm) at lower concentrations of ONOO(−). At higher concentration of ONOO(−) (125 mM), there was no further shift in the absorption maxima and the chromophore was almost completely bleached. The scavenging of ONOO(−) by phycocyanin and its bilin chromophore was also evaluated using competitive kinetics of pyrogallol red bleaching assays.[31] Pyrogallol red is one of the more efficient dyes that can be used to evaluate the ONOO(−) scavenging activity of any compound in aqueous solution. Phycocyanin is an efficient scavenger of ONOO(−); at 70 mM concentration it inhibited pyrogallol red bleaching to the extent of nearly 90%. However, both bilin chromophore and glutathione (a known ONOO(−) scavenger) appeared to be more efficient scavengers of ONOO(−) at lower concentrations than phycocyanin. It was also noticed that phycocyanin, its bilin chromophore, and glutathione, inhibited bleaching of pyrogallol red in a concentration-dependent manner with an IC_{50} value of 21.8 ± 2.6 mM, 30.5 ± 0.8 mM and 4.8 ± 1.2 mM respectively. The relative antioxidant activity ratios calculated for phycocyanin, its bilin group and glutathione were 3.9, 1.8, and 5.2 respectively. The relative antioxidant ratio as well as IC_{50} value clearly suggested that phycocyanin is more efficient ONOO(−) scavenger than its bilin chromophore. This result was attributed to the interaction of ONOO(−) with tyrosine and tryptophan residues present

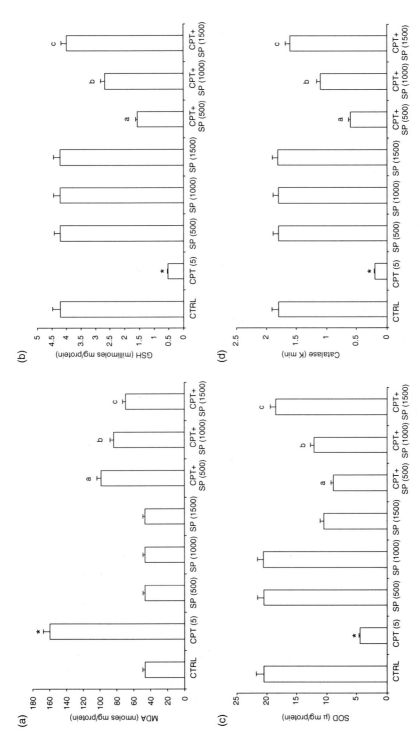

FIGURE 5.6 Effect of *Spirulina* (SP) (500, 1000, 1500 mg kg^{-1}, p.o.) on renal (a) lipid peroxidation, (b) reduced glutathione, (c) superoxide dismutase (SOD), and (d) catalase (CAT) in cisplatin (100 mg kg^{-1}, p.o.) treated rats. *$p < .05$ as compared to the control group (CTRL); [a,b,c] $p < .05$ as compared to the CPT group and with one another. (Kuhad et al., 2006.)

in the apoprotein moiety. The authors also proved that the bilin chromophore significantly inhibits the ONOO(−)-mediated single-strand breaks in supercoiled plasmid DNA in a dose-dependent manner with an IC_{50} value of 2.9 ± 0.6 mM.[26,42]

SPIRULINA AND HEPATOTOXIN-INDUCED OXIDATIVE DAMAGE

There are certain chemicals that are supposed to be hepatotoxic owing to the formation of the free radicals. Carbon tetrachloride (CCl_4) and R-(+)-pulegone-induced hepatotoxicity in rats are few examples of these. Vadiraja et al.,[43] studied the effect of c-phycocyanin from *S. platensis* on carbon tetrachloride and R-(+)-pulegone-induced hepatotoxicity in rats. In this study, a single dose (200 mg/kg) of phycocyanin administered intraperitoneally to rats one or 3 h before R-(+)-pulegone (250 mg/kg) or carbon tetrachloride (0.6 mL/kg) challenge, significantly reduced the different oxidative stress parameters and resultant hepatotoxicity caused by these chemicals. The hepatoprotective effect of phycocyanin was therefore attributed to the inhibition of reactions involved in the formation of reactive metabolites and possibly to its radical scavenging activity.[43] Similar hepatoprotective effect was seen in experiments where rats were fed an oil extract of *Spirulina* or its defatted fraction. Recently, Bhat and Madayastha[28] reported that c-phycocyanin from *Spirulina* effectively inhibited CCl_4-induced lipid peroxidation in rat liver *in vivo*. Extract from *S. fusiformis* also provides protection against mercuric chloride-induced hepatic toxicity.[40]

SPIRULINA AND NEURONAL OXIDATIVE DAMAGE

A recent interesting and elaborate study shows that oral administration of c-phycocyanin (100 mg/kg) in rats prevents kainic-acid-induced behavioral and glial reactivity in the rat hippocampus suggesting a corresponding protective effect on neurons. The study showed that phycocyanin reduced experimental status epilepticus, suggesting possible therapeutic intervention in the treatment of some forms of epilepsy. According to the authors, kainic acid (KA) triggered excitotoxicities resulted in the production of ROS. It is therefore postulated that the protective effect of phycocyanin in neuronal damage may be due to its free-radical scavenging and antioxidant properties.[26,44] An interesting aspect of this study is the finding that oral administration of phycocyanin exerts its effect in the hippocampus, crossing the hematoencephalic barrier. According to the authors, these findings and the virtual lack of toxicity of phycocyanin suggest that this phytochemical could be used in the treatment of neurodegenerative diseases such as Alzheimer's and Parkinsonism.[44]

Phycocyanin (1–3 mg/mL) prevents cell death caused by 24 h potassium and serum withdrawal in rat cerebellar granule cell (CGC) cultures. After 4 h potassium and serum deprivation, phycocyanin inhibited ROS formation measured as 2′,7′-dichlorofluorescein fluorescence, showing its scavenging capability.[45] Also pretreatment of CGC cultures with phycocyanin reduced thymidine incorporation into DNA below control values and reduced dramatically apoptotic bodies as visualized by propidium iodide, indicating inhibition of apoptosis induced by potassium and serum deprivation. Flow cytometry studies indicated that 24 h potassium and serum deprivation acts as a proliferative signal for CGC, which show an increase in S-phase percentage, and cells progressed into the apoptotic pathway. Phycocyanin protected

CGC from apoptosis induced by potassium and serum deprivation. Equivalent results were found when the neuronal damage in the hippocampus was evaluated through changes in peripheral benzodiazepine receptors (microglial marker) and heat shock protein 27 kD expression (astroglial marker).[45] Recently, it is also reported that *Spirulina*-enriched diets enhance striatal dopamine recovery and induce rapid, transient microglia activation after injury of the rat nigrostriatal dopamine system.[46] *Spirulina*-enriched diets had a significant reduction in the volume of infarction in the cerebral cortex and an increase in poststroke locomotor activity as well as it also resulted in decrease expression in caspase enzyme activity.[47]

At present, the mechanisms by which phycocyanin exerts its neuroprotective effects are not clear. However, growing evidence supports the hypothesis that the phycobiliprotein, acting as an antioxidant, inhibits neuronal death by a mechanism that involves free radical scavenging and therefore phycocyanin may be useful for the treatment of neurodegenerative disorders such as Alzheimer's, Parkinson's, and Huntington's diseases.

OTHERS

Phycocyanin, a water soluble protein of alga, was first reported as a powerful antioxidant by Romay et al., who demonstrated that phycocyanin was able to scavenge hydroxyl and alkoxyl radicals with activity equal to 0.125 mg/mL of dimethyl sulfoxide and 0.038 μg/mL of trolox, specific scavengers of these radicals respectively. Phycocyanin also inhibited liver microsomal lipid peroxidation. It is interesting to note that oxygen scavenging activity of c-phycocyanin was only 3 times lower than that of superoxide dismutase (SOD).[27] Recently, they also reported that phycocyanin inhibited 2,2'-azobis (imidinoprapane) dihydroxychloride (AAPH)-induced erythrocyte haemolysis in the same way as trolox and ascorbic acid, well-known antioxidants. On the basis of IC_{50} values (concentration of the additive that gave the 50% inhibition of peroxidative damage), phycocyanin was found to be 16 times more efficient as an antioxidant than trolox and about 20 times more efficient than ascorbic acid. These findings were supported by a more recent study that showed that the antioxidant activity of phycocyanobilin (a component of phycocyanin) was greater than that of alpha-tocopherol on a molar basis.[30] The antioxidant effect of phycocyanobilin was evaluated against oxidation of methyl linoleate in a hydrophobic system or with phosphatidylcholine liposomes. The study also showed that phycocyanin from spray-dried *Spirulina* had a similar antioxidant activity as phycocyanin from fresh *Spirulina*. The results suggest that the antioxidant activity of phycocyanin is attributable to phycocyanobilin, a prosthetic group in phycocyanin, since the apoprotein component may be denatured upon drying. The fact that the dried phycocyanin showed the same level of activity as the intact protein makes the preparation and utilization of phycocyanin commercially feasible.[48–50]

FUTURE IMPLICATIONS AND CONCLUSION

On reviewing the antioxidant studies of *Spirulina* it can thus be concluded that *Spirulina* is a unique blend of carotenoids, zeaxanthin, polyphenols, phycocyanin, and polysaccharides as well as superoxide dismutase. With accumulating epidemiological interventions and clinical evidence regarding strong association between antioxidant intake and incidence of chronic diseases, *Spirulina* has a potential application in prevention and mitigation of cancer, heart disease, inflammation, and premature aging. An efficacious approach to protect the body against consequences of oxidative stress consists in improving the antioxidant nutrition. Scientific studies have shown that the synergistic action of a wide spectrum of antioxidants is better than the activity of a single antioxidant and that antioxidant from the natural sources have a higher bioavailability and therefore higher protective efficacy than synthetic antioxidants. Thus well-planned human trials of *Spirulina* and its important constituents can provide a conclusive evidence of using it as a possible therapeutic option.

REFERENCES

1. Dangeard, P. Sur une algue bleue alimentaire pourl'homme: *Arthrospira platensis* (Nordst.) Gomont. *Actes Soc. Linn. Boreaux Extr. Proces-verbaux*. 91, 39–41, 1940.
2. Chamorro, G. et al. Update on the pharmacology of *Spirulina* (*Arthrospira*), an unconventional food. *Arch. Latinoam Nutr.* 52(3), 232–40, 2002.
3. Rich, F. Notes on *Arthrospira platensis*. *Rev. Algol.* 6, 75–79, 1931.
4. Marty, F., and Busson, F. Donnees cytologique, et systematiques sur *Spirulina platensis* (Gom.) Geitler et *Spirulina* Geitleri J. de Toni (Cyanophyceae-Oscillatoriaceae). *C. R. Acad. Sci. Ser. D* 270, 786–789, 1970.
5. Venkataraman, L. V. Algae as food/feed: a critical appraisal based on Indian experience, 83–134, 1980 (In National Workshop on Algal Systems. Indian Society for Biotechnology, New Delhi).
6. Drews, G., and Weckesser, J. The biology of cyanobacteria. *Bot. Monogr.* 19, 333–357, 1982.
7. Ciferri, O. *Spirulina*, the edible microorganism. *Microbiol. Rev.* 47(4), 551–578, 1983.
8. Kenyon, C. N., and Stanier, R. Y. Possible evolutionary significance of poly-unsaturated fatty acids in blue-green algae. *Nature* (*London*) 227, 1164–1166, 1970.
9. Ogawa, T., and Terui, G. Studies on the growth of *Spirulina platensis*. (I) On the pure culture of *Spiruilina platensis*. *J. Ferment. Technol.* 48, 361–367, 1970.
10. Ho, K. K., and Krogmann, D. W. Cytochrome f from spinach and cyanobacteria. *J. Biol. Chem.* 255, 3855–3861, 1980.
11. Hall, D. O., Rao, K. K., and Cammack, R. A stable and easily extractable plant-type ferredoxin from the blue-green alga *Spirulina maxima*. *Biochem. Biophys. Res. Commun.* 47, 798–802, 1992.
12. Manoj, G., Venkataraman, L. V., and Srinivas, L. Antioxidant properties of *Spirulina* (*Spirulina platensis*). In: Seshadri and Bai. *Spirulina*. MCRC. 48–154, 1992.
13. Zhi-gang, Z., Zhi-li, L., and Xue-xian, L. Study on the isolation, purification, and antioxidation properties of polysaccharides from *Spirulina maxima*. *Acta Botanica Sinica*. 39, 77–81, 1997.
14. Miranda, M. S. et al. Antioxidant activity of the microalga *Spirulina maxima*. *Braz. J. Med. Biol. Res.* 31, 1075–1079, 1998.
15. Belay, A. The potential application of *Spirulina* (*Arthrospira*) as a nutritional and therapeutic supplement in health management. *J. Am. Nutraceut. Assn.* 5, 2, 2002.

16. Herrero, M. et al. Pressurized liquid extracts from *Spirulina platensis* microalga. Determination of their antioxidant activity and preliminary analysis by micellar electrokinetic chromatography. *J. Chromatogr. A.* 27; 1047(2), 195–203, 2004.
17. Miranda, M. S., Sato, S., and Mancini-Filho, J. Antioxidant activity of the microalga *Chlorella vulgaris* cultured on special conditions. *Boll. Chim. Farm.* 140(3), 165–168, 2001.
18. Lee, H. S. et al. Attenuating effect of chlorella supplementation on oxidative stress and NF kappa B activation in peritoneal macrophages and liver of C57BL/6 mice fed on atherogenic diet. *Biosci. Biotech. Biochem.* 67, 2083–2090, 2003.
19. Wu, L. C. et al. Antioxidant and antiproliferative activities of *Spirulina* and Chlorella water extracts. *J. Agric. Food Chem.* 53(10), 4207–4212, 2005.
20. Fairchild, C. D., and Glazer, A. N. Nonenzymatic bilin addition to the alpha subunit of an apophycoerythrin. *J. Biol. Chem.* 269, 28988–28996, 1994.
21. Turner, L., Houghton, J. D., and Brown, S. B. Purification and identification of apophycocyanin alpha and beta subunits from soluble protein extracts of the red alga Cyanidium caldarium. Light exposure is not a prerequisite for biosynthesis of the protein moiety of this photosynthetic accessory pigment. *Planta* 201, 78–83, 1997.
22. Neufeld, G. J., and Riggs, A. F. Aggregation properties of c-phycocyanin from *Anacystis nidulans*. *Biochem. Biophys. Acta.* 181, 234–243, 1969.
23. MacColl, R., Berns, D. S., and Koven, N. L. Effect of salts on c-phycocyanin. *Arch. Biochem. Biophys.* 146, 477–482, 1971.
24. Stocker, R. et al. Antioxidant activities of bile pigments: biliverdin and bilirubin. *Methods Enzymol.* 186, 301–309, 1990.
25. Neuzil, J., and Stocker, R. Free and albumin-bound bilirubin are efficient co-antioxidants for alpha-tocopherol, inhibiting plasma and low density lipoprotein lipid peroxidation. *J. Biol. Chem.* 269, 16712–16719, 1994.
26. Romay, C. et al. c-Phycocyanin: a biliprotein with antioxidant, anti-inflammatory and neuroprotective effects. *Curr. Protein Pept. Sci.* 4(3), 207–216, 2003.
27. Romay, C. et al. Antioxidant and anti-inflammatory properties of c-phycocyanin from blue-green algae. *Inflamm. Res.* 47, 36–41, 1998.
28. Bhat, V. B., and Madyastha, K. M. c-Phycocyanin: a potent peroxyl radical scavenger *in vivo* and *in vitro*. *Biochem. Biophys. Res. Commun.* 18, 275(1), 20–25, 2000.
29. Lissi, E. A. et al. Kinetics of phycocyanin bilin groups destruction by peroxyl radicals. *Free Rad. Biol. Med.* 28, 1051–1055, 2000.
30. Romay, C., and Gonzalez, R. Phycocyanin is an antioxidant protector of human erythrocytes against lysis by peroxyl radicals. *J. Pharm. Pharmacol.* 52, 367–368, 2001.
31. Bhat, V. B., and Madyastha, K. M. Scavenging of peroxynitrite by phycocyanin and phycocyanobilin from *Spirulina platensis*: protection against oxidative damage to DNA. *Biochem. Biophys. Res. Commun.* 13, 285(2), 262–266, 2001.
32. Pinero Estrada, J. E., Bermejo Bescos, P., and Villar del Fresno, A. M. Antioxidant activity of different fractions of *Spirulina platensis* protean extract. *Farmaco.* 56(5–7), 497–500, 2001.
33. Dasgupta, T. et al. Chemomodulation of carcinogen metabolising enzymes, antioxidant profiles and skin and forestomach papillomagenesis by *Spirulina platensis*. *Mol. Cell. Biochem.* 226(1–2), 27–38, 2001.
34. Khan, M. et al. *Spirulina* attenuates cyclosporine-induced nephrotoxicity in rats. *J. Appl. Toxicol.* 26(5), 444–51, 2006.
35. Kuhad, A. et al. Renoprotective effect of *Spirulina fusiformis* on cisplatin-induced oxidative stress and renal dysfunction in rats. *Ren. Fail.* 28(3), 247–54, 2006.

36. Khan, M. et al. c-Phycocyanin ameliorates doxorubicin-induced oxidative stress and apoptosis in adult rat cardiomyocytes. *J. Cardiovasc. Pharmacol.* 47(1), 9–20, 2006

37. Khan, M. et al. Protective effect of *Spirulina* against doxorubicin-induced cardiotoxicity. *Phytother. Res.* 19(12), 1030–1037, 2005.

38. Jeyaprakash, K., and Chinnaswamy, P. Effect of *spirulina* and Liv-52 on cadmium induced toxicity in albino rats. *Indian J. Exp. Biol.* 43(9), 773–781, 2005.

39. Upasani, C. D., Khera, A., and Balaraman, R. Effect of lead with vitamin E, C, or *Spirulina* on malondialdehyde, conjugated dienes and hydroperoxides in rats. *Indian J. Exp. Biol.* 39(1), 70–74, 2001.

40. Kumar, M., Sharma, M. K., and Kumar, A. *Spirulina fusiformis*: a food supplement against mercury induced hepatic toxicity. *J. Health Sci.* 51(4), 421–430, 2005.

41. Lu, H. K. et al. Preventive effects of *Spirulina platensis* on skeletal muscle damage under exercise-induced oxidative stress. *Eur. J. Appl. Physiol.* 98(2), 220–226, 2006.

42. Desai, K. N., Wei, H., and Lamartiniere, C. A. The preventive and therapeutic potential of the squalene-containing compound, Roidex, on tumor promotion and regression. *Cancer Lett.* 101, 93–96, 1996.

43. Vadiraja, B., Gaikwad, N., and Madyastha, K. Hepatoprotective effect of c-phycocyanin: protection for carbontetrachloride and R-(+)-pulegone-mediated hepatotoxicity in rats. *Biochem. Biophys. Res. Commun.* 249, 428–431, 1998.

44. Rimbau, V. et al. Protective effect of c-phycocyanin against kainic acid induced neuronal damage in rat hippocampus. *Neurosci. Lett.* 276, 75–78, 1999.

45. Rimbau, V. et al. Naunyn-Scmiedeberg's. *Arch. Pharmacol.* 364, 96–104, 2001.

46. Stromberg, I. et al. Blueberry- and *spirulina*-enriched diets enhance striatal dopamine recovery and induce rapid, transient microglia activation after injury of the rat nigrostriatal dopamine system. *Exp. Neurol.* 196(2), 298–307, 2005.

47. Wang, Y. et al. Dietary supplementation with blueberries, spinach, or *spirulina* reduces ischemic brain damage. *Exp. Neurol.* 193(1), 75–84, 2005.

48. Hirata, T. et al. Antioxidant activities of phycocyanobillin prepared from *Spirulina platensis*. *J. Appl. Phycol.* 12(3–5), 435–439, 2000.

49. Jaime, L. et al. Separation and characterization of antioxidants from *Spirulina platensis* microalga combining pressurized liquid extraction, TLC, and HPLC-DAD. *J. Sep. Sci.* 28(16), 2111–2119, 2005.

50. Mendiola, J. A. et al. Characterization via liquid chromatography coupled to diode array detector and tandem mass spectrometry of supercritical fluid antioxidant extracts of *Spirulina platensis* microalga. *J. Sep. Sci.* 28(9–10), 2005.

6 Antioxidative and Hepatoprotective Effects of *Spirulina*

Li-chen Wu and Ja-an Annie Ho

CONTENTS

Algae can be regarded as the first photosynthetic life-form. Three-and-a-half billion years ago, blue-green microalgae, called cyanobacteria, created our atmosphere of oxygen, enabling other life to evolve. Since then, they have helped to regulate our planet's biosphere. This microalgae *Spirulina* has a spiral cellular structure, which is similar to that of a simple prokaryote. This alga has an extraordinary capacity to survive under conditions that are much too harsh for other algae. Habitats with extensive *Spirulina* growth include the Pacific Ocean near Japan and Hawaii, large

119

fresh water lakes, including Lake Chad in Africa, Klamath Lake of North America, Lake Texcoco in Mexico, and Lake Titikaka in South America.[1]

The blue-green microalgae *Spirulina* has been an important source of protein in the traditional diet of natives of Africa and Mexico. The species of *Spirulina* that are most commonly used in nutritional supplements are *Spirulina platensis* (*S. platensis*) and *Spirulina maxima* (*S. maxima*). It has been sold as commercial products in many countries, such as Japan and Taiwan, for use as a healthy functional food and for therapeutic purposes.[2] This tiny aquatic plant, *Spirulina*, contains large amounts of all-vegetable protein (70% dry weight),[3] carotenoid (4000 mg/kg),[4] *omega*-3 and *omega*-6 polyunsaturated fatty acids (such as rare essential fatty acid gamma linolenic acid), sulfolipids, glycolipids, polysaccharides, provitamins; other nutrients such as vitamin A,[5] vitamin E,[6] various B vitamins; and minerals, including calcium, iron, magnesium, manganese, potassium, zinc,[1] and selenium.[7] It is also a rich and inexpensive source of such pigments as phycocyanin (Pc), an accessory photosynthetic pigment of the phycobiliprotein family. Phycocyanin is commonly utilized in the food industry as a food colorant,[8] an emulsifier, a thickening agent, and a gelling agent. It can also be used in cosmetics colorants[9] and fluorescent markers in bio-medical research.[10] Various investigations have verified that various components of *Spirulina*, including phycocyanin, selenium, carotenoids, and fatty acid γ-linolenic acid (GLA) have significant antioxidant and radical scavenging characteristics.[11–14] It is, therefore, a potential therapeutic agent for treating oxidative stress-induced diseases, inflammations, allergies or even cancer.[13] This chapter summarizes recent findings concerning the antioxidant, anti-inflammatory, immunoenhancing, antiviral, anticancer, and hepatoprotection properties of *Spirulina*, with reference to the potential advantages of *Spirulina* as a regular nutritious supplement in the prevention of various disorders that are associated with oxidative stress, inflammation, cancer, and liver-malfunctioning diseases.

ANTIOXIDANT PROPERTIES OF *SPIRULINA*

Numerous disease development processes are caused or accompanied by oxidative stress, which refers to cellular damage that is caused by reactive oxygen intermediates (ROI)—especially in age-related disorders. Since oxidative stress is an important factor in the beginning of several pathologies, from cancer to cardiovascular and other neurodegenerative diseases,[15–21] an effective approach is sought to improve antioxidant nutrition to protect the body against the harmful consequences of oxidative stress. In this respect, antioxidants from natural sources are believed to have higher bioavailability and greater protective efficacy than synthetic antioxidants.[22] Restated, *Spirulina* is attracting more interest because of its potential pharmaceutical and neutraceutical value.

The antioxidant property of *Spirulina* or phycocyanin has been examined *in vitro*.[13–14,23–26] Since then, *Spirulina* or its specific component, phycocyanin, has been studied with reference to the role of antioxidants in improving health and preventing diseases.[27] Experimental investigations have established the importance of antioxidant activity of *Spirulina* in decreasing lead-induced lipid peroxidation and brain lead deposition.[23] Moreover, they have the following properties: efficacy in anti-inflammation,[28] inhibit zymosan-induced arthritis,[29] protects against heavy metal caused hepatic toxicity,[30] reverses age-induced increases in concentrations of proinflammatory cytokines, and declines in cerebellar β-adrenergic function.[24] *Spirulina* also inhibits tumor development and reduces incidence,[31,32] and helps to prevent chronic diffusion associated with liver disease.[33]

Our group[14] has devoted considerable effort to determining the antioxidant activity of *Spirulina* and *chlorella*, and their antiproliferative effect on liver cancer cells (Hep G2) and hepatic stellate cells (HSCs). Accordingly, the free radical scavenging activity of *Spirulina* and *chlorella* water extracts was determined using the DPPH• method and the ABTS•+ method, respectively. Experimental results revealed that the patterns of antioxidant activity of *Spirulina* and *chlorella* determined by the ABTS•+ and the DPPH• methods were similar. The results of DPPH• assay, in which ascorbic acid was used as a standard reference compound, demonstrated that 50% effective concentration (EC_{50}) was 19.39 ± 0.65 μmol of ascorbic acid equivalent/g of *Spirulina* extract and 14.04 ± 1.06 μmol of ascorbic acid equivalent/g of *chlorella* extract. The free radical scavenging ability of *Spirulina* was better than that of *chlorella* according to the ABTS•+ method using trolox as a standard reference compound (EC_{50}: 72.44 ± 0.24 μmol of trolox equivalent/g of *Spirulina* extract vs. 56.09 ± 1.99 μmol of trolox equivalent/g of chlorella extract).

Romay's group[25,26] applied a chemiluminescence (CL) assay to determine the scavenging capacity of phycocyanin to remove alkoxyl and hydroxyl radicals. They assayed the decrease in the CL intensity, by reacting *tert*-butyl hydroperoxide reacted with ferrous ions in the presence of luminol, while a water-soluble analogue of vitamin E (6-hydroxy-2,5,7,8-tetramethylchroman-2-carhoxylic acid) was used as the standard reference. The IC_{50} of 0.1 μM of trolox had approximately the same effect as 2 μM of phycocyanin at 50% inhibition of the produced CL intensity. In addition, the hydroxyl radical scavenging capacity of phycocyanin could be determined from the protection against 2-deoxyribose damage; phycocyanin inhibited deoxyribose damage in a dose-dependent manner.[11,25,26] The same method has been used to determine the IC_{50} values of phycocyanin as 19 μM and 28 μM, respectively.[25,26] Since free radicals are important to the pathogenesis of inflammation, a powerful antioxidant may also be a potential anti-inflammation candidate. Parij et al. (1995)[34] obtained a reaction rate constant of approximately 1.9 to 3.5×10^{11} $M^{-1}S^{-1}$ for the interaction of phycobiliprotein with hydroxyl radicals, and 1.8×10^{10} for the interaction between ibuprofen and indomethacin, which are nonsteroidal anti-inflammatory drugs (NSAIDs), suggesting that phycobiliprotein may be an alternative anti-inflammatory therapeutic agent.

STRUCTURE OF PHYCOCYANIN

Padyana et al. (2001)[35] solved the crystal structure of phycocyanin, a phycobiliprotein, by molecular replacement. Complexes of phycobiliprotein, constituting the main light-harvesting antenna in blue-green microalgae for oxygenic photosynthesis, form supermolecules known as phycobilisome assemblies. In phycobiliproteins, the chromophore, a linear tetrapyrrole (bilin), is covalently attached to the apoprotein

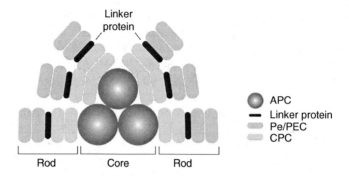

FIGURE 6.1   Schematic representative of one type of phycobilisome. (Modified from MacColl, R., *Biochimica et biophysica acta*, 1657, 73–81, 2004; L.-N. Liu et al., *Biochimica et biophysica acta*, 1708, 133–142, 2005.)

by thioether bonds to the cysteine residues. Allophycocyanin (APC), phycocyanin (pc), phycoerythrin (PE), and phycoerythrocyanin (PEC) are the four basic classes of phycobiliproteins in supermolecular phycobilisomes. Electron microscopic and crystallographic studies have elucidated the general architecture of this macromolecular assembly. It comprises high affinity α- and β-subunit polypeptides, which commonly associate with each other to form $(\alpha\beta)_3$ or $(\alpha\beta)_6$-monomers. Figure 6.1 schematically depicts one phycobilisome with a three-cylinder core. The antennae rods of phycobilisomes consist of APC at the core, C-phycocyanin (Cpc) in the middle (blue), and PE/PEC at the tip (pink).[35,36] Their collective range of absorption covers the entire visible spectrum of sunlight, with an overall energy transduction efficiency that exceeds 95%, such that the energy proceeds in the direction from tip to the core through PE/PEC, Cpc, APC, and finally to the reaction center.

Effect of Phycocyanin on Lipid Peroxidation

Lipid peroxidation can be defined as the oxidative deterioration of lipids that contain carbon–carbon double bonds. Lipid hydroperoxides are nonradical intermediates that are derived from unsaturated fatty acids, phospholipids, glycolipids, and cholesterol esters. Lipid hydroperoxides may be formed in enzymatic or nonenzymatic reactions that are mediated by "reactive oxygen species" (ROS), which are responsible for the destruction and damage of cell membranes. These ROS include hydroxyl radicals, lipid oxyl or peroxyl radicals, as well as singlet oxygen and peroxinitrite that are formed from nitrogen oxide (NO). All of these groups of atoms are frequently byproducts of oxygen metabolism, behaving as a unit, called a free radical.

Various investigations have verified that phycocyanin scavenges free radicals because its open chain tetrapyrroles structure. Phycocyanin has been observed to be able to inhibit liver microsomal lipid peroxidation that is induced by Fe^{+2}-ascorbic acid.[25,26] The group[25,26] that presented that observation also reported that phycocyanin reduced significantly ($p < .05$) and in a dose-dependent manner ear edema in mice that was induced by arachidonic acid and tetradecanoylphorbol acetate, as well as carrageenan-induced rat paw edema (both in intact and adrenalectomized animals).[25,26] Furthermore, C-phycocyanin (from *S. platensis*) effectively inhibited

CCl_4-induced lipid peroxidation in rat liver *in vivo*. Both native and reduced phycocyanin substantially suppressed peroxyl radical-induced lipid peroxidation in rat liver microsomes. The inhibition depended on the concentration, with an IC_{50} of 11.35 and 12.7 μM, respectively.[11] Several works have clearly suggested that phycocyanin exhibits anti-inflammatory activity in experimental animal models of inflammation, and its antioxidative and oxygen free radical-scavenging properties may contribute, at least partially, to its anti-inflammatory activity.[25,26]

ANTI-INFLAMMATORY ACTIVITY OF *SPIRULINA*

Cyclooxygenase-2 (COX-2) has an important role in catalyzing the conversion of arachidonic acid to prostaglandins and other eicosanoids.[37] The overexpression of COX-2 is associated with high levels of prostaglandin E_2 (PGE_2) that are observed in various malignancies of the colon, breast, lung, prostrate, skin, cervix, pancreas, and bladder.[38] Excess prostaglandin levels cause inflammation, influence cell proliferation, and the mediation of immune suppression.[39,40] Many investigations have confirmed that nonsteroidal anti-inflammatory drugs and selective COX-2 inhibitors can induce apoptosis in colon cancer cell lines and transformed fibroblasts.[41,42] Phycocyanin, present in *Spirulina*, has been claimed to have a selectively inhibitory effect on COX-2.[28] Restated, phycocyanin is a natural COX-2 inhibitor, which controls inflammation that is caused by the presence of the enzyme COX-2. Studies have been conducted to examine the involvement of phycocyanin in inducing apoptosis in tumor cells and the mechanisms of the apoptotic process. Pardhasaradhi et al. (2003)[43] reveals that phycocyanin activated the caspase that is involved in the apoptotic death process. Phycocyanin induced the generation of ROS by the tumor cells, subsequently inducing apoptosis. In addition, phycocyanin down-regulates Bcl-2, which is known to participate importantly in the apoptotic death processes.[43] The high phycocyanin content in *Spirulina* has specific anti-inflammatory properties. The amount of carotenoids in *Spirulina* (including β-carotene, lycopene, and lutein), is almost 10 times more than that in carrots, causing it to have good antioxidant properties. As they quench ROS, antioxidants have the intrinsic anti-inflammatory characteristics.

Phycocyanin, a photoharvesting pigment, belongs to the class of phycobilliproteins that are found in blue-green algae. All phycobiliproteins are water-soluble and therefore, unlike carotenoids, cannot exist within a membrane. Rather, phycobiliproteins cluster and adhere to the membrane, forming phycobilisomes. Phycocyanin normally represents up to 20% of the dry weight of a blue-green algae harvest. Bhat and Madyastha[11,13] examined C-phycocyanin, which is responsible for the deep bluish color of *Spirulina*, and found that it was able to not only scavenge free radicals, but also exhibited significant hepatoprotective effects.[44] As stated above,[25,26] phycocyanin can inhibit inflammation in mouse ears.[26] An *in vivo* study has verified that the blue-green algae can reduce the level of arachidonic acid in plasma because it contains considerable amounts of omega-3-α-linolenic acid.[45]

IMMUNOENHANCING EFFECTS OF *SPIRULINA*

Numerous natural products have an immunoenhancing effect.[46] Experimental works have shown that *Spirulina* products positively affect innate immune functions and

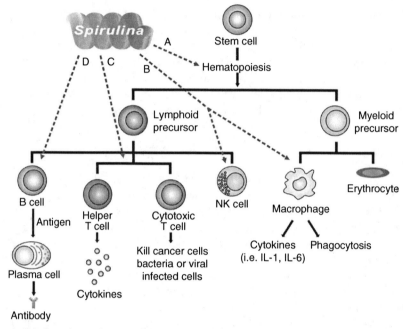

A. *Spirulina* enhances hematopoiesis to produce more erythrocytes and lymphocytes
B. *Spirulina* shows diredct effect on innate immunity by activating macrophages and NK cells
C. *Spirulina* activates T-helper cells and T-cytotoxic cells
D. *Spirulina* induces the maturity of B-cells for the production of antibodies

FIGURE 6.2   Effects of *Spirulina* on immunomodulation.

build up both the humoral and the cellular immune system (summarized in Figure 6.2). Sulfated-polysaccharides isolated from a water extract of *Spirulina*, called calcium-spirulan (Ca-Sp), exhibit immunomodulatory and antiviral activities.[47–50] Furthermore, immolina, a high-molecular-weight polysaccharide fraction of *Spirulina*, promotes chemokine expression in human monocytic THP-1 cells.[51] Other investigations have studied the use of the *Spirulina* in improving immune response.[52–55] Polysaccharides and phycocyanin from *Spirulina* enhance bone marrow reproduction, thymus growth, and spleen cell proliferation, increasing immunity in the animal model, such as mice. Studies have also demonstrated that *Spirulina* up-regulates the immune system by improving their ability to function in spite of stress from environmental toxins, bacteria, and virus.[47–51,53,54,56] The literature states that phycocyanin from *Spirulina* stimulates hematopoiesis, and especially erythropoiesis, by inducing the release of erythropoietin hormone (EPO).[1] Phycocyanin and polysaccharides from *Spirulina* promote antibody and white blood cell production.[53–56] According to Qureshi and Ali (1996),[53] the percentage of phagocytic macrophages in cats increased when they were administered a water-soluble extract of *S. platensis*. Moreover, the water-soluble extract of *S. platensis* caused the secretion of interleukins, such as IL-1, from murine peritoneal macrophages,[55] and the proliferation of thymocytes. In addition, the effect of *Spirulina* on nonspecific immunity has been measured at the level of natural killer (NK) cell activity. Leukocytes taken from the spleen of chickens fed with *Spirulina* had greater antitumor cell activity than those of control animals, perhaps because of the production of such cytokines as interferon.[54,57] Studies of a chicken model have demonstrated increased activity of NK cells in terminating tumor cells.[53,54] The capacity of peritoneal macrophages to ingest latex particles has been evaluated in another study,[55] in which peritoneal macrophages were removed from mice that had been fed on a *Spirulina*-supplemented diet (10% of the food by dry weight) for 10 weeks: a slight increase in the percentage of phagocytes from 91.3 to 95.9% was found *in vitro*. This work also found that phycocyanin of *Spirulina* inhibited release of histamine, a bioactive molecule involved with allergy.[49,58]

ANTIVIRAL EFFECTS OF *SPIRULINA*

Soon after the discovery of the human immunodeficiency virus (HIV) as the causative agent of acquired immune deficiency syndrome (AIDS) in 1984, heparin and other sulfated polysaccharides were found to be potential inhibitors of HIV-1 replication in cell culture. As a potent anti-HIV drug candidate, sulfated polysaccharides had several promising advantages, including their ability to block HIV replication in cell culture at rather low concentrations (0.1–0.01 µg/mL) without observable side-effects or cytotoxicity to the host cells at concentrations of up to 2.5 mg/mL. They could also inhibit the cytopathic effect of HIV, and prevent HIV-induced giant cell (syncytium) formation.[59–63]

As mentioned above, this important component of *Spirulina*, sulfated polysaccharides (calcium spirulan, Ca-SP) consists of rhamnose, ribose, mannose, fructose, galactose, xylose, glucose, glucuronic acid, galacturonic acid, sulfate, and calcium. Ca-SP inhibits the replication of various enveloped viruses, including herpes simplex virus, influenza virus, measles virus, mumps virus, and HIV,[48,60,62,63] by selectively inhibiting the penetration of the virus into host cells. Its antiviral effect[60] depends on the retention of its molecular conformation by chelating calcium ions with sulfate groups.[60,62,63]

In 1998, Ayehunie et al.[59] investigated an aqueous extract of the blue-green algae, *S. platensis*, and found that it inhibited HIV-1 replication in human T-cell lines, peripheral blood mononuclear cells (PBMC), and Langerhans cells (LC). The 50% effective concentration (EC_{50}) of the extract for reducing HIV-1 production in PBMCs ranged between 0.3 and 1.2 µg/mL, while the 50% inhibitory concentration (IC_{50}) of algae extract for PBMC growth ranged between 0.8 and 3.1 mg/mL. HIV-1 contagion was directly inactivated when the algae extract was preincubated with virus before it was added to human T-cell lines or other cells.

ANTICANCER EFFECTS OF *SPIRULINA*

Spirulina is one of the richest natural sources of β-carotene and phycocyanin. Since both β-carotene and phycocyanin exhibit anticancer activity,[64] *Spirulina* has also been claimed to be a potent cancer-fighting phytonutrient. *Spirulina* not only has antioxidant and immune-enhancing effects but also has anticancer properties that have been demonstrated in numerous studies of laboratory animals by preventing the development of experimentally produced cancers.[57,65–68] The administration of phycocyanin to mice with liver cancer markedly increased their survival rate, perhaps because of the powerful antioxidant activity of phycocyanin, which prevented cancer and reduced DNA damage that is caused by free radicals. Subhashini et al. (2004)[67] revealed that molecular mechanisms in C-phycocyanin induced apoptosis in human chronic myeloid leukemia cell line-K562. They observed a substantial decline (49%) in the proliferation of myeloid leukemia cell upon treatment with phycocyanin (50 μM) for 48 h. C-Phycocyanin induced apoptosis in K562 cells by the following mechanism; (1) the release of cytochrome c from mitochondria into the cytosol, (2) the cleavage of poly(ADP-ribose) polymerase (PARP), and (3) the down regulation of Bcl-2. Phycocyanin induced apoptotic death in histiocytic tumor AK-5 cells, which process is inhibited by Bcl-2 expression through the regulation of the generation of free radicals. Phycocyanin, a natural product, may therefore be a chemotherapeutic agent based on its apoptotic activity against tumor cells.[43]

The hematopoietic function of *Spirulina* is very important to its anticancer effect, which increases the population of immune cells, and thereby immunoboosts natural resistance against cancer, and other diseases.[53–55,68] Mishima et al. (1998)[65] studied the inhibition of tumor invasion and metastasis by calcium spirulan (Ca-SP), a novel sulfated polysaccharide that is derived from *Spirulina*.[68] Hirahashi et al. (2004)[57] elucidated a possible mechanism by which *Spirulina* activates the human innate immune system. *Spirulina* promotes the production of interferon and tumor necrosis factor alpha (TNF-α) as well as NK cells when a hot water extract of *S. platensis* was orally administered. In other experimental animal studies, when extracts of *Spirulina* were injected directly into cancerous tumors, the tumor stopped growing.[66] One human study involved individuals who had oral leukoplakia, a condition of the mouth that normally develops into cancer if it is untreated. The oral intake of *Spirulina* for 1 year prevented the progression of cancer in 45% of the study participants. More clinical investigations of humans must be conducted to verify the exact anticancer effects of *Spirulina*.

Apart from the positive effects of *Spirulina* on health discussed above (and summarized in Figure 6.3), *Spirulina* has potential neutraceutical and pharmaceutical characteristics, including hepatoprotective effects. Alcohol-medicated liver injury has been linked to oxidative stress that is caused by the production of ROI. Apoptotic cells can be observed in animal models with acute alcohol intoxication following glutathione depletion. Antioxidants reduce the rate of apoptosis in experimental animals.[69,70] A study conducted by our group demonstrated that an aqueous extract of *Spirulina* significantly ($p < .01$) inhibits the proliferation of HepG2 and HSC, perhaps because of its antioxidative activity. The properties of *Spirulina* in Hepatic Protection are discussed below.

HEPTOPROTECTIVE EFFECT OF *SPIRULINA*

ANTIOXIDATIVE EFFECT AND HEPATOPROTECTION

Several studies[11,13,25] have examined the use of Cpc, one of the major biliproteins of *S. platensis*, in hepatoprotection. This protection derives mostly from its ability to scavenge reactive radicals.[13] In a study of liver injury, the intraperitoneal

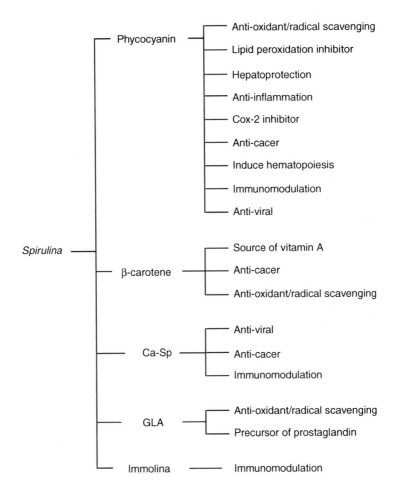

FIGURE 6.3   Effects of *Spirulina* on the promotion of health.

administration of C-phycocyanin (200 mg/kg body weight) 3 h prior to treatment with carbon tetrachloride and R-(+)-pulegone substantially reduced the hepatotoxicity and the serum glutamate pyruvate transaminase (SGPT) activity, and lower levels of toxic intermediates formed (haloalkane free radicals and menthofuran).[44] Furthermore, the activities of microsomal cytochrome P450, glucose-6-phosphatase, and aminopyrine-*N*-demethylase were restored.[44] This protection effect may come from either the inhibition by phycocyanin of cytochrome P450-mediated reactions that are involved in converting toxic metabolites or scavenging reactive metabolites. Another investigation demonstrated that the hepatoprotective effect of *Spirulina* derives primarily from its radical scavenging ability.[13]

   Phycocyanin has been reported to be able to scavenge hydroxyl, alkoxyl, and peroxyl radicals[71,72] with IC_{50} values of 0.91 mg/mL, 76 μg/mL, and 5 μM, respectively, as determined by CL assay, as described earlier.[25] The free radical scavenging capacity reduces the generation of lipid peroxides, disrupting the membrane structure and the biochemical functions. Pycocyanin markedly reduces the peroxidation of lipids that is induced by the Fenton-type reaction[25] and amount of peroxyl radicals[13] on rat liver microsomes. The addition of phycocyanin to isolated microsomes in the Fe^{+2}-ascorbate and azo-initiated lipid peroxidation resulted in a concentration-dependent decrease in the concentrations of thiobarbituric acid reactive substances (TBARS), an index of lipid peroxidation, with IC_{50} values of 327 and 11.35 μM, respectively.[13,25] The scavenging of reactive radicals therefore reduces hepatotoxicity caused by carbon tetrachloride.[13] The chromophore (bilin), rather than the apoprotein of phycocyanin, is primarily responsible for the scavenging of reactive radicals.[73] The chromophore of phycocyanin is phycocyanobilin, which is an analog of biliverdin and can be reduced by $NaBH_4$ to a bilirubin-like structure.[74] The native and the reduced forms of phycocyanin had similar scavenging abilities.[13] Apart from its scavenging effect, phycocyanin inhibits lipid peroxidation by chelating metal ions, such as the ferrous ion, in the Fenton-type reaction.

METALLOPROTECTION AND HEPATOPROTECTION

A more beneficial effect of *Spirulina* has been discussed.[75–80] Several studies[75–79] have demonstrated that *Spirulina* possesses the metalloprotective effects. As is well established, heavy metals, such as lead and cadmium, impact the cellular growth, diminish cellular productivity, and induce toxicity in cells by accelerating iron dependent lipid peroxidation, ultimately leading to cellular death.[75–80] Heavy metal decreases DNA synthesis. Microalgae, including *Spirulina*, was found to increase the DNA synthesis and repair.[81] Heavy metals by microorganisms can be removed through several mechanisms, such as adsorption, enzymatic synthesis, or through the production of extracellular polymers.[77] Japanese researchers found the modulatory effect of *Spirulina*, which significantly reduced kidney toxicity caused by heavy metal mercury.[82] Kumar et al. (2005)[80] also demonstrated the protection of *S. fusiformis* extract against mercury in Swiss albino mice. The modulatory effects of lead toxicity by *S. fusiformis* (Oscillatoreaceae) were observed as well on the testes of Swiss albino mice at a dose level of 800 mg/kg body weight.[78] In this study, the survival time was significantly enhanced in the pre- and post-treated *Spirulina* group over that of the control (lead treated) group. According to previously reported results, lead-induced toxicity was reduced with respect to testes weight, animal weight, and tubular diameter in the pre-*Spirulina* treated group. The modulatory effects may be owing to the antioxidants, β-carotene, and SOD enzyme in *Spirulina*. Collective evidence further suggested that *Spirulina* benefits human, especially those inflicted with heavy metal poisoning.

Air pollution endangers a growing number of areas, as evidenced by exposure of the air, water, and food supply to several toxic chemicals. Humans require a mechanism for continuously eliminating such accumulated toxins. *Spirulina* possesses a unique combination of phytonutrients, including phycocyanin, polysaccharides (Ca-Sp), Vitamin A and E, and essential GLA. Such nutrients can not only help cleanse human bodies, but also provide antioxidant, radical scavenging, anticancer, antiviral, anti-inflammation, hepatoprotection, and immunomodulation capabilities.

EFFECT OF *SPIRULINA* ON FATTY LIVER

FATTY LIVER

Fatty liver is a common cause of chronic liver disease and refers to accumulation of excess fat in the liver. It is diagnosed that if fat exceeds 5% of the total weight of normal liver or when more than 30% of the hepatocytes in a liver lobule have lipid deposits, most of the fat that accumulates in the liver is triacylglycerols and fatty acids; other forms of fat, such as cholesterol, cholesterol ester, and phospholipids, are also present. Fatty liver is often associated with alcoholic liver disease, hyperinsulinemia, and insulin-resistance. Accordingly, it is most often observed in alcoholics, obese persons, and diabetic patients. It is also frequently caused by drugs,[83] viral hepatitis,[84] chemical intoxication,[85] pregnancy,[86] intestinal bypass surgery,[87] and malnutrition.[88] Histological findings reveal that fat deposits in the liver may vary in size and distribution. Hepatocytes may contain large fat droplets with an anomalously displaced nucleus (macrovesicular type) or multiple small droplets with a central nucleus (microvesicular type). Macrovesicular type steatosis is typically seen in metabolic syndrome, while the microvesicular type is observed in acute fatty liver during pregnancy, chemical intoxication, and Rey's syndrome. In acute alcoholic hepatic steatosis, mixed macrovesicular and foamy-type fatty degeneration (cell swelling with a massive accumulation of microvesicular fat droplets) in the perivenular region occurs.[89] Most fatty liver patients are asymptomatic. However, an enflamed fatty liver may lead to cirrhosis and finally hepatocellular carcinoma.

A fatty liver that was caused by excessive alcohol intake may result in liver inflammation (alcoholic hepatitis) and scarring (alcoholic cirrhosis), causing alcoholic liver disease. The development of an enflamed fatty liver in the absence of pregnancy and alcoholism is referred to as nonalcoholic steatohepatitis (NASH). The term nonalcoholic fatty liver disease (NAFLD) refers to fatty liver, NASH, and cirrhosis. Although NASH may occur in all ages and both genders, it is commonly found in middle-aged (40–60 year-old) women, many of whom are obese, or may have type 2 diabetes mellitus (insulin resistance) or hyperlipidemia.[90] People who are neither overweight nor have diabetes mellitus or hyperlipidemia have been recently reported as suffering from NASH.[91]

NASH develops for various reasons, and proceeds by several poorly understood biochemical mechanisms. The causes of steatosis may involve the reduced synthesis of very low density lipoprotein (VLDL) and elevated levels of hepatic triacylglycerols, because of the reduced levels of fatty acid oxidation or an increase in the amount of lipids that circulate to the liver. As lipids accumulate, lipid peroxidation is likely to occur in the presence of free radicals, causing cell damage, which results in inflammation. These changes will activate HSCs, causing fibrosis, cirrhosis, and portal hypertension, if NASH is advanced, up to 40% of NASH patients develop liver fibrosis or 5–10% cirrhosis.[92]

Hepatic steatosis is diagnosed nowadays by noninvasive imaging tests, such as ultrasonographic examination, CT, and MRI. The abnormality that can be detected in the laboratory is usually an increased aminotransferase level. For fatty liver associated with obesity, SGPT commonly exceeds SGOT, while SGPT is smaller than SGOT in alcoholic liver disease.[93] In addition, serum alkaline phosphatase and γ-glutamyl transpeptidase (GGT) are elevated in alcoholic liver disease and are within normal ranges in obesity-related hepatic steatosis.

No known treatment exists for fatty liver. The widely accepted treatment goal is to eliminate the potential causes and risk factors, since fatty liver due to obesity or alcoholism is reversible. Such actions as the discontinuation of drugs or toxins, body weight control and the prescription of hyperlipidemia and hyperglycemia help to reach this goal. Many other treatments have also been tested, including ursodeoxycholic acid (UDCA),[94] metformin,[95] rosiglitazone,[96] betaine,[97] and vitamins E and C.[98] Although more investigations are required before recommendations can be made for NAFLD patients, UDCA and metformin seem promising. UDCA is a non-toxic natural bile acid that is initially used to dissolve gallstone and is now used to reduce liver fat deposition. Metformin, an antidiabetic drug and an insulin-sensitizing agent, is potentially useful for the fatty liver caused by insulin resistance and hyperisulinemia.[95]

A recent study indicated that patients with fatty liver disease should be encouraged to take vitamin E and C supplements.[98] This treatment was claimed to be safe and affordable. Patients were randomly prescribed either oral vitamin E (600 IU/day) plus vitamin C (500 mg/day) or ursodeoxycholic acid (10 mg/kg/day). Clinical data suggested that at the end of 6 months of therapy, vitamin E plus C combination treatment yielded results that were comparable to those obtained with ursodeoxycholic acid. Serum alanine aminotransferase levels declined to normal levels in 17 of the 27 (63%) patients who received vitamin E plus C, and 16 of the 29 (55%) patients who received ursodeoxycholic acid. Antioxidants such as vitamin E and C appear to have a beneficial effect on fatty liver. In this regard, *Spirulina* seems to be a candidate for the attenuation of fatty liver.

REGULATION OF LIPID METABOLISM AND OXIDATIVE STRESS BY *SPIRULINA* ON FATTY LIVER

As reported elsewhere, *Spirulina* prevents the formation of fatty liver in animal models[99–105] and in humans.[106–109] The effectiveness of *Spirulina* against fatty liver may follow from its antioxidants, which include GLA, selenium, phycobilins, vitamins and carotenoids (β-carotene). In addition, essential fatty acids like GLA can prevent the accumulation of cholesterol in the body.[109]

In an animal model, fatty liver has been reported to be induced by a high cholesterol diet,[100] a 60% fructose diet,[101] carbon tetrachloride,[102,103] and alloxan-induced experimental diabetes.[105] The high fructose diet induces fatty liver because the rapid conversion of fructose to acyl-CoA or α-glycerophosphoric acid elevates plasma lipid level.[110] Fructose has been reported to have less effect on lipoprotein lipase (LPL) activation[111] and to promote the activities of fatty acid synthesis-related enzymes such as acetyl-CoA carboxylase,[112,113] fatty acid synthetase,[112–114] and malic enzyme.[112] The effectiveness of administering *Spirulina* to an animal with high fructose diet-induced hyperlipidemia (probably fatty liver) appears to be demonstrated in hypolipidemic effect,[115,116] reduced liver triacylglycerol, and hypocholesterolemia.[101] The beneficial effect of *Spirulina* may derive from the activated LPL activities, which are determined using postheparin serum.[116]

Carbon tetrachloride-induced hepatocyte injury and fatty liver have been suggested to be caused by an increase in the synthesis of liver fatty acids, elevated lipoperoxidation and altered release of hepatic lipoprotein.[102–119] The prevention by *S. maxima* of carbon tetrachloride-induced fatty liver is evidenced by restored lipoprotein levels and hypocholesterolemic, and hypotriacylglycerolemic effects.[102–103] It has a similar protective effect on a high fructose[101,115] and hypercholesterolemic diet-induced[120] fatty liver. In an animal study of fatty liver induced by the administering of simvastatin (75 mg/kg body weight), ethanol (20%) and a hypercholesterolemic diet (1% cholesterol) to male CD-1 mice for 5 days, significant measured liver total lipids (40%), liver triacylglycerols (50%), serum high-density lipoprotein (HDL) (45%), and serum triacylglycerols (50%) all markedly decreased when animals received *Spirulina* treatment (10% of diet) 2 weeks prior to the onset of the fatty liver.[120]

Different extracts of *Spirulina* (5% of diet composition) were investigated to determine the preventative effects on hypercholesterolemia and hypertriacylglycerolemia.[103,121] Oil extracts and defatted extracts were fed to male rats before a single intraperitoneal injection of carbon tetrachloride. The total liver lipids differed significantly, by 28% between the group that had not (50 mg/g wet weight) and the group that had (36.2 mg/g wet weight) been given *Spirulina* defatted-extracts. It differed by 30% between the former group and the group that had been treated with an oil fraction. Liver total triacylglycerols (defatted: 80%; oil: 54%) and cholesterol (defatted: 74.5%; oil: 71%) were similarly reduced. Liver total lipid, triacylglycerol, and cholesterol levels fell to normal ranges following the treatment.[102,103] However, hypotriacylglycerolemic and hypocholesterolemic effects in serum vary among studies, because of variations among the fractions of *Spirulina*, the dosage effect, the causes of fatty liver, gender, and the experimental schedule.[101–103,105,116] The hypoglycemic action of *S. maxima* in rats has been examined using a water-soluble fraction.[121] A study was conducted to measure the effect of *S. maxima* on serum glucose levels in diabetic rats. It was suggested that the water-soluble fraction suppressed serum glucose levels at fasting, while the water-insoluble fraction was found to be effective in reducing glucose levels at glucose loading.[121]

Studies have reported that the relief of accumulated liver lipids in a *Spirulina*-treated animal model is probably caused by increasing LPL activity,[116] increasing the level of serum HDL and restoring LDL and VLDL levels.[103,105] Moreover, the reduced hepatic lipoperoxidation contributes to the attenuation of the carbon tetrachloride-induced fatty liver.[103,105] *Spirulina* treatment caused liver microsomal TBARS, a lipoperoxidation product, to drop to a normal level,[103,122] probably because of the antioxidant constituents, such as selenium, chlorophyll, carotene, γ-linolenic acid, vitamins E and C, and phycocyanins.[13,123]

The fatty liver is also commonly associated with Type II diabetes, which is related to the variation in insulin resistance and hyperinsulinemia. One study indicated that the dietary administering of 5% *S. maxima* (SM) dried powder for 4 weeks to alloxan-induced (250 mg/kg body weight, intraperitoneal) diabetes in CD-1 mice prevented the formation of fatty liver in male and female animals.[105] The glucose, cholesterol, triacylglycerol, total lipid, and TBARS levels in the serum and the liver were measured. Serum lipoprotein, HDL-cholesterol and LDL plus VLDL levels were also determined. The hypoglycemia effect was seen in *Spirulina*-treated diabetic male mice but not in female mice. No significant change in serum and liver cholesterol levels was observed among the animals that received SM. The major effect by which *Spirulina* reduces the level of fat in the liver is by reducing triacylglycerol levels in the serum and the liver. Having received SM, female mice exhibited reduced liver triacylglycerol and a significant decline ($p < .05$) in serum triacylglycerol. Male mice, however, exhibited a significant decrease ($p < .05$) in the triacylglycerol level in the liver rather than in the serum. Reduced triacylglycerol accumulation relieves the formation of fatty liver. The hypotriacylglycerolemic effect of *Spirulina* may help to reduce liver total lipid and thereby lower the risk of hepatic steatosis.

Gonadectomized female animals reportedly are more likely to develop diabetes because of the effect of female sex steroids on glucose metabolism.[124] However, female CD-1 mice were more resistant to alloxan-induced diabetes, but more responsive to the beneficial effects of *S. maxima*, such as the hypotriglycerolemic effect, reduced liver lipids, lowered liver microsomal TBARS levels, and elevated HDL.[105] The benefit of *Spirulina* is also evident in the appearance of liver lobes. Round liver lobules were observed in mice with diabetes that had not undergone *Spirulina* treatment, while normal liver lobes were observed in treated diabetic mice.

The hypocholesterolemic effect of *Spirulina* in humans has been reported.[107,125] Reduced serum cholesterol (4.5%), triacylglycerol and LDL were observed when *Spirulina* (4.2 g/day) was added for 8 weeks to the diet of thirty Japanese males with high cholesterol, mild hypertension, and hyperlipidemia. Serum cholesterol returned to its initial level if the intake of *Spirulina* was discontinued after 4 weeks. In addition, the hypocholesterolemic effect was greater in men with a higher cholesterol diet.[125] Becker et al. (1986)[107] evaluated clinical and biochemical outcomes following the application of *Spirulina* to treat obesity. They found weight loss accompanied by reduced cholesterol level.

Similar lipid lowering effects were observed on long-term studies of *Spirulina* supplementation in patients with hyperlipidemic nephrotic syndrome[109] and type 2 diabetes mellitus.[108,126] *Spirulina* improved long-term regulation of blood sugar in nephrotic and NIDDM patients. In the study, 23 patients (age 2–13 years) with hyperlipidemic nephrotic syndrome received medication plus *Spirulina* supplementation (1 g/day) for 2 months markedly reduced serum total cholesterol (TC). Other beneficial effects included increased ratio of HDL-cholesterol (HDL-C):LDL-C and decreased ratio of LDL-C:HDL-C and TC:HDL-C. Samuel (2002)[109] concluded that the lipid-lowering effects in patients with hyperlipidemic nephrotic syndrome were due to the large amount of GLA contained in *Spirulina*. GLA, an essential *omega*-6 fatty acid and a potential precursor of arachidonic acid (AA), has been proven to prevent fatty liver induced by ethanol, carbon tetrachloride, and *omega*-6 fatty acid deficiency[127,128] through up-regulated PGE_2 production.[129,130] PGE_2 and its precursor, arachidonic acid, have been reported to be associated with lipoprotein and triacylglycerol secretion by liver.[127] In addition, in the NIDDM study carried out by Parikh (2001),[108] lipid lowering effects of *Spirulina* were demonstrated in the reduced content of triacylglycerols and LDL-C, and the lowered indices of TC:HDL-C and LDL-C:HDL-C as observed in nephrotic patients. Besides, elevated level of HDL-C and apolipoprotein ratio of A1:B was also observed.

TABLE 6.1

The Hepatoprotective Effects of *Spirulina* on Fatty Liver in Laboratory Animals

Model	Inducer	*Spirulina* dose	Effects	Reference
Rats	1% cholesterol diet	16%	Hypocholesterolemic, hypoglycemic effects; reduced arteriosclerosis and fatty liver	Kato and Takemoto, 1984
Wistar rats (male)	High-fructose diet (68%)	5%, 10%, 15%, 4 weeks	Hypolipidemic effect; increased lipoprotein lipase activity	Iwata et al., 1990
Wistar rats	60% of fructose	5%, 3 weeks	Hypocholesterolemic effect; reduced liver triacylglycerol	González de Rivera et al., 1993
Rats	Carbon tetrachloride (i.p. 1 mL/kg, single dose)	5%	Reduced liver triacylglycerol	Torres-Durán et al., 1998
Rats	Carbon tetrachloride (i.p. 1 mL/kg)	5%, 5 days	Reduced liver total lipids, triacylglycerol, cholesterol; increased HDL; restored VLDL, LDL, and TBARS	Torres-Durán et al., 1999
CD-1 mice (female, male)	Alloxan induced diabetes	5%, 4 weeks	Hypoglycemic, hypotriacylglycerolemic, hypolipidemic effects; restored VLDL + LDL; improved HDL, TBARS	Rodríguez-Hernández et al., 2001
CD-1 mice (male)	Hypercholesterol diet, ethanol and simvastatin	10%, 2 weeks	Reduced liver cholesterol and triacylglycerol; hypotriacylglycerolemic effect; increased HDL	Blé-Castillo et al., 2002

Spirulina also attenuates alcohol-induced fatty liver through ALDH activity, which is inactive in subjects intoxicated by alcohol, especially in Asian populations.[131,132] In an experimental model, the Km value of ALDH decreased from 0.91 to 0.70 mM after treating with *Spirulina*. However, the activity of alcohol dehydrogenase (ADH) did not change.[133] Apparently, *Spirulina* facilitates alcohol metabolism through enhanced clearance of accumulated aldehyde, which may increase susceptibility to alcoholic liver disease (ALD), such as fatty liver and fibrosis. Summary of numerous reports, which studied the effect of *Spirulina* on fatty liver, is listed in Tables 6.1 and 6.2.

EFFECT OF *SPIRULINA* ON LIVER FIBROSIS

LIVER FIBROSIS AND ACTIVATION OF HEPATIC STELLATE CELLS

Hepatic fibrosis is a common outcome of the progressive accumulation of connective tissue in the liver in response to hepatocellular damage. It is a complex and dynamic

TABLE 6.2

The Hepatoprotective Effects of *Spirulina* on Fatty Liver in Human Studies

Model	Inducer	*Spirulina* dose	Effects	Reference
Human (30 male)	High cholesterol, mild hypertension and hyperlipidemia	4.2 g/day for 4 weeks	Hypocholesterolemic, hypoglycemic and hypotriacylglycer-olemic effects; reduced LDL	Nayaka et al., 1988
Obese subjects	Obesity	2.8 g/three times daily for 4 weeks	Hypocholesterolemic effect; weight loss	Becker et al., 1986
Human (25 patients)	Type-2 diabetes mellitus	2 g/day for 2 months	Hypoglycemic and hypolipidemic effects; reduced HbA-Ic	Parikh et al., 2001
Human (23 patients, age 2–13)	Hyperlipidemic nephritic syndrome	1 g/day for 2 months	Hypoglycemic and hypocholesterolemic effect	Samuels et al., 2002

process that follows a repeated or chronic insult of sufficient intensity to begin a "wound healing"-like reaction.[134,135] The fibrotic process arises from excessive production of the extracellular matrix (ECM). Various cells and factors participate in fibrogenesis. HSC, Kupffer cells, and the recruited mononuclear cells are the main cells that are responsible for the process. In addition, transforming growth factor $\beta 1$ (TGF$\beta 1$) is essential for the fibrotic diseases.[136–138]

Activated fibroblasts with myofibroblast characteristics are central in hepatic fibrosis.[139] Both animal models and human studies indicate three subpopulations of myofibroblasts—in the portal area or fibrous septal, at interface between the liver cells and the stroma of the portal area, and the perisinusoidal HSC.[135] The amplification of ECM production by activated HSC is the primary cause of hepatic fibrosis.[140–142] Most HSC, formerly called Ito cells, lipocytes, perisinusoidal cells, and fat-storing cells are present in the Disse's space, which is between the hepatocytes and the sinusoidal endothelial cells; they are also present in the perivascular space around portal area.[134,135,143] The major functions of quiescent HSC in normal liver include the secretion of cytokines, the production of ECM, the storage of vitamin A in lipid vacuoles, and the regulation of blood flow.[144] HSC transforms from a quiescent phenotype to the activated state following a fibrogenic stimulus. The activation results in multitudinous changes in cellular morphology, metabolism, and gene expression. The changes in the morphology of activated HSC that are observed in animal models are also seen in tissue culture models. One of the most significant changes appears to be the transformation from quiescent HSC to myofibroblast-like cells. The modified myofibroblast-like HSC are characterized by enhanced expression of smooth muscle α-actin and desmin, proliferation, contractility, and migration, as well as altered ECM synthesis (a drastic increase in type I collagen level) and loss of retinol stores.[134,135,145–148]

The early progress of the activation of stellate cells is recognized as initiation, which develops later into perpetuation. Significant changes in phenotype and induction of early genes[149] during the initiation of activation of stellate cells are responses to a series of profibrogenic stimuli, including an imbalanced redox state, altered early ECM composition and paracrine stimulation from injured hepatocytes, sinusoidal endothelial cells, and Kupffer cells. The initiation stage is also associated with an up-regulated kruppel-like transcription factor (Zf9)[150] and adhesion molecule (ICAM-1).[151] Injured sinusoidal endothelial cells activate HSC by producing variant fibronectins (EIIIA isoform).[152] Furthermore, the activation of Kupffer cells and the up-regulated redox-sensitive transcription factors, such as activator protein-1 (AP-1) and nuclear factor κB (NF-κB), intensify this stage.[153,154] In the perpetuation stage, accelerated fibrosis proceeds with amplified cellular events through enhanced paracrine and autocrine activities and continued ECM remodeling.[135,140] Events in perpetuation of transdifferentiated HSC include proliferation, fibrogenesis, contractility, matrix disruption, and inflammation. Many of these responses are associated with RTK-mediated interactions between cytokines and corresponding up-regulated receptors.[155]

Expression of platelet-derived growth factor (PDGF) receptor appears to be important in HSC proliferation,[156] in which the ERK/mitogenic-activated protein kinase (MAPK) pathway[156] and the activation of phosphatidylinositol 3-kinase (PI 3K)[156,157] are involved. Moreover, heightened activities of PDGF-regulated Na^+/H^+ and Na^+/Ca^{2+} exchangers are reported in activated HSC[158] and injured liver,[159] sustaining extracellular calcium intake and altered pH for proliferation. Recent evidence reveals that proteinase-activated receptor agonists, thrombin, and MC tryptase also regulate HSC proliferation and collagen production.[160]

Another predominant mediator in fibrogenesis is the up-regulated transforming growth factor β1 (TGFβ1), which induces ECM genes like collagen and fibronectin.[161,162] TGFβ1 knockout mice with acute liver injury that exhibit a marked reduction in collagen accumulation reveal the essential role of TGFβ1 in fibrosis.[163] Most TGFβ1 in normal liver are from Kupffer cells, while some are from endothelial cells. However, in fibrotic rat liver, elevated autocrine TGFβ1 expression in HSC is evident.[142,164] The injury-induced activity occurs not only at the transcriptional level but also through proteolysis by a urokinase-type plasminogen activator.[165] Enhanced TGFβ1 results in the strengthened response of activated HSC to injury by interaction with receptors to produce type I collagen, which is low in normal liver ECM.[165] The collagen type III content increases before that of collagen type I following liver injury.[134] The accumulated collagen subsequently switches from type III to type I, becoming fibril-forming. The fibrosis further proceeds to sclerosis and cirrhosis when 60–70% of all of the collagen is type I.[166,167] The deposition of excessive collagen in fibrotic liver impairs the exchange of nutrients and metabolites between parenchymal cells and blood flow (capillarization). The altered fibrillar ECM interacts with integrins and RTKs on the plasma membrane, further activating HSC.

As the amount of fibril-forming collagen in ECM increases, the normal matrix is decomposed by several enzymes such as matrix metalloproteinase-2 (gelatinase A), 3 (stromelysin 1) and 9 (gelatinase B) (MMP-2, 3 and 9),[168–172] and membrane-type MMPs.[134] HSC expresses MMP-2, MMP-3 and the recently reported

MMP-9, disrupting basement-membrane collagen IV and subendothelial ECM. Furthermore, as fibrosis progresses, fully activated HSC releases TIMP1 and 2, inhibiting the activity of MMP, leading to advanced collagen accumulation and scar formation.[169,173-175]

Portal vein resistance, an important event in advanced fibrosis, results from the contractility of activated myofibroblast-like HSC, through the stimulation of autocrine-derived endothelin-1 (ET-1).[176] This enzyme also stimulates the proliferation of quiescent HSC and inhibits the growth of activated HSC.[177] Increased portal resistance compresses the fibrillar ECM, reducing the blood supply to hepatocytes through the bypassing effect of the connection of afferent portal veins and efferent hepatic veins.[178] The retraction of fibrotic tissue results in hepatocyte ischemia and portal hypertension, which have been seen in typical sclerosis and cirrhosis. Accelerated fibrosis can be induced through the migration of activated HSC to the site of injury. This chemotaxis effect is mediated by PDGF and monocyte chemotactic protein-1 (MCP-1).[179,180] The recruitment of leukocytes, which is critical to the perpetuation of HSC activation, together with up-regulated adhesion molecules and HSC-released autocrine cytokines and chemokines like colony-stimulating factor and MCP-1, amplify inflammation and accelerate fibrosis.[181] The ROS generated by Kupffer cells and hepatocytes promotes inflammation.

The role of hepatic macrophages in hepatic fibrosis has recently been emphasized. The activation of macrophages have been proposed to exhibit two distinct mechanisms: (1) the classic macrophages are activated by T_H 1 lymphokines, bacteria, and fungal cell wall components and (2) the alternatively activated macrophages are activated by T_H 2 lymphokines, apoptotic cells, and corticorsteroids.[182,183] The classic macrophages release proinflammatory mediators and are involved in matrix decomposition,[184] whereas the alternative activated macrophages produce anti-inflammatory cytokines such as IL-10 and TGF-β, and promote matrix accumulation upon incubation with myofibroblasts.[185,186] These two characteristics of macrophages are evident in injured tissues.[187] CD11b-DTR transgenic mice injured by carbon tetrachloride were selectively subject to depletion of macrophages during fibrosis and recovery,[183] to clarify the duality of macrophages in liver injury and repair. The antifibrotic effect was significant during the depletion of macrophages during liver injury. On the contrary, a substantial matrix accumulated during depletion in the early recovery phase. This investigation demonstrates the opposite role of hepatic macrophages in liver inflammatory scaring. In addition, whether this difference in behavior resulted from the same or different subpopulations remains unclear. However, the evidence suggests that one subset undergoes phenotype switching during the progressing and recovery phases.[188,189] Figure 6.4 shows a summary of recent studies on liver fibrosis.

OXIDATIVE STRESS AND LIVER FIBROSIS

Liver fibrosis is usually associated with variations in the extent of oxidative stress.[134] Oxygen-derived reactive species from hepatocyte lipid peroxidation trigger cultured HSC proliferation and collagen type I synthesis.[190] Administering of antioxidants, such as vitamin E, carotenoids and flavonoids reduces fibrosis, often repairing

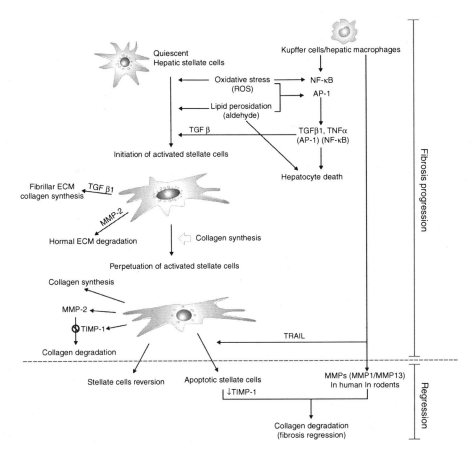

FIGURE 6.4 Summary of hepatic fibrosis and regression.

injury by scavenging free radicals. ROS mainly released from Kupffer cells and hepatocytes,[191] initiate HSC activation and further cause fibrosis through the regulation of autocrine cytokines by redox-sensitive transcription factors like AP-1 and NF-κB. AP-1 is important to the transcription of liver fibrosis-related factors such as TGFβ1, collagen type I and matrix metalloproteinases.[192,193] NF-κB, mostly regulated at the post-translational level, assist in the transcription of inflammatory mediators (TNFα, IL-2, IL-6, IL-8), and adhesion molecules (intercellular, endothelial, and vascular cell adhesion molecules; ICAM, ECAM, and VCAM).[134] Furthermore, NF-κB behaves differently from AP-1 in response to 4-hdroxy-2-nonenal (HNE),[194,195] a lipid peroxidation-derived aldehyde. Significantly increased AP-1 nuclear binding rather than NF-κB is observed after Kupffer and stellate cells are treated with HNE. This fact is indicative of the fact that ROS and HNE trigger different mechanisms for enhancing fibrosis. ROS promotes inflammation, while HNE may contribute to the initiation of HSC activation.

Oxidative stress is also caused by alcohol, in a process that is catalyzed by cytochrome P450 2E1 (CYP2E1), an isoform of P450 in hepatocytes. This enzyme generates more ROS than cytochrome P450 by reducing O_2 to $O_2^{\bullet-}$, and the subsequent converting of $O_2^{\bullet-}$ to H_2O_2 through superoxide dismutases. The enhanced expression of CYP2E1 in HSC promotes the generation of ROS and collagen I.[196] Antioxidant treatment suppresses the collagen I gene (COL1A2) expression. Furthermore, acetaldehyde, an alcohol metabolite, produced by alcohol metabolism through hepatic CYP2E1, activates collagen synthesis in activated HSC in a paracrine manner. The phagocytosis of alcohol-induced hepatocyte apoptotic bodies by Kupffer cells and HSC may lead to elevated expression of TGFβ1 and activation of HSC. The activation of HSC may also result from the stimulation of ROS and TGFβ1, which are released by Kupffer cells.[197]

The progress of fibrosis depends not only on the autocrine effects of cytokines and chemokines, but also on such reactive species as H_2O_2 and HNE, which can permeate the cell plasma menbrane.[198]

SPIRULINA AND POTENTIAL RESOLUTION OF LIVER FIBROSIS

Liver fibrosis may resolve by the reversion of the normal matrix, the attenuation of inflammation or the reversion/apoptosis of HSCs.[140] Whether HSC can revert to the quiescent state is unknown. However, the evidence indicates that HSC remains quiescent when cultured on a normal matrix.[199] Moreover, IL-10, secreted as a negative feed back signal to down-regulate inflammation, increases interstitial collagenase activity, to reduce fibrosis through modifying the collagen structure.[200,201] Recently, α-melanocyte-stimulating hormone (α-MSH) gene therapy has demonstrated that the reversion of carbon tetrachloride-induced liver fibrosis in mice by regulating collagen metabolism, including reducing the mRNA expression of liver TGFβ1, collagen α1, and adhesion molecules; attenuating the activities of α-smooth muscle actin (α-SMA) and COX-2; increasing the activity of MMP, and deactivating TIMP.[202] The induction of HSC apoptosis associated with attenuated TIMP-1 expression during the recovery phase of liver injury is another approach for reducing fibrosis.[203] Furthermore, HSC apoptosis with elevated levels of Fas ligand, NF-κB, p53 and Bcl-2 during spontaneous activation, has been documented.[204–206]

Innate immunity, including Kupffer cells/macrophages, natural killer (NK) cells, and NKT cells, together with interferon-α and γ (IFN-α, γ), has been indicated to regulate fibrosis progression and development.[197] Macrophages and NK cells have been reported to kill activated HSC and attenuate fibrosis through matrix degradation during recovery.[189,207] Besides, IFN-α and γ inhibit fibrosis by means of blocking TGFβ1 signaling and HSC activation.[208]

Spirulina has been reportedly associated with the attenuation of fibrosis by the induction of HSC apoptosis and the antioxidative activity, which is involved in the reduction of oxidative stress[25] and a decrease in proinflammatory cytokine gene expression.[209] In addition, Cpc, a pigment from blue-green algae including *Spirulina*, reduces the extent of Kupffer cell phargocytosis.[209]

Oxidative stress promotes the activation of HSC, whereas antioxidants may suppress this process.[210,211] Antioxidants such as the natural phenolic compounds resveratrol and quercetin markedly inhibit HSC proliferation.[211] *Spirulina*, which contains many antioxidants such as phycocyanins, carotenoids, selenium, and some phenolics,[212] suppresses oxidative stress and the up-regulation of proinflammatory cytokine expression. It may further attenuate the progress of liver fibrosis. The administration of a suitable antioxidant supplement has been established to prevent significantly lipid peroxidation and fibrotic autocrine cytokine expression in rat liver, induced by CCl_4.[213]

Natural phenolics modulate the activity of receptor tyrosine kinases and the expression of cell cycle protein cyclin D1, thereby modulating the functions of stellate cells.[211] In addition, sulfhydryl antioxidants regulate stellate cells by exhibiting reducing activity.[210] Natural phenolic compounds such as resveratrol and quercetin have been suggested to be potent inhibitors of the growth of stellate cells by perturbing the signal transduction pathway and the expression of the cell cycle protein.[211] Furthermore, quercetin selectively inhibits growth and causes apoptosis in hepatic tumor cells rather than in normal cells.[214] *Spirulina* extracts are likely to constitute compounds, such as phenolics or phycocyanin, that are potential anticancer or antifibrosis agents.

Pycocyanin, like Cpc, has been reported to reduce significantly carbon phagocytosis and carbon-induced O_2 uptake on perfused rat liver by exploiting its antioxidant and anti-inflammatory capacities.[209] Cpc also reduces 3,3′,5-triiodothyronine (T_3)-induced (thyroid calorigenesis) serum nitrite and TNF-α levels and hepatic nitric oxide synthase (NOS) activity. TNF-α, a profibrogenic factor that is released from activated macrophages, up-regulates in response to a net increase of ROS.[215] The hepatoprotective/antifibrosis effect of Cpc corresponds to the decline in the formation of reduced ROS and proinflammatory cytokine.

The apoptosis of key cells of fibrogenesis may also have the antifibrosis effect. Hepatic macrophages and stellate cells are central to fibrosis. Hepatic macrophages play different roles in fibrosis or antifibrosis during liver injury and the recovery stage.[183] Hepatic macrophages have been suggested to secrete tumor necrosis factor (TNF)-related apoptosis-inducing ligand (TRAIL) and other stimuli to provoke the apoptosis of activated stellate cells.[216] Activated HSC also undergoes apoptosis during spontaneous activation that is associated with Bcl, NF-κB, and p53/p21 WAF1 system.[206] Accordingly, a possible means of recovering from liver fibrosis is to trigger the apoptosis of activated HSC.[140,217]

Hepatic macrophage apoptosis at an early specific stage of fibrosis may help to attenuate the progress of fibrosis due to the reduced level of profibrotic cytokine, such as TGFβ1. Cpc has been reported to induce macrophage apoptosis in a cultured LPS-stimulated RAW 264.7 macrophage cell line.[28] Cpc not only selectively inhibits COX-2 activity, but also inhibits the growth and multiplication of RAW 264.7 macrophages in an arresting cell cycle at sub-G_0/G_1 phase. Moreover, Cpc apoptosis is independent of Bcl-2 and mediated by the release of cytochrome c.

Our earlier study demonstrated the apoptosis of rat-activated HSC and Hep G2, a human hepatocellular carcinoma cell line, by treating it with *Spirulina* aqueous extract.[14] The algae extract-treated cells underwent pronounced morphological changes such as cell shrinkage, the formation of membrane blebs, and DNA fragmentation. The dose-dependent suppression of cell proliferation by treatment of both sets of cells with *Spirulina* aqueous extract suggests that *Spirulina* may have the potential to reduce liver fibrosis and probably liver tumors. The data herein are

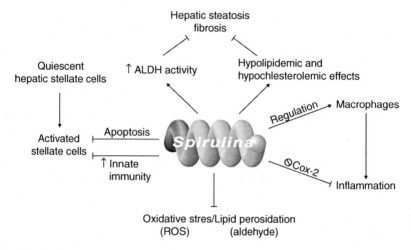

FIGURE 6.5   Effects of *Spirulina* on liver fibrosis.

consistent with the results of clinical and laboratory studies,[33] which have found that administering *Spirulina* is a valid treatment for chronic diffuse liver conditions because of its hepatoprotective properties. The results herein also show that aqueous *Spirulina* extract arrests the HSC cell cycle in the G2/M phase, suppressing proliferation and further inducing apoptosis, as verified by annexin-V analysis and the hypodiploid peak. Moreover, activation of innate immunity is an alternative approach to kill activated HSC. *Spirulina* may kill activated HSC through the enhanced innate immunity by means of activating NK cells and macrophages; increasing production of interferons.[53,57] In conclusion, these findings are evidences of the potential antifibrotic action of *Spirulina*, which may partially explain the beneficial effects of *Spirulina* on liver diseases. The effects of *Spirulina* on liver fibrosis are illustrated in Figure 6.5.

CONCLUDING REMARKS

Collective research results explore numerous effects of *Spirulina*, including antioxidative, anti-inflammatory, anticancer, antiviral, neuroprotective, hepatoprotective and immunoenhancing. Many of the effects are associated with the antioxidative effect, which appears to be involved in synergistic effects of a series of phytochemicals, such as selenium, carotenoids, phenolics, phycocyanins, and essential fatty acid GLA. The oxidative stress and subsequent induced inflammation substantially lead to liver damages such as hepatic steatosis, fibrosis, and carcinoma. Considerable results suggest that *Spirulina* is able to control hepatic steastosis through its antioxidative and anti-inflammatory effects, induction of PGE_2 production by GLA, hypolipidemic and hypochlesterolemic effects, and activated ALDH activity. In addition, ROS and related oxidative intermediates have been recognized as the potential stimuli for the accumulation of connective tissue in the liver. Various types of cells are involved in liver fibrosis. Kupffer cells and HSC are mainly responsible for the fibrosis process by exerting several paracrine and autocrine signalings. However *Spirulina* can be used to attenuate fibrotic process through antioxidative effect, anti-inflammation, induction of apoptosis of HSC and probably enhanced innate immunity. *Spirulina* enhances the activity of endonuclease and repair DNA synthesis, which makes it promising for cancer therapy. On the basis of the findings from many studies, the supplement of *Spirulina* as an adjunct could benefit the treatment of several chronic diseases.

ACKNOWLEDGMENTS

The authors would like to thank Mr. Nien-Chu Fanfor his assistance with the preparation of all art work. This work was supported in part by the Taiwan National Science Council under Contract No. NSC 94-2113-M-260-008.

REFERENCES

1. Khan, Z., Bhadouria, P., and Bisen, P.S., Nutritional and therapeutic potential of *Spirulina*, *Curr. Pharm. Biotechnol.*, 6, 373, 2005.
2. Venkataraman, L.V. et al., Simplified method of raising inoculums of blue green algae *Spirulina platensis* for rural application in India, *Phykos*, 21, 56, 1982.
3. Dillon, J.C. and Phan, P.A., *Spirulina* as source of protein in human nutrition, *Bull. Inst. Oceanogr.*, 12, 103, 1993.
4. Kapoor, R. and Mehta, U., Utilization of beta-carotene from *Spirulina platensis* by rats, *Plant Foods Hum. Nutr.*, 43, 1, 1993.
5. Annapurna, V.V., Deosthale, Y.G., and Bamji, M.S., *Spirulina* as a source of vitamin A, *Plant Foods Hum. Nutr.*, 41, 125, 1991.
6. Mitchell, G.V. et al., Effects of graded dietary levels of *Spirulina maxima* on vitamins A and E in male rats, *J. Nutr.*, 120, 1234, 1990.
7. Cases, J. et al., Assessment of selenium bioavailability from high-selenium *Spirulina* subfractions in selenium-deficient rats, *J. Agric. Food Chem.*, 50, 3867, 2002.
8. Yoshida, A., Takagaki, Y., and Nishimume, T., Enzyme immunoassay for phycocyanin as the main component of *Spirulina* color in foods, *Biosci. Biotechnol. Biochem.*, 60, 57, 1996.
9. Cohen, Z., Products from microalgae, in *Handbook of Microalgal Mass Culture*, Richmond, A., Ed., CRC Press Inc, Boca Raton, FL, 1986, 421.
10. Glazer, A.N., Phycobiliproteins—a family of valuable, widely used fluorophores, *J. Appl. Phycol.*, 6, 105, 1994.
11. Bhat, V.B. and Madyastha, K.M., Scavenging of peroxynitrite by phycocyanin and phycocyanobilin from *Spirulina platensis*: protection against oxidative damage to DNA, *Biochem. Biophys. Res. Commun.*, 285, 262, 2001.
12. Miranda, M.S. et al., Antioxidant activity of the microalga *Spirulina maxima*, *Braz. J. Med. Biol. Res.*, 31, 1075, 1998
13. Bhat, V.B. and Madyastha, K.M., C-Phycocyanin: a potent peroxyl radical scavenger in vivo and in vitro, *Biochem. Biophys. Res. Commun.*, 275, 20, 2000.
14. Wu, L.C. et al., Antioxidant and antiproliferative activities of *Spirulina* and *Chlorella* water extracts, *J. Agric. Food Chem.*, 53, 4207, 2005.
15. Benedetti, S. et al., Antioxidant properties of a novel phycocyanin extract from the blue-green alga *Aphanizomenon flos-aquae*, *Life Sci.*, 75, 2353, 2004.

16. Galli, F., Canestrari, F., and Bellomo, G., Pathophysiology of oxidative stress and its implication in uremia and dialysis, *Contrib. Nephrol.*, 127, 1, 1999.

17. Parthasarathy, S. et al., Oxidative stress in cardiovascular disease, *J. Nucl. Cardiol.*, 8, 379, 2001.

18. Cooke, M.S. et al., Oxidative DNA damage: mechanisms, mutation, and disease, *FASEB J.*, 17, 1195, 2003.

19. Beal, M.F., Aging, energy, and oxidative stress in neurodegenerative diseases, *Ann. Neurol.*, 38, 357, 1995.

20. Markesbery, W.R., Oxidative stress hypothesis in Alzheimers disease, *Free. Radic. Biol. Med.*, 23, 134, 1997.

21. LeBel, C.P. and Bondy, S.C., Oxidative damage and cerebral aging, *Prog. Neurobiol.*, 38, 601, 1992.

22. Gey, K.F., Vitamins E plus C and interacting conutrients required for optimal health. A critical and constructive review of epidemiology and supplementation data regarding cardiovascular disease and cancer, *Biofactors*, 7, 113, 1998.

23. Upasani, C.D. and Balaraman, R., Protective effect of *Spirulina* on lead induced deleterious changes in the lipid peroxidation and endogenous antioxidants in rats, *Phytother. Res.*, 17, 330, 2003.

24. Gemma, C. et al., Diets enriched in foods with high antioxidant activity reverse age-induced decreases in cerebellar beta-adrenergic function and increases in proinflammatory cytokines, *J. Neurosci.*, 22, 6114, 2002.

25. Romay, C. et al., Antioxidant and anti-inflammatory properties of C-phycocyanin from blue green algae, *Inflamm. Res.*, 47, 36, 1998.

26. Romay, C., Ledón, N., and González, R., Further studies on anti-inflammatory activity of phycocyanin in some animal models of inflammation, *Inflamm. Res.*, 47, 334, 1998.

27. Kehrer, J. P. and Smith, C.V., Free radical in biology: sources, reactivities, and roles in the etiology of human disease, in *Natural Antioxidants in Human Health and Disease*, Frei, B., Ed., Academic Press, San Diego, CA, 1994, 25.

28. Reddy, M.C. et al., C-Phycocyanin, a selective cyclooxygenase-2 inhibitor, induces apoptosis in lipopolysaccharide-stimulated RAW 264.7 macrophages, *Biochem. Biophys. Res. Commun.*, 304, 385, 2003.

29. Remirez, D. et al., Inhibitory effects of *Spirulina* in zymosan-induced arthritis in mice, *Mediators Inflam.*, 11, 75, 2002.

30. Kumar, M., Sharma, M.K., and Kumar, A., *Spirulina fusiformis*: a food supplement against mercury induced hepatic toxicity, *J. Health Sci.*, 51, 424, 2005.

31. Dasgupta, T. et al., Chemomodulation of carcinogen metabolising enzymes, antioxidant profiles and skin and forestomach papillomagenesis by *Spirulina platensis*, *Mol. Cell Biochem.*, 226, 27, 2001.

32. Mathew, B. et al., Evaluation of chemoprevention of oral cancer with *Spirulina fusiformis*, *Nutr. Cancer*, 24, 197, 1995.

33. Gorban, E.M. et al., Clinical and experimental study of *Spirulina* efficacy in chronic diffuse liver diseases, *Lik. Sprava.*, 6, 89, 2000.

34. Parij, V.B., Bagym, A.N., and Neve, J., Linear and non-linear competition plots in the deoxyribose assay for determination of rate constants for reaction of non steroidal anti-inflammatory drugs with hydroxyl radicals, *Free Rad. Res.*, 23, 571, 1995.

35. Padyana, A.K. et al., Crystal structure of a light-harvesting protein C-phycocyanin from *Spirulina platensis*, *Biochem. Biophys. Res. Commun.*, 282, 893, 2001.

36. MacColl, R., Allophycocyanin and energy transfer, *Biochim. Biophys. Acta (Bioenergetics)*, 1657, 73, 2004.

37. Williams, C.S., Mann, M., and DuBois, R.N., The role of cyclooxygenases in inflammation, cancer, and development, *Oncogene*, 18, 7908, 1999.

38. Dannenberg, A.J. et al., Cyclooxygenase 2: a pharmacological target for the prevention of cancer, *Lancet Oncol.*, 2, 544, 2001.

39. Bandoopadhyay, G.K. et al., Linoleate metabolites enhance the *in vitro* proliferative response of mouse mammary epithelial cells to epidermal growth factor, *J. Biol. Chem.*, 262, 2750, 1987.

40. Marnett, L.J., Aspirin and the potential role of prostaglandins in colon cancer, *Cancer Res.*, 52, 5575, 1992.

41. Sheng, H. et al., Modulation of apoptosis and Bcl-2 expression by prostaglandin E2 in human colon cancer cells, *Cancer Res.*, 58, 362, 1998.

42. Lu, X. et al., Nonsteroidal antiinflammatory drugs cause apoptosis and induce cyclooxygenases in chicken embryo fibroblasts, *Proc. Natl. Acad. Sci. USA*, 92, 7961, 1995.

43. Pardhasaradhi, B.V.V. et al., Phycocyanin-mediated apoptosis in AK-5 tumor cells involves down-regulation of Bcl-2 and generation of ROS, *Mol. Cancer Ther.*, 2, 1165, 2003.

44. Vadiraja, B.B., Gaikward, N.W., and Madyastha, K.M., Hepatoprotective effect of C-phycocyanin: protection for carbon tetrachloride and R-(+)-pulegone-mediated hepatotoxicity in rats, *Biochem. Biophys. Res. Commun.*, 249, 428, 1998.

45. Kushak, R.I., Drapeau, C., and Van Cott, E.M., Favorable effects of blue-green algae *Aphanizomenon flos-aquae* on rat plasma lipids, *JANA*, 2, 59, 2000.

46. Lee, A.V. and Werth, V.P., Activation of autoimmunity following use of immunostimulatory herbal supplements, *Arch. Dermatol.*, 140, 723, 2004.

47. Pugh, N. et al., Isolation of three high molecular weight polysaccharide preparations with potent immunostimulatory activity from *Spirulina platensis*, *aphanizomenon flos-aquae* and *Chlorella pyrenoidosa*, *Planta Med.*, 67, 737, 2001.

48. Hernandez-Corona, A. et al., Antiviral activity of *Spirulina maxima* against herpes simplex virus type 2, *Antiviral Res.*, 56, 279, 2002.

49. Mao, T.K., Van de Water, J., and Gershwin, M.E., Effects of a *Spirulina*-based dietary supplement on cytokine production from allergic rhinitis patients, *J. Med. Food*, 8, 27, 2005.

50. Balachandran, P. et al., Toll-like receptor 2-dependent activation of monocytes by *Spirulina* polysaccharide and its immune enhancing action in mice, *Int. Immunopharmacol.*, 6, 1808, 2006.

51. Grzanna, R. et al., Immolina, a high-molecular-weight polysaccharide fraction of *Spirulina*, enhances chemokine expression in human monocytic THP-1 cells, *J. Altern. Complement. Med.*, 12, 429, 2006.

52. Jensen, G.S. et al., Consumption of *Aphanizomenon flos-aquae* has rapid effects on the circulation and function of immune cells in humans, *JANA*, 2, 50, 2002.

53. Qureshi, M. and Ali, R., *Spirulina platensis* exposure enhances macrophage phagocytic function in cats, *Immunopharmacol. Immunotoxicol.*, 18, 457, 1996.

54. Qureshi, M.A., Garlich, J.D., and Kidd, M.T., Dietary *Spirulina platensis* enhances humoral and cell-mediated immune function in chickens, *Immunopharmacol. Immunotoxicol.*, 18, 465, 1996.

55. Hayashi, O., Katoh, T., and Okuwaki, Y., Enhancement of antibody production in mice by dietary *Spirulina platensis*, *J. Nutr. Sci. Vitaminol.*, 40, 431, 1994.

56. Al-Batshan, H.A. et al., Enhancement of chicken macrophage phagocytic function and nitrite production by dietary *Spirulina platensis*, *Immunopharmacol. Immunotoxicol.*, 23, 281, 2001.

57. Hirahashi, T. et al., Activation of the human innate immune system by *Spirulina*: augmentation of interferon production and NK cytotoxicity by oral administration of hot water extract of *Spirulina platensis*, *Int. Immunopharmacol.*, 2, 423, 2002.

58. Kim, H.M. et al., Inhibitory effect of mast cell-mediated immediate-type allergic reactions in rats by *Spirulina*. *Biochem. Pharmacol.*, 55, 1071, 1998.

59. Ayehunie, S. et al., Inhibition of HIV-1 replication by an aqueous extract of *Spirulina platensis* (*Arthrospira platensis*), *J. Acquir. Immune. Defic. Syndr. Hum. Retrovirol.*, 18, 7, 1998.

60. Hayashi, T. et al., Calcium spirulan, an inhibitor of enveloped virus replication, from a blue-green alga *Spirulina platensis*, *J. Nat. Prod.*, 59, 83, 1996.

61. Witvrouw, M. and De Clercq, E., Sulfated polysaccharides extracted from sea algae as potential antiviral drugs, *Gen. Pharmacol.*, 29, 497, 1997.

62. Hayashi, K., Hayashi, T., and Kojima, I., A natural sulfated polysaccharide, calcium spirulan, isolated from *Spirulina platensis*: *in vitro* and *ex vivo* evaluation of anti-herpes simplex virus and anti-human immunodeficiency virus activities, *AIDS Res. Hum. Retroviruses*, 12, 1463, 1996.

63. Hayashi, K. et al., An extract from *Spirulina platensis* is a selective inhibitor of *Herpes simplex* virus type 1 penetration into HeLa cells, *Phytother. Res.*, 7, 76, 1993.

64. Peto, R. et al., Can dietary beta-carotene materially reduce human cancer rates? *Nature*, 290, 201, 1981.

65. Mishima, T. et al., Inhibition of tumor invasion and metastasis by calcium spirulan (Ca-SP), a novel sulfated polysaccharide derived from a blue-green alga, *Spirulina platensis*, *Clin. Exp. Metastasis*, 16, 541, 1998.

66. Schwartz, J. and Shklar, G., Regression of experimental hamster cancer by beta carotene and algae extracts, *J. Oral. Maxillofac. Surg.*, 45, 510, 1987.

67. Subhashini, J. et al., Molecular mechanisms in C-phycocyanin induced apoptosis in human chronic myeloid leukemia cell line-K562, *Biochem. Pharmaco.*, 68, 453, 2004.

68. Zhang, H.Q. et al., Chemo- and radio-protective effects of polysaccharide of *Spirulina platensis* on hemopoietic system of mice and dogs, *Acta. Pharmacol. Sin.*, 22, 1121, 2001.

69. Kurose, I. et al., Oxidative stress-mediated apoptosis of hepatocytes exposed to acute ethanol intoxication, *Hepatology*, 25, 368, 1997.

70. Lieber, C., Cytochrome P450 2E1: its physiological and pathophysiological role, *Physiol. Rev.*, 77, 517, 1997.

71. Kobayashi, H. et al., Quality control of reactive oxygen species measurement by alcohol-dependent chemiluminescence assay, *J. Androl.*, 22, 568, 2001.

72. Huang, D., Ou, F., and Prior, R.L., The chemistry behind antioxidant capacity assays, *J. Agric. Food Chem.*, 53, 1841, 2005.

73. Stocker, R. and Ames, B., Potential role of conjugated bilirubin and copper in the metabolism of lipid peroxides in bile, *Proc. Natl. Acad. Sci. USA*, 84, 8130, 1987.

74. Trull, F.R., Ibars, O., and Lightner, D.A., Conformation inversion of bilirubin formed by reduction of the biliverdin-human serum albumin complex: evidence from circular dichroism, *Biochem. Biophys.*, 298, 710, 1992.

75. Saxena, P.S. and Kumar, M., Modulatory potential of *Spirulina fusiformis* on testicular phosphatases in Swiss albino mice against mercury intoxication, *Indian J. Exp. Biol.*, 42, 998, 2004.

76. Sharma, M.K., Kumar, M., and Kumar, A., Modulatory influence of *Ocimum sanctum* and *Spirulina fusiformis* against mercury induced toxicity in liver, *Bull. Environ. Sci.*, 19, 85, 2001.

77. Costa, A.C.A.d. and Franca, F.P.d., Cadmium uptake by *Spirulina maxima*: toxicity and mechanism, *J. Microbiol. Biotech.*, 14, 579, 1998.
78. Shastri, D., Kumar, M., and Kumar, D.A., Modulation of lead toxicity by *Spirulina fusuformis*, *Phytother. Res.*, 13, 258, 1999.
79. Kumar, M., Kumar, M., and Kumar, A., *Spirulina fusiformis*: a food supplement against mercury induced hepatic toxicity, *J. Health Sci.*, 51, 424–430, 2005.
80. Rana, S.V.S., Singh, R., and Verma, S., Protective effects of few antioxidants on liver function in rats treated with cadmium and mercury, *Indian J. Exp. Biol.*, 34, 177, 1996.
81. Pang, Q.S., Guo, B.J., and Ruan, J.H., Enhancement of endonuclease activity and repair DNA synthesis by polysaccharide of *Spirulina platensis*, *Acta. Genet. Sinica (Chinese Journal of Genetics)*, 15, 374, 1988.
82. http://www.febico.com.tw/faq_e_0402.htm (accessed December, 2006)
83. Yu, A.S. and Keeffe, E.B., Nonalcoholic fatty liver disease, *Rev. Gastroenterol. Disord.*, 2, 11, 2002.
84. Altlparmak, E. et al., Viral and host causes of fatty liver in chronic hepatitis B. *World J. Gastroenterol.*, 11, 3056, 2005.
85. Guha Mazumder, D.N., Arsenic and liver disease, *J. Indian Med. Assoc.*, 99, 311, 2001.
86. Riely, C.A. et al., Acute fatty liver of pregnancy, *Semin. Liver Dis.*, 7, 47, 1987.
87. Adams, L.A. and Talwalkar, J.A., Diagnostic evaluation of nonalcoholic fatty liver disease, *J. Clin. Gastroenterol.*, 40, S34, 2006.
88. Doherty, J.F., Golden, M.H., and Brooks, S.E., Peroxisomes and the fatty liver of malnutrition: an hypothesis, *Am. J. Clin. Nutr.*, 54, 674, 1991.
89. Uchida, T. et al., Alcoholic foamy degeneration—a pattern of acute alcoholic injury of the liver, *Gastroenterology*, 84, 683, 1983.
90. Davea, R.A. et al., Severe combined hyperlipidemia and retinal lipid infiltration in a patient with Type 2 diabetes mellitus, *Lipids Health Dis.*, 5, 29, 2006.
91. Fan, J.G. et al., Experiment study of steatohepatitis with obesity and hyperlipidemia, *Chinese Science*, 6, 515, 2000.
92. Mehta, K. et al., Nonalcoholic fatty liver disease: pathogenesis and the role of antioxidants, *Nutr. Rev.*, 60, 289, 2002.
93. Matloff, D.S., Selinger, M.J., and Kaplan, M.M., Hepatic transaminase activity in alcoholic liver disease, *Gastroenterology*, 78, 1389, 1980.
94. Fan, J.G. et al., Influence of ursodeoxycholic acid on the therapeutic effects of low-calorie diet in obesity and hyperlipidemia rats with steatohepatitis, *Zhonghua. Gan. Zang. Bing. Za. Zhi.*, 10, 43, 2002.
95. Lin, H.Z. et al., Metformin reverses fatty liver disease in obese, leptin-deficient mice, *Nat. Med.*, 6, 998, 2000.
96. Turmellel, Y.P. et al., Rosiglitazone inhibits mouse liver regeneration, *FASEB J.*, 20, 2609, 2006.
97. Cheng, R.Y. et al., Study on preventive effect of betaine on experimental hyperlipidemia and fatty liver in mice, *China Pharmacist.*, 7, 411, 2004.
98. Ersoz, G. et al., Management of fatty liver disease with vitamin E and C compared to ursodeoxycholic acid treatment, *Turk. J. Gastroenterol.*, 16, 124, 2005.
99. Devi, M.A. and Venkataraman, L.V., Hypocholesterolemic effect of blue-green algae *spirulina platensis* in albino rats, *Nutr. Rep. Int.*, 28, 519, 1983.
100. Kato, T. and Takemoto, K., Effects of *Spirulina* on hypercholesterolemia and fatty liver in rats. *Saitama Med. College, Japan. Japan Nutr. Foods Assoc. Jour.*, 37, 321, 1984.

101. González de Rivera, C. et al., Preventive effect of *Spirulina maxima* on the fatty liver induced by a fructose-rich diet in the rat, a preliminary report, *Life Sci.*, 53, 57, 1993.

102. Torres-Durán, R.V. et al., *Spirulina maxima* prevents induction of fatty liver by carbon tetrachloride in the rat, *Biochem. Mol. Biol. Int.*, 44, 787, 1998.

103. Torres-Durán, R.V. et al., *Spirulina maxima* prevents induction of fatty liver by carbon tetrachloride in the rat, *Biochem. Mol. Biol. Int.*, 44, 787, 1998.

104. Iwasa, M. et al., *Spirulina*-associated hepatotoxicity, *Am. J. Gastroenterol.*, 97, 3212, 2002.

105. Rodríguez-Hernández, A. et al., *Spirulina maxima* prevents fatty liver formation in CD-1 male and female mice with experimental diabetes, *Life Sci.*, 69, 1029, 2001.

106. Nayaka, et al., Cholesterol lowering effect of *Spirulina*, *Nutr. Rep. Int.*, 37, 1329, 1988.

107. Becker, E.W. et al., Clinical and biochemical evaluations of *Spirulina* with regard to its application in the treatment of obesity, *Inst. Chem. Pfanz. Nutrition Reports Intl.*, 33, 565, 1986.

108. Parikh, P., Mani, U.V., Iyer, U.M., Role of *Spirulina* in the control of glycemia and lipidemia in type 2 diabetes mellitus, *J. Med. Food*, 2001, 4(4), 193–199.

109. Samuels, R. et al., Hypocholesterolemic effect of *Spirulina* in patients with hyperlipidemic nephritic syndrome, *J. Med. Food*, 5, 91, 2002.

110. Pereira, J.N. and Jangaard, N.O., Different rates of glucose and fructose metabolism in rat liver tissue *in vitro*, *Metabolism*, 20, 392, 1971.

111. Cryer, A. et al., Effects of fructose, sucrose and glucose feeding on plasma insulin concentrations and on adipose-tissue clearing-factor lipase activity in the rat, *Biochem. J.*, 140, 561, 1974.

112. Michaelis, O.E.I.V., Nace, C.S., and Szepesi, B., Determination of a specific metabolic effect of dietary disaccharides in the rat, *J. Nutr.*, 105, 1186, 1975.

113. Waterman, R.A. et al., Effects of dietary carbohydrate source on growth, plasma metabolites and lipogenesis in rats, pigs and chicks, *Proc. Soc. Exp. Biol. Med.*, 150, 220, 1975.

114. Volpe, J.J. and Vagelos, P.R., Regulation of mammalian fatty-acid synthetase. The roles of carbohydrate and insulin, *Proc. Natl. Acad. Sci. USA*, 71, 889, 1974.

115. Iwata, K., Inayama, T., and Kato, T., Effects of *Spirulina platensis* on fructose-induced hyperlipidemia in rats, *J. Japan Soc. Nutr. Food Sci.*, 40, 463, 1987.

116. Iwata, K., Inayama, T., Kato, T., Effects of *Spirulina* on plasma lipoprotein lipase activity in rats, *J. Nutr. Sci. Vitaminol.*, 36, 165, 1990.

117. Maling, H.M., Frank, A., and Horning, M.G., Effect of carbon tetrachloride on hepatic synthesis and release of triglycerides, *Biochim. Biophys. Acta.*, 64, 540, 1962.

118. Pencil, S.D. et al., Carbon tetrachloride-dependent inhibition of lipid secretion by isolated hepatocytes. Characterization and requirement for bioactivation, *Biochem. Pharmacol.*, 33, 2419, 1984.

119. Glende, E.A. Jr., and Recknagel, R.O., An indirect method demonstrating that CCl_4-dependent hepatocyte injury is linked to a rise in intracellular calcium ion concentration, *Res. Comm. Chem. Pathol. Pharmacol.*, 73, 41, 1991.

120. Blé-Castillo, J.L. et al., *Arthrospira maxima* prevents the acute fatty liver induced by the administration of simvastatin, ethanol and a hypercholesterolemic diet to mice, *Life Sci.*, 70, 2665, 2002.

121. Takai, Y., Hosoyamada, Y., and Kato, T., Effect of water soluble and water insoluble fractions of *Spirulina* over serum lipids and glucose resistance of rats, *J. Japan Soc. Nutr. Food Sci.*, 44, 273, 1991.

122. Mitchell, G.V., Jenkins, M.Y., and Grundel, E., Tissue alpha-tocopherol, thiobarbituric acid-reactive substances (TBARS), and glutathione levels in rats fed algal proteins, *Ann. N.Y. Acad. Sci.*, 570, 478, 1988.

123. Kay, R.A., Microalgae as food and supplement, *Crit. Rev. Food Sci. Nutr.*, 30, 555, 1991.

124. Godsland, I.F., The influence of female sex steroids on glucose metabolism and insulin action, *J. Intern. Med.*, 240(Suppl 738), 1, 1996.

125. Nayaka, N., Homma, Y., and Goto, Y., Cholesterol lowering effect of *Spirulina. Nutrition Reports Intl.*, 37, 1329, 1988.

126. Mani, U.V., Desai, S., and Iyer, U., Studies on the long-term effect of *spirulina* supplementation on serum lipid profile and glycated proteins in NIDDM patients, *J. Nutraceut.*, 2, 25, 2000.

127. Cunnane, S.C., Hepatic triacylglycerol accumulation induced by ethanol and carbon tetrachloride: interactions with essential fatty acids and prostaglandins, *Alcohol Clin. Exp. Res.*, 11, 25, 1987.

128. Murai, A., Furuse, M., and Okumura, J., Involvement of (n-6) essential fatty acids and prostaglandins in liver lipid accumulation in Japanese quail, *Am. J. Vet. Res.*, 57, 342, 1996.

129. Lukivskaya, O.Y., Maskevich, A.A., and Buko, V.U., Effect of ursodeoxycholic acid on prostaglandin metabolism and microsomal membranes in alcoholic fatty liver, *Alcohol*, 25, 99, 2001.

130. Nakanishi, T. et al., γ-Linolenic acid prevents conjugated linoleic acid-induced fatty liver in mice, *Nutrition*, 20, 390, 2004.

131. Chao, Y.C. et al., Alcoholism and alcoholic organ damage and genetic polymorphisms of alcohol metabolizing enzymes in Chinese patients, *Hepatology*, 25, 112, 1997.

132. Tanaka, F. et al., High incidence of ADH2*1/ALDH2*1 gene among Japanese alcohol dependents and patients with alcoholic liver disease, *Hepatology*, 23, 234, 1996.

133. Kato, T., Saiki, I., and Nishino, H., Cancer prevention and inhibition of tumor metastasis by *Spirulina* components, *Dic. Tech Rev.*, 1, 57, 1995.

134. Poli, G., Pathogenesis of liver fibrosis: role of oxidative stress, *Mol. Aspect Med.*, 21, 49, 2000.

135. Ijzer, J. et al., Morphological characterization of portal myofibroblasts and hepatic stellate cells in the normal dog liver, *Comp. Hepatol.*, 5, 7, 2006.

136. Border, W.A. and Noble, N.A., Transforming growth factor-β in tissue fibrosis, *New Engl. J. Med.*, 331, 1286, 1994.

137. Bedossa, P. and Paradis, V., Transforming growth factor-β (TGF-β): a key role in liver fibrogenesis, *J. Hepatol.*, 22(Suppl. 2), 37, 1995.

138. Poli, G. and Parola, M., Oxidative damage and fibrogenesis, *Free Radic. Biol. Med.*, 22, 287, 1997.

139. Crawford, J.M., Liver cirrhosis, in *Pathology of the Liver*, MacSween, R.N.M. et al., Eds., Churchill Livingstone, Edinburg, 2002, 575.

140. Friedman, S.L., Molecular regulation of hepatic fibrosis, an integrated cellular response to tissue injury, *J. Biol. Chem.*, 275, 2247, 2000.

141. Gressner, A.M., Liver fibrosis: perspectives in pathobiochemical research and clinical outlook, *Eur. J. Clin. Chem. Clin. Biochem.*, 32, 225, 1991.

142. Gressner, A.M., Cytokines and cellular crosstalk involved in the activation of fat-storing cells, *J. Hepatol.*, 22(Suppl. 2), 28, 1995.

143. Suematsu, M. et al., Intravital and electronomicroscopic observation of Ito cells in rat hepatic microcirculation, *Microvascular Res.*, 46, 28, 1993.

144. Friedman, S.L., Hepatic stellate cells, *Prog. Liver Dis.*, 14, 101, 1996.
145. Burt, A.D., Review pathobiology of hepatic stellate cells, *J. Gastroenterol.*, 34, 299, 1999.
146. Safadi, R. and Friedman, S.L., Hepatic fibrosis–role of stellate cell activation, *Med. Gen. Med.*, 4, 27, 2002.
147. Reeves, H.L. and Friedman, S.L., Activation of hepatic stellate cells—a key issue in liver fibrosis, *Front Biosci.*, 7, 808, 2002.
148. Sato, M., Suzuki, S., and Senoo, H., Review hepatic stellate cells: unique characteristics in cell biology and phenotype, *Cell. Struct. Funct.*, 28, 105, 2003.
149. Lalazar, A. et al., Early genes induced in hepatic stellate cells during wound healing, *Gene*, 195, 235, 1997.
150. Ratziu, V. et al., Zf9, a Kruppel-like transcription factor up-regulated *in vivo* during early hepatic fibrosis, *Proc. Natl. Acad. Sci. USA*, 95, 9500, 1998.
151. Hellerbrand, C. et al., Expression of intracellular adhesion molecule 1 by activated hepatic stellate cells, *Hepatology*, 24, 670, 1996.
152. Jarnagin, W.R. et al., Expression of variant fibronectins in wound healing: cellular sources nd biological activity of the EIIIA segment in rat hepatic fibrogenesis, *J. Cell Biol.*, 127, 2037, 1994.
153. Lindros, K.O., Zonation of cytochrome P450 expression, drug metabolism and toxicity in liver, *Gen. Pharmacol.*, 28, 191, 1997.
154. Arrigo, A.P., Gene expression and the thio redox state, *Free Radic. Biol. Med.*, 27, 936, 1999.
155. Ankoma-Sey, V. et al., Coordinated induction of VEGF receptors in mesenchymal cell types during rat hepatic wound healing, *Oncogene* 17, 115, 1998.
156. Pinzani, M., Milani, F., and Carloni, V., Signal transduction in hepatic stellate cells, *Liver*, 18, 2, 1998.
157. Marra, F. et al., Phosphatidyl-inositol 3-kinase is required for platelet-derived growth factors actions on hepatic stellate cells, *Gastroenterology*, 112, 1297, 1997.
158. Di Sario, A. et al., Intracellular pathways mediating Na^+/H^+ exchange activation by platelet-derived growth factor in rat hepatic stellate cells, *Gastroenterology*, 116, 1155, 1999.
159. Nakamura, T. et al., Expression of the Na^+/Ca^{2+} exchanger emerges in hepatic stellate cells after activation in association with liver fibrosis, *Proc. Natl. Acad. Sci. USA*, 95, 5389, 1998.
160. Gaca, M.D., Zhou, X., and Benyon, R.C., Regulation of hepatic stellate cell proliferation and collagen synthesis by proteinase-activated receptors, *J. Hepatol.*, 36, 362, 2002.
161. Warana, J.L., Transforming growth factor-β signaling and cirrhosis, *Hepatology* 29, 1909, 1999.
162. Roberts, A.B. and Sporn, M.B., Physiological actions and clinical applications of transforming growth factor β, *Growth Factor*, 8, 1, 1993.
163. Hellerbrand, C., Stefanovic, B., and Giordano, F., The role of TGF betal in initiating hepatic stellate cell activation *in vivo*, *J. Hepatol.*, 30, 77, 1999.
164. Pieter, J. et al., Glutathione levels discriminate between oxidative stress and transforming growth factor-beta signaling in activated rat hepatic stellate cells, *J. Biol. Chem.*, 274, 33881, 1999.
165. Friedman, S.L., Cytokines and fibrogenesis, *Semin. Liver Dis.*, 19, 129, 1999.
166. Milani, S. et al., Cellular localization of types I, III, and IV procollagen gene transcripts in normal and fibrotic human liver, *Am. J. Pathol.*, 137, 5, 1990.

167. Ramadori, G., Knittel, T., and Saile, B. Fibrosis and altered matrix synthesis, *Digestion*, 59, 372, 1998.
168. Arthur, M.J. et al., Secretion of 72-kDa type IV collagenase/gelatinase by cultured human lypocytes: analysis of gene expression protein synthesis and proteinase activity, *Biochem. J.*, 287, 701, 1992.
169. Arthur, M.J., Collagenases and liver fibrosis, *J. Hepatol.* 22(Suppl. 2), 43, 1995.
170. Iredale, J.P. et al., Tissue inhibitor of metalloproteinase-1 messenger RNA expression is enhanced relative to interstitial collagenase messenger RNA in experimental liver injury and fibrosis, *Hepatology*, 24, 176, 1996.
171. Han, Y.P. et al., Essential role of matrix metalloproteinases in interleukin-1-induced myofibroblastic activation of hepatic stellate cell in collagen, *J. Biol. Chem.*, 279, 4820, 2004.
172. Vyas, S.K. et al., Transin (stromelysin) is expressed in early rat lipocyte primary culture, *Gastroenterology*, 109, 889, 1995.
173. Maruyama, K. et al., Mammalian collagenase increases in early alcoholic liver disease and decreases with cirrhosis, *Life Sci.*, 30, 1379, 1982.
174. Okazaki, I. and Maruyama, K., Collagenase activity in experimental hepatic fibrosis, *Nature*, 252, 49, 1974.
175. Iredale, J.P. et al., Tissue inhibitor of metalloproteinase-1 and interstitial collagenase expression in auto immune chronic active hepatitis and activated human hepatic lipocytes, *Clin. Sci.*, 89, 75, 1995.
176. Rockey, D.C. et al., Cellular localization of endothelin-1 and increased production in liver injury in the rat: potential for autocrine and paracrine effects on stellate cells, *Hepatology*, 27, 472, 1998.
177. Pinani, M. et al., Endothelin 1 is overexpressed in human cirrhotic liver and exerts multiple effects on activated hepatic stellate cells, *Gastroenterology*, 110, 534, 1996.
178. Le Couteur, D.G. et al., Hepatic artery flow and propranolol metabolism in perfused cirrhotic rat liver, *J. Pharmacol. Exp. Ther.*, 289, 1553, 1999.
179. Marra, F. et al., Expression of monocyte chemotactic protein 1 precedes monocyte recruitment in a rat model of acute liver injury: modulation by vitamin E pretreatment, *J. Invest. Med.*, 47, 66, 1999.
180. Ikeda, K. et al., *In vitro* migratory potential of rat quiescent hepatic stellate cells and its augmentation by cell activation, *Hepatology*, 29, 1760, 1999.
181. Knittel, T. et al., Expression and regulation of cell adhesion molecules by hepatic stellate cells (HSC) of rat liver, *Am. J. Pathol.*, 154, 153, 1999.
182. Goerdt, S. and Orfanos, C.E., Other functions, other genes: alternative activation of antigen-presenting cells, *Immunity*, 10, 137, 1999.
183. Duffield, J.S. et al., Selective depletion of macrophages reveals distinct, opposing roles during liver injury and repair, *J. Clin. Invest.*, 115, 56, 2005.
184. Pierce, R.A. et al., Monocytic cell type-specific transcriptional induction of collagenase, *J. Clin. Invest.*, 97, 1890, 1996.
185. Mantovani, A. et al., Macrophage polarization: tumor-associated macrophages as a paradigm for polarized M2 mononuclear phagocytes, *Trends Immunol.*, 23, 549, 2002.
186. Raes, G. et al., FIZZ1 and Ym as tools to discriminate between differentially activated macrophages, *Dev. Immunol.*, 9, 151, 2002.
187. Duffield, J.S. et al., Suppression by apoptotic cells defines tumor necrosis factor-mediated induction of glomerular mesangial cell apoptosis by activated macrophages, *Am. J. Pathol.*, 159, 1397, 2001.

188. Duffield, J.S., The inflammatory macrophage: a story of Jekyll and Hyde, *Clin. Sci.*, 104, 27, 2003.

189. Friedman, S.L., Mac the knife? Macrophages-the double-edged sword of hepatic fibrosis, *J. Clin. Invest.*, 115, 29, 2005.

190. Svegliati Baroni, G. et al., Fibrogenic effect of oxidative stress on rat hepatic stellate cells, *Hepatology*, 27, 720, 1998.

191. Maher, J.J., Leukocytes as modulators of stellate cell activation, *Alcohol Clin. Exp. Res.*, 23, 917, 1999.

192. Lo, Y.Y. and CruZ, T.F., Involvement of reactive oxygen species in cytokine and growth factor induction of c-fos expression in chondrocytes, *J. Biol. Chem.*, 270, 11727, 1995.

193. Feinberg, M.W. et al., TGF-beta 1 inhibits cytokine-mediated induction of MMP-12 in macrophages, *J. Biol. Chem.*, 275, 25766, 2000.

194. Camandola, S. et al., Biogenic 4-hydroxy-2-nonenal activates transcription factor AP-1. but not NF-kappa B in cells of the macrophage lineage, *Biofactors*, 6, 173, 1997.

195. Parola, M. et al., HNE interacts directly with JNK isoforms in human hepatic stellate cells, *J. Clin. Invest.*, 102, 1942, 1998.

196. Nieto, N., et al., CYP2E1-mediated oxidative stress induces collagen type I expression in rat hepatic stellate cells, *Hepatology*, 30, 987, 1999.

197. Purohit, V. and Brenner, D.A., Mechanisms of alcohol-induced hepatic fibrosis: a summary of the Ron Thurman symposium, *Hepatology*, 43, 87, 2006.

198. Poli, G. et al., Separation and characterization of the aldehydic products of lipid peroxidation stimulated by carbon tetrachloride or ADP-iron in isolated rat hepatocytes and rat liver microsomal suspensions, *Biochem. J.*, 227, 629, 1985.

199. Olaso, E. et al., Proangiogenic role of tumor-activated hepatic stellate cells in experiment melanoma metastasis, *Hepatology*, 37, 674, 2003.

200. Wang, et al., Electroporative alpha-MSH gene transfer attenuates thioacetamide-induced hepatic fibrosis by MMP and TIMP modulation, *Gene Ther.*, 13, 1000, 1998.

201. Hung, K.S. et al., Interleukin-10 gene therapy reverses thioacetamide-induced liver fibrosis in mice, *Biochem. Biophys. Res. Commun.*, 336, 324, 2005.

202. Lee, T.H. et al., Alpha-melanocyte-stimulating hormone gene therapy reverses carbon tetrachloride induced liver fibrosis in mice, *J. Gene Med.*, 8, 764, 2006.

203. Iredale, J.P. et al., Mechanisms of spontaneous resolution of rat liver fibrosis. Hepatic stellate cell apoptosis and reduced hepatic expression of metalloproteinase inhibitors, *J. Clin. Invest.*, 102, 538, 1998.

204. Gong, W.R. et al., Transformation-dependent susceptibility of rat hepatic stellate cells to apoptosis induced by soluble fas ligand, *Hepatology*, 28, 492, 1998.

205. Gressner, A.M., The cell biology of live fibrogenesis-an imbalance of proliferation, growth arrest and apoptosis of myfibroblasts, *Cell Tissue Res.*, 292, 447, 1998.

206. Saile, B. et al., The bcl, NF-κB and p53/p21 WAF1 system are involved in spontaneous apoptosis and in the anti-apoptosis effects on TGF-β or TNF-α on activated hepatic stellate cells, *Eur. J. Cell Biol.*, 80, 554, 2001.

207. Radaeva, S. et al., Natural killer cells ameliorate liver fibrosis by killing activated stellate cells in NKG2D-dependent and tumor necrosis factor-related apoptosis-inducing ligand-dependent manners, *Gastroenterology*, 130, 435, 2006.

208. Ingaki, Y. et al., Interferon-alfa down-regulates collagen gene transcription and suppresses experimental hepatic fibrosis in mice, *Hepatology*, 38, 890, 2003.

209. Remirez, D. et al., Influence of C-phycocyanin on hepatocellular parameters related to liver oxidative stress and Kupffer cell functioning, *Inflamm Res.*, 51, 351, 2002.

210. Kim, K.Y. et al., *N*-acetylcysteine induces cell cycle arrest in hepatic stellate cells through its reducing activity, *J. Biol. Chem.*, 276, 40591, 2001.

211. Kawada, N. et al., Effect of antioxidants, resveratrol, quercetin, and *N*-acetylcysteine, on the functions of cultured rat hepatic stellate cells and Kupffer cells, *Hepatology*, 27, 1265, 1998.

212. Miranda, M.S. et al., Antioxidant activity of the microalga *Spirulina maxima*, *Braz. J. Med. Biol. Res.*, 31, 1075, 1998.

213. Parola, M. et al., Vitamin E dietary supplementation inhibits transforming growth factor $\beta 1$ gene expression in the rat liver, *FEBS Lett.*, 308, 267, 1992.

214. Son, Y.O. et al., Selective effects of quercetin on the cell growth and antioxidant defense system in normal versus transformed mouse hepatic cell lines, *Eur. J. Pharmacol.*, 502, 195, 2004.

215. Marok, R. et al., Activation of the transcription factor nuclear factor-kappaB in human inflamed synovial tissue, *Arthritis Rheum.*, 39, 583, 1996.

216. Fischer, R. et al., Caspase 9-dependent killing of hepatic stellate cells by activated Kupffer cells, *Gastroenterology*, 13, 845, 2002.

217. Murphy, F.R. et al., Inhibition of apoptosis of activated hepatic stellate cells by tissue inhibitor of metalloproteinase-1 is mediated via effects on matrix metalloproteinase inhibition: implications for reversibility of liver fibrosis, *J. Biol. Chem.*, 227, 11069, 2002.

7 Drug-Induced Nephrotoxicity Protection by *Spirulina*

Vijay Kumar Kutala, Iyyapu Krishna Mohan, Mahmood Khan, Narasimham L. Parinandi, and Periannan Kuppusamy

CONTENTS

INTRODUCTION

DRUG TOXICITY

Drugs and their reactive metabolites cause toxicity at the organ level in animals including humans. Depending on the nature of a specific drug and its metabolite, the toxicity manifests in one or many target organs. Organ-specific drug toxicities such as hepatotoxicity, renal toxicity, cardiotoxicity, pulmonary toxicity, and gastrointestinal toxicity, to name a few, have been well recognized. Adverse effects of drugs at the cellular level in an organ lead to cytotoxicity involving cell necrosis and apoptosis. Systemic toxicities of drugs, in association with the organ toxicities including the immunotoxicity and hematotoxicity, result in immunosuppression and hypersensitivity reactions. Genotoxicity of certain drugs is also known, which leads to mutagenesis, carcinogenesis, and teratogenesis owing to the interaction of drugs or their reactive metabolites with the genetic machinery (DNA, transcription, and translation). Drugs undergo metabolic detoxification in the body for effective elimination (clearance) of the drug from the body in the form of metabolites to minimize or abolish the adverse actions of drugs. An imbalance between the formation of reactive metabolites of a drug and their detoxification results in drug toxicity. Hypersensitivity and subsequent tissue damage result if the metabolite acts as a hapten and transforms into a neoantigen. The reactive metabolites of drugs uncouple selective biochemical processes, interfere with the structure and function of various macromolecules like proteins, DNA and RNA, and cause a multitude of adverse actions of drugs. A drug may directly or indirectly cause adverse actions of a drug. Again, it should be emphasized that such adverse actions of drugs may be individual-specific involving sudden death, cancer, and inheritable mutations.

Hypersensitivity reaction, one of the major adverse actions arise from drug toxicity, is recognized to be associated with significant morbidity and mortality among the human subjects.[1,2] The major adverse actions of drugs include thrombocytopenia, hemolytic anemia, toxic erythema, and toxic epidermal necrolysis. A substantial body of evidence currently available indicates that the adverse actions of drugs are often caused by the drug metabolites rather than by the parent drug itself. For example, the primary amines (β-naphthylamine, aminobiphenyl), the acetyl derivatives of primary amines (2-acetylaminofluorene), and the secondary amines (*N*-methyl-4-aminoazobenzene) are N-hydroxylated by either cytochrome P-450 enzymes or amine *N*-oxidase. Under certain conditions, the metabolites are further activated by their metabolic conversion to N–O-sulfate esters.[3,4] Owing to the variations in inherent metabolic nature among different individuals of a population (apparently determined by their genetic makeup), the drug toxicity mainly depends upon the body's ability to protect itself against such toxicity through the upregulation of defense or repair mechanisms and the involvement of immune system. However, the clinical use of protective drugs to combat severe toxicity caused by drugs and toxicants has been limited.[5–7]

DRUG-INDUCED NEPHROTOXICITY

Kidney is the major site of action in the removal of toxic drugs and their reactive metabolites from the body through urinary excretion. As a result of this, the kidney is routinely exposed to high concentrations of these drugs and their active metabolites, leading to the manifestation of nephrotoxicity. Kidney, rich in vasculature, is capable of accumulating nephrotoxins.[8–10] As most of the drugs cause nephrotoxicity directly or indirectly, the clinical use of several important life-saving drugs has been limited. Some of the important drugs such as antibiotics, nonsteroidal anti-inflammatory drugs (NSAIDS), angiotensin converting enzyme (ACE) inhibitors, anticancer agents, immunosuppressants, and radiographic contrast agents are known to cause nephrotoxicity.[11–14] Antibiotics like aminoglycosides, amphotericin B, tetracyclines, acyclovir, and pentamidine have been reported to cause renal failure through different mechanisms including direct toxicity to the renal tubules, allergic interstitial nephritis, and crystallization of the antibiotic within the renal tubules.[11,12] NSAIDS (aspirin and COX-2 inhibitors) have been identified to cause hypertension, congestive heart failure (CHF), and acute or chronic renal failure.[13] Certain ACE inhibitors have been shown to cause uremia, hyperkalemia, decreased glomerular filtration rate (GFR, an index of kidney function), and dialysis dependence.[15]

Cisplatin, a heavy metal chemotherapeutic drug, is effective in treating a variety of malignancies in the experimental animals and humans. However, cisplatin is a potent nephrotoxin causing renal failure in 25–36% of patients after a single dose of administration.[16–18] Lithium, used for therapy against bipolar disorder in patients, has been known to cause renal abnormalities such as nephrogenic diabetes insipidus, chronic interstitial nephritis, and minimal change glomerulonephropathy.[19] Cyclosporine (CsA) and tacrolimus (FK-506 or Fujimycin) have been widely used as immunosuppressive drugs to prevent allograft rejection in heart, liver, and kidney transplantation and to treat autoimmune diseases. CsA and tacrolimus therapies have been known to lead to thrombotic microangiopathy and functional and structural changes in the kidney of the experimental animals and transplant patients, ultimately causing renal dysfunction.[20,21] Radiographic contrast dye has been shown to cause severe vasospasm in the afferent arteriole and acute renal failure in individuals with risk factors including diabetes, chronic renal failure, diuretic therapy, myeloma, and CHF.[14,22] Drugs of abuse such as cocaine have been reported to induce renal damage including the acute tubular necrosis due to rhabdomyolsis and allergic interstitial nephritis.[23]

Apart from the administration of nephrotoxic drugs, prolonged use of Chinese herbs as alternative medicines has been implicated in the manifestation of 35% of all the cases of acute renal failure in some countries.[24] Several reports have been made on the progressive kidney failure leading to the end-state renal disease among women taking diet pills containing Chinese herbs. Aristolochic acid has been identified as the toxicant in the Chinese herbs, and the resulting nephropathy due to the consumption of those Chinese herbs was characterized by an extensive fibrosis of the renal interstitium. Toxic metals such as mercury, lead, arsenic, and bismuth present in certain drugs and herbal medicines have been shown to cause renal dysfunction. The combined use of more than one nephrotoxic drug tends to cause possible additive toxic effects. Acute tubular necrosis results due to the administration of statins in combination with immunosuppressive agents such as cyclosporine. Similarly, nephrotoxicity arising from the combined treatment of cisplatin and aminoglycosides may be more severe than that induced by either of the agents alone.

THERAPEUTIC OPTIONS TO PREVENT AND TREAT DRUG-INDUCED NEPHROTOXICITY

In most cases, the ability of hydration pretreatment to reduce the nephrotoxicity of many drugs has been recognized. Fluid volume replacement, dialysis therapy, drug dosage adjustment, and steroid usage in the treatment of acute interstitial nephritis, while avoiding the repeated administration of the same drug(s), have been recognized as the important strategies to prevent or attenuate the nephrotoxicity of some routinely used drugs in clinical practice. Nephrotoxicity of cisplatin can be attenuated by intravenous saline administration at a dose of 150–250 mL/h before, during, and after cisplatin chemotherapy. Discontinuation of administration of the nephrotoxic drug, introduction of oral prednisone therapy (1–2 mg/kg/day for 4–6 weeks), and plasmapheresis appear to be beneficial to patients with the drug-induced acute allergic interstitial nephritis and thrombotic microangiopathy. Hydration therapy with the intravenous saline infusion and prophylactic mucomyst has been shown to reduce the contrast agent-induced nephrotoxicity.[22,25] Correction of hyperkalemia and acidosis and supplementation with insulin-like and hepatocyte-type growth factors have been shown to offer recovery among the patients with intrinsic acute renal failure. In patients with acute renal failure, the use of osmotic agent, mannitol, which induces hypervolemia, is avoided.[26]

CISPLATIN-INDUCED NEPHROTOXICITY

Cisplatin is a water-soluble planar member of the platinum coordination complex class of anticancer drugs. Structurally, the drug consists of an atom of platinum surrounded by chloride and ammonium atoms in the *cis* position of a horizontal plane. Cisplatin still remains as a preferred antineoplastic drug for the treatment of a variety of solid tumors such as metastatic bladder and testicular and ovarian carcinomas.[27] In circulation, cisplatin binds to serum proteins up to 90%, gets distributed to most of the tissues, and is cleared in the intact parent form by the kidney.[28] Cisplatin and their analogs have been shown to interact with the thiols and macromolecules.[29] The nephrotoxicity of cisplatin is associated with the actions of reactive oxygen species (ROS). Glutathione (GSH) detoxifies cisplatin by rapid complexation (binding) as the reactivity (affinity) of platinum complexes is greater with the cysteine residue of GSH.[30] The enhanced production of tumor necrosis factor-α (TNF-α) has been suggested to mediate the cisplatin nephrotoxicity[31] through the activation of p38 mitogen-activated protein kinase (p38 MAPK).[32] Light microscopic and ultrastructural studies have shown that the cisplatin-induced kidney injury and necrosis in rat are predominantly confined to the S3 segment of proximal tubules in the corticomedullary region without or with accompaniment of distal changes.[33] Recent studies have shown that nedaplatin, a second generation platinum complex, is less nephrotoxic than cisplatin.[10,34] Despite the intensive prophylactic measures, irreversible renal damage is encountered among nearly one-third of the cisplatin-treated patients.[27,35] Cisplatin treatment also induces extensive cell death in the proximal and distal tubules and loop of henle.[27,36] Deoxyribonuclease I has been shown to be involved in the cisplatin nephrotoxicity.[37] Multiple studies have demonstrated that cisplatin nephrotoxicity is associated with DNA fragmentation, activation of the MAPK cascade, and molecular responses typical to stress responses.[9] Increased Bax and decreased senescence marker protein-30 (SMP)-30 gene expression has been observed during the cisplatin-induced nephrotoxicity as analyzed by the Microarray Technology[38] indicating apoptosis and perturbation of the intracellular calcium homeostasis. Oxidative stress has emerged as one of the crucial mechanisms of cisplatin-induced nephrotoxicity as it is associated with the elevated generation of ROS and induction of lipid peroxidation in the kidney as a result of decline in the antioxidant levels and antioxidant enzyme activities.[39,40] Cisplatin treatment also has been shown to cause significant oxidant generation in the kidney through both the xanthine oxidase activation and impaired antioxidant defense system, thus contributing to the accelerated oxidative stress-mediated reactions in the tissue.[41]

NEPHROPROTECTIVE AGENTS

Several strategies have been sought after to alleviate the nephrotoxic effects of cisplatin during the anticancer therapy including the use of less intensive treatment and replacement with less toxic analog of cisplatin, carboplatin. Identification of specific cytochrome P450 isoenzymes in the human renal tubular cells and the development of specific inhibitors appear to be promising in either the protection or amelioration of cisplatin nephrotoxicity. Several studies have demonstrated that dietary antioxidants apparently detoxify the ROS and also enhance the anticancer efficacy of chemotherapy while minimizing certain adverse effects (reviewed by Conklin, 2000).[42] Various antioxidants also have been shown to protect against cisplatin-induced nephrotoxicity.[43,44] Radical scavengers and antioxidants such as vitamin E, vitamin C,[45] manganese superoxide dismutase (SOD),[44] selenium,[46] caffeic acid phenylethylester,[47] melatonin,[48] N-acetyl cysteine,[49] erdosteine,[50] edarabone,[51] have been reported to attenuate cisplatin-induced nephrotoxicity. Recent studies have suggested that the combination of tomato juice and dried black grapes ameliorate the cisplatin nephrotoxicity.[41] Agents such as amifostine (a cytoprotector),[52] recombinant human erythropoietin,[53] quercitin,[54] and desferrioxamine (iron chelator)[55] have also been reported to attenuate the drug-induced toxicity.

Nitric Oxide (NO) plays a crucial role in maintaining normal renal function.[56] The nitric oxide synthase (NOS) inhibitors (NG-nitro-L-arginine methyl ester and 2-amino-4-methylpyridine) have been shown to effectively mitigate lipid peroxidation and other biochemical alterations associated with the cisplatin nephrotoxicity.[57] On the other hand, the NOS inhibition has been observed to aggravate the cisplatin-induced nephrotoxicity.[58] The essential amino acid and a precursor of NO, L-arginine, has been shown to offer nephroprotection, while the NOS inhibitor, L-NAME, exerts the opposite effect.[59]

Both the animal and human studies have demonstrated that the use of diuretics (furosemide and mannitol) and hydration have markedly decreased the nephrotoxicity caused by cisplatin, carboplatin, and ormaplatin.[35,60,61] Procaine (local anesthetic drug)[62] and procainamide (antiarrhythmic drug)[63] have been shown to enhance the therapeutic index of cisplatin and to reduce its nephrotoxicity without compromising its antitumour action. The methylxanthine derivative, pentoxifylline, and the nonselective adenosine receptor antagonist, theophylline, are reported to decrease the concentration of adenosine and severity of renal dysfunction induced by the nephrotoxic drugs.[64] Several other studies have demonstrated that the compounds such as lycopene,[65] edarabone,[51] bismuth subnitrate,[66] serum thymic factor,[67] salicylate,[68] and gum Arabica[69] ameliorate the cisplatin nephrotoxicity.

Naturally occurring antioxidants of medicinal plant origin have been tested for their protective effect against cisplatin nephrotoxicity.[70] Several natural plant products (phytochemicals) such as the extracts of a polypore fungus, *Phellinuns rimosus*,[71] *Cassia auriculata*,[72] and the flowers of *Pongamia pinnata* and *Aerva lanata*,[73,74] lupeol, an antioxidant from the medicinal plant, *Crataeva nurvala*,[75] xanththorrhizol, a protein kinase inhibitor from *Curcuma xanthorrhiza*,[76] and capsaisin, a major pungent ingredient of hot red peppers,[77] have been shown to offer protection against the cisplatin nephrotoxicity. Also, the gentamycin-induced nephrotoxicty has been shown to be ameliorated by *Ginkgo biloba* in the experimental animals.[78]

Reports have also been made on the protection against the cyclosporine-induced chronic nephrotoxicity by several natural antioxidants, nutrients, and drugs including colchicines,[79] tea polyphenols,[80] lazaroid,[81] vitamins E and C,[82] and calcium channel blocker, lacidipine.[83] Melatonin, a pineal hormone,[84] carvedilol, a beta blocker,[85] and probucol[86] have been reported to protect against the gentamycin-induced nephrotoxicity in rats.

SPIRULINA—A MEDICINAL BLUE-GREEN ALGA

Among several known medicinal plants at present, *Spirulina*, a microscopic fila-mentous blue-green alga, is emerging as a promising therapeutic aquatic microphyte. *Spirulina*, the simplest members among algae, are widely distributed both as the ter-restrial and aquatic forms. They are referred in the literature by different names such as Cyanophyta, Myxophyta, Cyanochloronta, Cyanobacteria, blue-green algae, and blue-green bacteria. Blue-green algae are either unicellular or filamentous forms.[87] *Spirulina* belongs to the kingdom Monera and division Cyanophyta. *Spirulina* is a genus of the phylum Cyanobacteria ("Cyano" from the Greek meaning blue). *Spirulina* is a freshwater blue-green alga found in most lakes and ponds. The word *Spirulina* originates from Latin denoting the helix or spiral nature (whorl) of the alga. The German scientist, Deurben had named it "*Spirulina*" in 1927. *Spirulina* has been orally consumed for thousands of years by humans among the Mexican (Aztecs, May-ans), African, and Asian societies and also is a popular food and nutritional supplement in Japan and the United States. *Spirulina*, wheat grass, barley grass, and *Chlorella* are often referred to as "green foods." Among several occurring species of *Spirulina*, the most commonly used in nutritional supplements are *Spirulina platensis* (also called *Arthrospira platensis*) and *Spirulina maxima*. Although the nutritional importance of *Spirulina* is greatly recognized, studies on its pharmacological and therapeutic prop-erties are limited. Here, we present a comprehensive overview on the therapeutic effects of *Spirulina* in protection against the drug-induced nephrotoxicity.

CHEMICAL COMPOSITION OF SPIRULINA

Spirulina adds to the list of the most enriched nutrient foods currently known. The alga is rich in all the three broad categories of essential nutrients including mac-ronutrients (proteins, lipids, and carbohydrates), minerals such as zinc, magnesium, calcium, iron, managanese, selenium, micronutrients, provitamin A (β-carotene), riboflavin, cyanocobalamin, α-tocopherol, α-linoleic acid, the most potent antiox-idant enzyme, SOD, phytopigments including chlorophyll and the characteristic phycobilin pigments[88,89] in an greater bioavailable state. The typical phycobilin pigments of *Spirulina* include C-phycocyanin and allophycocyanin. The pigments,

C-phycocyanin and chlorophyll, give *Spirulina* their bluish tinge, and hence the species are classified under blue-green algae. Phycobilins, in structure, are similar to the bile pigments such as bilirubin. In *Spirulina*, phycobilins are intracellularly attached to proteins and the phycobilin–protein complex is called phycobiliprotein. *Spirulina* contains high amounts of bioavailable iron, which has been shown to be easily absorbed in the gastrointestinal tract.[90]

PHARMACOLOGY AND TOXICOLOGY OF *SPIRULINA*

The pharmacokinetics and pharmacodynamics of *Spirulina* in humans have not been thoroughly investigated. However, the proteins, lipids, and carbohydrates in *Spirulina* are digested, absorbed, and metabolized by the humans upon oral consumption. *Spirulina* can be consumed at a dose of 3–20 g/day without manifestation of any adverse effects.[91] Studies on the acute, subchronic, and chronic toxicity and mutagenicity of *Spirulina* have revealed no specific body or organ toxicity or genotoxicity.[92,93] Studies in animals fed with large quantities of *Spirulina* have shown that the alga is neither toxic nor causes adverse health effects.[94] Dietary ingestion of very high levels of *Spirulina* during pregnancy has not caused any fetal abnormalities or birth defects.[95] Independent feeding tests have shown no toxic or adverse effects in the humans, rats, pigs, and chickens.[92,96,97] Feeding experiments with rats conducted in Japan have revealed no acute or chronic toxicity or reproductive toxicity of *Spirulina*.[94] To date, there are no drug interactions reported with *Spirulina*. The United Nations Organization (UNO) has recommended *Spirulina* as the ideal food for mankind and the World Health Organization (WHO) has also declared *Spirulina* as a safe food with excellent nutritional value.

THERAPEUTIC USES OF *SPIRULINA*

Spirulina and its active constituents have specific therapeutic uses beyond general nutritional values. *In vitro* and *in vivo* studies have shown that either *Spirulina* or its active constituent, C-phycocyanin is promising in chemoprevention and cancer protection,[98] neuroprotection,[99] antiviral action,[100] cardiovascular protection,[87] immunomodulation,[101] hepatoprotection,[102] anti-inflammatory action,[103] antioxidant action,[104] and protection against chemical- and drug-induced toxicities.[87,105–107]

SPIRULINA AS AN ANTIOXIDANT

Currently, *S. platensis* is gaining a tremendous attention not only for its nutritional values but also for its potential antioxidant properties. Experimental and epidemiological evidences suggest that oxidative stress characterized by excessive generation of ROS is a critical player in many pathological states including the inflammatory diseases, neurodegenerative diseases, atherosclerosis, cardiovascular diseases, diabetes mellitus, cancer, and reperfusion injury.[108–112] Therefore, the therapeutic use of natural antioxidants appears to be promising in either prevention or protection or both from those diseases among humans. Many algal products appear to improve thenutritional quality of foods because of their ability to combat oxidative damage to cells.[113] *Spirulina* and C-phycocyanin have been shown to protect against the oxidative stress-mediated pathological conditions.[104,106,114,115] Studies have shown that *Spirulina* has potent antioxidant activity [105,106] and scavenges hydroxyl and peroxyl radicals both *in vitro* and *in vivo* through its C-phycocyanin constituent.[116] C-phycocyanin has been reported not only to scavenge the hydroxyl, peroxyl,[114] and superoxide radicals,[87] and peroxynitrite[117] but also to act as a potent antioxidant by inhibiting the membrane lipid peroxidation.[102,118–120] Hence, C-phycocyanin, one of the major biliproteins of *Spirulina*, is regarded as an effective antioxidant and a free radical scavenger.[116]

PROTECTION OF DRUG-INDUCED NEPHROTOXICITY BY *SPIRULINA*

Studies have revealed that *Spirulina* offers protection against the drug- and chemical-induced toxicity.[87,106,121,122] Earlier, we have demonstrated the nephroprotective effects of *Spirulina* in a rat model of cisplatin-induced nephrotoxicity.[40] In our study, *Spirulina* pretreatment in rats significantly attenuated the cisplatin-induced elevation of the levels of plasma urea, creatinine, and urinary β-NAG (a marker of renal tubular damage) (Figure 7.1). The cisplatin-impaired renal function also

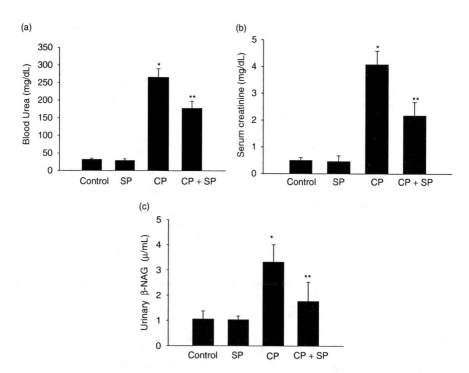

FIGURE 7.1   Effect of *Spirulina* (SP) on cisplatin (CP)-induced nephrotoxicity as measured by (a) plasma urea; (b) plasma creatinine; and (c) urinary β-NAG. Nephrotoxicity in rats was induced by CP (6 mg/kg b.w. single dose, i.p) and *Spirulina* (1 g/kg) was administered orally, 3 days prior to CP treatment and continued till end of the experiment. Values are expressed as mean $\pm$ SD ($n = 6$), $^*p < .05$ vs. control; $^{**}p < .05$ vs. CP.

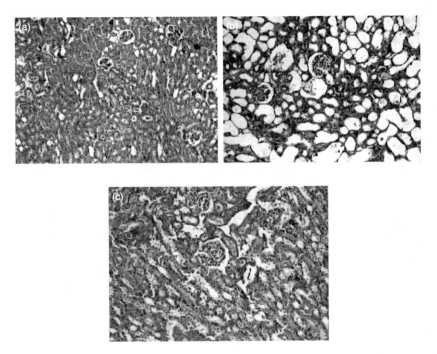

FIGURE 7.2 Histological examination of rat kidney (40X). (a) Control rat show normal morphology; (b) cisplatin-treated rat show renal tubules with hyaline casts, swelling, and vacuolization and proximal tubular necrosis; and (c) Cisplatin + *Spirulina*-treated rat show minimal tubular necrosis.

has been confirmed by the histological examination of kidney in the regions of cortex and corticomedullary junctions (Figure 7.2). While the control rats have shown no signs of abnormality in the kidney, in the cisplatin-treated animals, a marked proximal tubular necrosis, extensive epithelial vacuolization, swelling and tubular dilation, and renal tubules with hyaline casts have been clearly evident (Figure 7.2b). The alterations in glomerulus and tubular epithelium are less severe in the animals treated with cisplatin and *Spirulina* together when compared with that in the animals treated with cisplatin alone (Figure 7.2c), further revealing that *Spirulina* offers protection against the cisplatin-induced nephrotoxicity. *Spirulina* pretreatment has significantly attenuated the cisplatin-induced increase in the extent of lipid peroxidation (malondialdehyde, (MDA) formation) in the plasma and kidney and decrease in the activities of SOD, catalase and glutathione peroxidase (Figures 7.3 and 7.4). Though the results of this study suggest that *Spirulina* offers protection against the cisplatin-induced nephrotoxicity through the inhibition of oxidative stress, the involvement of other possible mechanim(s) cannot be ruled out. Studies reported by others reveal that apoptosis is involved in the cisplatin-induced renal injury.[123,124] Recently, we have demonstrated that *Spirulina* and C-phycocyanin have significantly inhibited the doxorubicin-induced free radical generation and apoptosis by attenuating caspase-3 activity in the isolated rat cardiomyocytes[125] and also have ameliorated the ischemia-reperfusion injury in isolated rat heart model.[126] Another

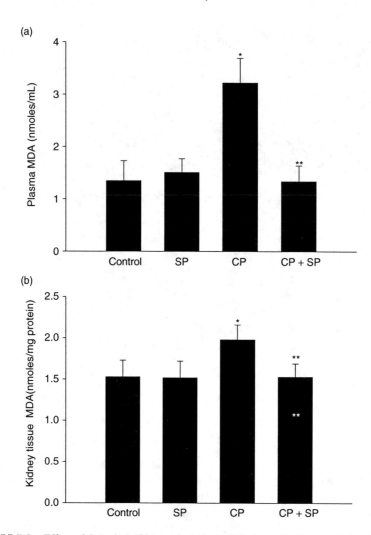

FIGURE 7.3 Effect of *Spirulina* (SP) on cisplatin (CP)-induced lipid peroxidation (MDA). Rats were treated CP (6 mg/kg b.w. single dose, i.p) and *Spirulina* (1 g/kg) was administered orally, 3 days prior to CP treatment and continued till end of the experiment. Values are expressed as mean $\pm$ SD ($n = 6$), *$p < .05$ vs. control; **$p < .05$ vs. CP. The results show that *Spirulina* treatment attenuated the CP-induced increase in lipid peroxidation.

recent study has demonstrated that the treatment with a *Spirulina*-enriched diet has lowered the ischemia-reperfusion-induced apoptosis and cerebral infarction by inhibiting the caspase-3 activity.[99] *Spirulina* treatment does not appear to interfere with the anticancer efficacy of cisplatin treatment.[40] One possible crucial mechanism that needs further investigation is the attenuation of the cisplatin-induced oxidative stress and apoptosis by *Spirulina*.

Spirulina has been also shown to protect against the cyclosporine-induced nephrotoxicity in rats.[107] In this study, pretreatment with *Spirulina* has significantly

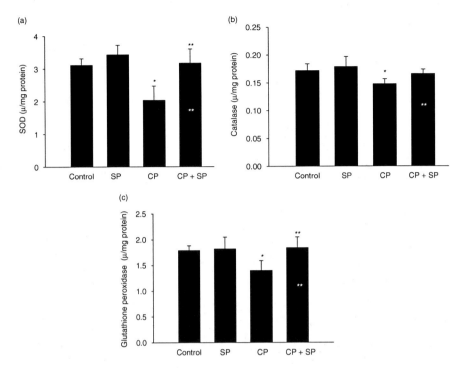

FIGURE 7.4 Effect of *Spirulina* (SP) on cisplatin (CP)-induced changes in SOD (a), catalase (b), and glutathione peroxidase (c). Rats were treated CP (6 mg/kg b.w. single dose, i.p) and *Spirulina* (1000 mg/kg) was administered orally, 3 days prior to CP treatment and continued till end of the experiment. Values are expressed as mean ± SD ($n = 6$), *$p < .05$ vs. control; **$p < .05$ vs. CP. The results show that *Spirulina* treatment attenuated the CP-induced decrease in SOD, catalase, and glutathione peroxidase.

attenuated the cyclosporine-induced nephrotoxicity and this effect has been attributed to its antioxidant property. Pretreatment of rats with *Spirulina* has resulted in significant attenuation of cyclosporine-induced increase in plasma urea and creatinine (Figure 7.5). Histological study of the kidney in the cyclosporine-treated rats reveals severe isometric vacuolization and widening of interstitium (Figure 7.6). Rats treated with cyclosporine and *Spirulina* together have shown a normal tubulo-interstitial pattern with fewer isometric vacuolization. In the cyclosporine-treated rats, there has been a significant increase in the extent of lipid peroxidation (MDA) of plasma and kidney as compared to that in the control animals (Table 7.1). *Spirulina* pretreatment has caused a significant attenuation of the cyclosporine-induced decrease in the activities of SOD, catalase and glutathione peroxidase in the kidney (Table 7.1). Also, it should be emphasized that *Spirulina* offers protection against the cyclosporine-induced nephrotoxicity without interfering with the metabolism of cyclosporine.[107] Several reports have established that apoptosis is involved in the cyclosporine-induced renal injury.[115,127] Our earlier investigation revealing that *Spirulina* attenuates the doxorubicin-induced apoptosis and

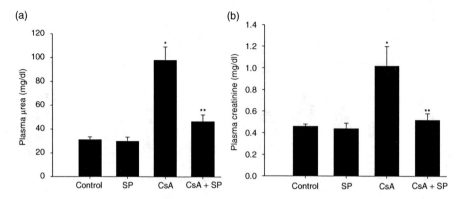

FIGURE 7.5 Effect of *Spirulina* (SP) on cyclosporine (CsA)-induced nephrotoxicity as measured by (a) plasma urea and (b) plasma creatinine. Nephrotoxicity in rats was induced by CsA (50 mg/kg b.w. orally for 14 days) and *Spirulina* (500 mg/kg) was administered orally, 3 days prior to CsA and continued till end of the experiment. Values are expressed as mean ± SD ($n = 6$), *$p < .05$ vs. control; **$p < .05$ vs. CsA.

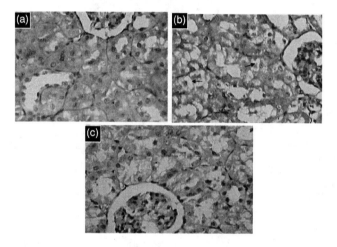

FIGURE 7.6 Histological examination of rat kidney. Left panel shows cortical region (H&E 60X); (a) Control rat show normal morphology; (b) Cyclosporine-treated rat shows severe isometric vacuolization (indicated by arrow) and widening of interstitium. (c) Csa + *Spirulina* treated rat show minimal tubular necrosis.

ischemia-reperfusion injury through the inhibition of caspase-3 activity[125] further suggests that through the inhibition of the apoptotic pathway, *Spirulina* probably offers protection against the cyclosporine-induced nephrotoxicity. However, this requires further investigation.

The mechanisms by which oxalate causes deleterious effects on kidneys have not yet been clearly established, however, some of the toxic effects of oxalate have been attributed to the induction of oxidative stress.[128] The oxalate-induced membrane lipid peroxidation leads to the loss of renal cell membrane integrity and ultimately calcium

TABLE 7.1

Effect of *Spirulina* on Cyclosporine (CsA)-Induced Changes in Lipid Peroxidation (MDA) and Activities of Antioxidant Enzymes

Parameter	Control	*Spirulina*	CsA	CsA + *Spirulina*
Plasma MDA (nm)	1.41 ± 0.06	1.43 ± 0.04	$2.74 \pm 0.58^*$	$1.87 \pm 0.19^{**}$
Kidney tissue MDA (nm/mg protein)	2.56 ± 0.18	2.48 ± 0.18	$4.31 \pm 0.58^*$	$2.87 \pm 0.51^{**}$
SOD U/mg protein	2.15 ± 0.19	2.19 ± 0.08	$1.32 \pm -0.43^*$	$2.32 \pm 0.20^{**}$
Catalase U/mg protein	0.35 ± 0.02	0.33 ± 0.02	$0.21 \pm 0.40^*$	$0.29 \pm 0.05^{**}$
Glutathione peroxidase U/mg protein	0.53 ± 0.09	0.51 ± 0.04	$0.37 \pm 0.04^*$	$0.55 \pm 0.03^{**}$

Values are expressed as mean $\pm$ SD ($n = 7$). $^*p < .05$ vs. control; $^{**}p < .05$ vs. CsA.

oxalate crystal deposition in the kidney. C-phycocyanin has also been shown to protect against the oxalate-mediated renal injury in rats.[129] Experimental observations reveal that C-phycocyanin administration causes a significant restoration in the thiol content of the renal tissue and red blood cells (RBCs) through the elevation of the GSH levels, a marked decrease in the extent of lipid peroxidation (MDA) in the plasma, and a significant enhancement of the activities of antioxidant enzymes (catalase and glucose-6-phosphate dehydrogenase) in the RBCs of oxalate-treated animals, suggesting that C-phycocyanin not only ameliorates oxidative stress but also acts as a free radical scavenger.[129]

Collectively, various studies have confirmed that *Spirulina* offers protection against the drug- and chemical-induced renal toxicity. Gentamycin, an aminoglycoside antibiotic used in the treatment of Gram-negative infections, has been shown to enhance the generation of oxidants including the superoxide anion, peroxynitrite, hydrogen peroxide, and hydroxyl radical in the renal cortical mitochondria.[130,131] Recent studies have established that *Spirulina fusiformis*, significantly and dose dependently, protects against the gentamycin-induced oxidative stress, renal histological alterations, and renal dysfunction in rats.[132] Reports have been made on the characteristic morphological changes such as tubular necrosis, tubular regeneration, and tubulointestinal mononuclear cell filtration in the kidneys of the gentamycin-treated rats, which are significantly attenuated by *Spirulina*, further supporting the active role of antioxidants and β-carotene present in *Spirulina* in such protection.[104,133] An enhanced generation of NO by the inducible NOS (iNOS) is shown to cause injury to the kidney through several mechanisms. Elevated levels of NO leads to the depletion of cellular ATP through inactivation of the enzymes of the Krebs cycle and mitochondrial electron transport chain.[134] Gentamicin has been observed to enhance glomerular NO production.[135] *Spirulina* has been noticed to significantly and dose dependently attenuate the gentamycin-induced nitrosative stress and this probably is due to the inhibition of the iNOS activity.[132]

The involvement of heavy metals has been emphasized in a variety of pathological states such as hypertension and renal, neural and hepatic disorders.[136] MDA provides an index of lipid peroxidation of cell membranes. *Spirulina* has been reported to effectively decrease the extent of lipid peroxidation and restore the levels of various

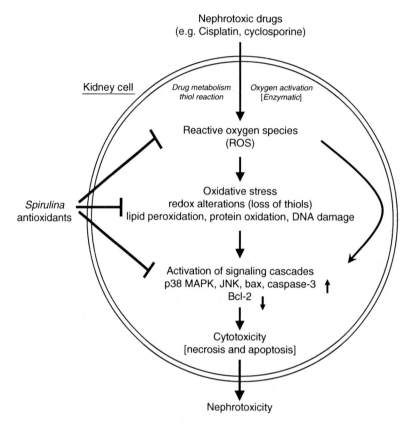

SCHEMA 1 Proposed mechanism of protection against drug-induced nephrotoxicity protection by *Spirulina* and its antioxidants. Drugs entering the kidney cells undergo metabolism by the drug-metabolizing enzymes and get transformed into their respective metabolites. Either the parent drugs (e.g., cisplatin and cyclosporine) or their metabolites activate molecular oxygen through oxygenases such as the xanthine oxidase or the mitochondrial electron transport system into the ROS, which cause oxidative stress. The ROS thus formed induce intracellular oxidative stress involving lipid peroxidation, protein oxidation, and DNA damage. The oxidative stress also triggers activation of the stress-activated kinases (p38 MAPK and JNK), which in turn activate caspase-3 and down-regulate Bcl-2. These signaling cascades induce the renal cell toxic events including necrosis and apoptosis thus resulting in the nephrotoxicity. *Spirulina* and its antioxidants have been shown to inhibit the formation of ROS, attenuate oxidative stress, and inhibit the activation of signaling cascades and the resultant necrosis and apoptosis in the cells of the kidney exposed to the nephrotoxic drugs. Alternatively, the ability of *Spirulina* and its antioxidants to modulate the drug-metabolism and drug-induced enzymatic activation of molecular oxygen is also proposed as a possible mechanism of protection against the drug-induced nephrotoxicity.

endogenous antioxidants in several organs such as the kidney, liver, heart, lung, and brain of the experimental animals.[82,106,132] Reports have been made that *Spirulina* restores the activities of various membrane-bound enzymes including the Na^+–K^+ -ATPase, Ca^{++}-ATPase and Mg^{++}-ATPase and several lipids in the vital organs such as the liver, kidney, heart, and lung of rats exposed to lead.[106] Rats fed with *Spirulina* have shown amelioration of the kidney damage from cadmium toxicity.[137] The induction of oxidative stress by heavy metals in a wide variety of systems is also established. Therefore, from these studies it is conceivable to deduce that *Spirulina* offers a protective antioxidant effect against the renal injury (nephrotoxicity) caused by various toxicants, heavy metals, and drugs including the anticancer chemotherapeutic agents (Schema 1). Nevertheless, the molecular mechanisms behind protection of the chemical- and drug-induced nephrotoxicity by *Spirulina* through the mitigation of the oxidant reactions, modulation of the antioxidant enzymes, and the inhibition of apoptosis need to be thoroughly investigated and established in both *in vitro* and *in vivo* systems.

CONCLUSION

Spirulina is being considered as one of the nutritionally enriched naturally occurring foods consisting of proteins, minerals, and vitamins. The alga contains active phytochemicals possessing immense prophylactic and therapeutic properties without exerting any toxicity or adverse effects. *Spirulina*, as a rich source of antioxidants, combats oxidant damage and protects against drug-induced nephrotoxicity. Further, a thorough pharmacological characterization of the active phytochemical constitutents of *Spirulina* will establish the therapeutical potential of the natural products of the alga. Spriulina also offers a promising pharmacological intervention strategy in the humans encountering the clinical drug-induced nephrotoxicity caused by therapeutics during transplantation and cancer treatment. Needless to mention, extensive preclinical and clinical studies are warranted to establish the nutritional values, pharmacological uses, safety, efficacy, and nephroprotective role of *Spirulina* and its phytochemical constituents in scenarios of nephrotoxicity in patients receiving the nephrotoxic life-saving therapeutic drugs.

ACKNOWLEDGMENT

We thank M/s Parry Neutraceuticals, Chennai, India for providing pure powder of *Spirulina* for our studies. Dr.Vijay Kumar Kutala is on sabbatical from Nizam's Institute of Medical Sciences, Hyderabad, India.

REFERENCES

1. Lazarou, J., Pomeranz, B. H., Corey, P. N. Incidence of adverse drug reactions in hospitalized patients: a meta-analysis of prospective studies, *JAMA*, 279(15), 1200, 1998.
2. Pirmohamed, M., Breckenridge, A. M., Kitteringham, N. R., Park, B. K. Adverse drug reactions, *BMJ*, 316(7140), 1295, 1998.
3. Miller, E. C., Miller, J. A. Mechanisms of chemical carcinogenesis: nature of proximate carcinogens and interactions with macromolecules, *Pharmacol Rev*, 18, 805, 1966.

4. Weisburger, J. H., Weisburger, E. K. Biochemical formation and pharmacological, toxicological, and pathological properties of hydroxylamines and hydroxamic acids, *Pharmacol Rev*, 25(1), 1, 1973.

5. Lefrak, E. A., Pitha, J., Rosenheim, S., Gottlieb, J. A. A clinicopathologic analysis of adriamycin cardiotoxicity, *Cancer*, 32(2), 302, 1973.

6. Loehrer, P. J., Einhorn, L. H. Drugs five years later. Cisplatin, *Ann Intern Med*, 100(5), 704, 1984.

7. Singal, P. K., Iliskovic, N. Doxorubicin-induced cardiomyopathy, *N Engl J Med*, 339(13), 900, 1998.

8. Weinberg, J. M. The cellular basis of nephrotoxicity. In: Schrier RW, Gottschalk CW, editors. *Diseases of the Kidney*. Boston: Little Brown, 1031, 1993.

9. Arany, I., Safirstein, R. L. Cisplatin nephrotoxicity, *Semin Nephrol*, 23(5), 460, 2003.

10. Kawai, Y., Kohda, Y., Kodawara, T., Gemba, M. Protective effect of a protein kinase inhibitor on cellular injury induced by cephaloridine in the porcine kidney cell line LLC-PK(1), *J Toxicol Sci*, 30(3), 157, 2005.

11. Smith, C. R., Lipsky, J. J., Laskin, O. L., Hellmann, D. B., Mellits, E. D., Longstreth, J., Lietman, P. S. Double-blind comparison of the nephrotoxicity and auditory toxicity of gentamicin and tobramycin, *N Engl J Med*, 302(20), 1106, 1980.

12. Barza, M., Ioannidis, J. P., Cappelleri, J. C., Lau, J. Single or multiple daily doses of aminoglycosides: a meta-analysis, *BMJ*, 312(7027), 338, 1996.

13. Perazella, M. A., Eras, J. Are selective COX-2 inhibitors nephrotoxic? *Am J Kidney Dis*, 35(5), 937, 2000.

14. Barrett, B. J. Contrast nephrotoxicity, *J Am Soc Nephrol*, 5(2), 125, 1994.

15. Randomised placebo-controlled trial of effect of ramipril on decline in glomerular filtration rate and risk of terminal renal failure in proteinuric, non-diabetic nephropathy. The GISEN Group (Gruppo Italiano di Studi Epidemiologici in Nefrologia), *Lancet*, 349(9069), 1857, 1997.

16. Madias, N. E., Harrington, J. T. Platinum nephrotoxicity, *Am J Med*, 65(2), 307, 1978.

17. Heidemann, H. T., Muller, S., Mertins, L., Stepan, G., Hoffmann, K., Ohnhaus, E. E. Effect of aminophylline on cisplatin nephrotoxicity in the rat, *Br J Pharmacol*, 97(2), 313, 1989.

18. Lebwohl, D., Canetta, R. Clinical development of platinum complexes in cancer therapy: an historical perspective and an update, *Eur J Cancer*, 34(10), 1522, 1998.

19. Boton, R., Gaviria, M., Batlle, D. C. Prevalence, pathogenesis, and treatment of renal dysfunction associated with chronic lithium therapy, *Am J Kidney Dis*, 10(5), 329, 1987.

20. Andoh, T. F., Burdmann, E. A., Bennett, W. M. Nephrotoxicity of immunosuppressive drugs: experimental and clinical observations, *Semin Nephrol*, 17(1), 34, 1997.

21. Pham, P. T., Peng, A., Wilkinson, A. H., Gritsch, H. A., Lassman, C., Pham, P. C., Danovitch, G. M. Cyclosporine and tacrolimus-associated thrombotic microangiopathy, *Am J Kidney Dis*, 36(4), 844, 2000.

22. Tepel, M., van der Giet, M., Schwarzfeld, C., Laufer, U., Liermann, D., Zidek, W. Prevention of radiographic-contrast-agent-induced reductions in renal function by acetylcysteine, *N Engl J Med*, 343(3), 180, 2000.

23. Nzerue, C. M., Hewan-Lowe, K., Riley, L. J., Jr. Cocaine and the kidney: a synthesis of pathophysiologic and clinical perspectives, *Am J Kidney Dis*, 35(5), 783, 2000.

24. Kadiri, S., Arije, A., Salako, B. L. Traditional herbal preparations and acute renal failure in south west Nigeria, *Trop Doct*, 29(4), 244, 1999.

25. Solomon, R., Werner, C., Mann, D., D'Elia, J., Silva, P. Effects of saline, mannitol, and furosemide to prevent acute decreases in renal function induced by radiocontrast agents, *N Engl J Med*, 331(21), 1416, 1994.

26. Cosentino, F. Drugs for the prevention and treatment of acute renal failure, *Cleve Clin J Med*, 62(4), 248, 1995.

27. Taguchi, T., Nazneen, A., Abid, M. R., Razzaque, M. S. Cisplatin-associated nephrotoxicity and pathological events, *Contrib Nephrol*, 148, 107, 2005.

28. Royer, B., Guardiola, E., Polycarpe, E., Hoizey, G., Delroeux, D., Combe, M., Chaigneau, L., Samain, E., Chauffert, B., Heyd, B., Kantelip, J. P., Pivot, X. Serum and intraperitoneal pharmacokinetics of cisplatin within intraoperative intraperitoneal chemotherapy: influence of protein binding, *Anticancer Drugs*, 16(9), 1009, 2005.

29. Baliga, R., Ueda, N., Walker, P. D., Shah, S. V. Oxidant mechanisms in toxic acute renal failure, *Drug Metab Rev*, 31(4), 971, 1999.

30. Jansen, B. A., Brouwer, J., Reedijk, J. Glutathione induces cellular resistance against cationic dinuclear platinum anticancer drugs, *J Inorg Biochem*, 89(3–4), 197, 2002.

31. Ramesh, G., Reeves, W. B. Inflammatory cytokines in acute renal failure, *Kidney Int Suppl*, (91), S56, 2004.

32. Ramesh, G., Reeves, W. B. p38 MAP kinase inhibition ameliorates cisplatin nephrotoxicity in mice, *Am J Physiol Renal Physiol*, 289(1), F166, 2005.

33. Townsend, D. M., Deng, M., Zhang, L., Lapus, M. G., Hanigan, M. H. Metabolism of cisplatin to a nephrotoxin in proximal tubule cells, *J Am Soc Nephrol*, 14(1), 1, 2003.

34. Uehara, T., Watanabe, H., Itoh, F., Inoue, S., Koshida, H., Nakamura, M., Yamate, J., Maruyama, T. Nephrotoxicity of a novel antineoplastic platinum complex, nedaplatin: a comparative study with cisplatin in rats, *Arch Toxicol*, 79(8), 451, 2005.

35. Santoso, J. T., Lucci, J. A., 3rd, Coleman, R. L., Schafer, I., Hannigan, E. V. Saline, mannitol, and furosemide hydration in acute cisplatin nephrotoxicity: a randomized trial, *Cancer Chemother Pharmacol*, 52(1), 13, 2003.

36. Arany, I., Megyesi, J. K., Kaneto, H., Price, P. M., Safirstein, R. L. Cisplatin-induced cell death is EGFR/src/ERK signaling dependent in mouse proximal tubule cells, *Am J Physiol Renal Physiol*, 287(3), F543, 2004.

37. Basnakian, A. G., Apostolov, E. O., Yin, X., Napirei, M., Mannherz, H. G., Shah, S. V. Cisplatin nephrotoxicity is mediated by deoxyribonuclease I, *J Am Soc Nephrol*, 16(3), 697, 2005.

38. Huang, Q., Dunn, R. T., 2nd, Jayadev, S., DiSorbo, O., Pack, F. D., Farr, S. B., Stoll, R. E., Blanchard, K. T. Assessment of cisplatin-induced nephrotoxicity by microarray technology, *Toxicol Sci*, 63(2), 196, 2001.

39. Somani, S. M., Frank, S., Rybak, L. P. Responses of antioxidant system to acute and trained exercise in rat heart subcellular fractions, *Pharmacol Biochem Behav*, 51(4), 627, 1995.

40. Mohan, I. K., Khan, M., Shobha, J. C., Naidu, M. U., Prayag, A., Kuppusamy, P., Kutala, V. K. Protection against cisplatin-induced nephrotoxicity by *Spirulina* in rats, *Cancer Chemother Pharmacol*, 58(6), 802, 2006.

41. Cetin, R., Devrim, E., Kilicoglu, B., Avci, A., Candir, O., Durak, I. Cisplatin impairs antioxidant system and causes oxidation in rat kidney tissues: possible protective roles of natural antioxidant foods, *J Appl Toxicol*, 26(1), 42, 2006.

42. Conklin, K. A. Dietary antioxidants during cancer chemotherapy: impact on chemotherapeutic effectiveness and development of side effects, *Nutr Cancer*, 37(1), 1, 2000.

43. Antunes, L. M., Araujo, M. C., Darin, J. D., Bianchi, M. L. Effects of the antioxidants curcumin and vitamin C on cisplatin-induced clastogenesis in Wistar rat bone marrow cells, *Mutat Res*, 465(1–2), 131, 2000.

44. Davis, C. A., Nick, H. S., Agarwal, A. Manganese superoxide dismutase attenuates Cisplatin-induced renal injury: importance of superoxide, *J Am Soc Nephrol*, 12(12), 2683, 2001.

45. Appenroth, D., Frob, S., Kersten, L., Splinter, F. K., Winnefeld, K. Protective effects of vitamin E and C on cisplatin nephrotoxicity in developing rats, *Arch Toxicol*, 71(11), 677, 1997.

46. Antunes, L. M., Francescato, H. D., Darin, J. D., de Lourdes, P. B. M. Effects of selenium pretreatment on cisplatin-induced chromosome aberrations in wistar rats, *Teratog Carcinog Mutagen*, 20(6), 341, 2000.

47. Ozen, S., Akyol, O., Iraz, M., Sogut, S., Ozugurlu, F., Ozyurt, H., Odaci, E., Yildirim, Z. Role of caffeic acid phenethyl ester, an active component of propolis, against cisplatin-induced nephrotoxicity in rats, *J Appl Toxicol*, 24(1), 27, 2004.

48. Hara, M., Yoshida, M., Nishijima, H., Yokosuka, M., Iigo, M., Ohtani-Kaneko, R., Shimada, A., Hasegawa, T., Akama, Y., Hirata, K. Melatonin, a pineal secretory product with antioxidant properties, protects against cisplatin-induced nephrotoxicity in rats, *J Pineal Res*, 30(3), 129, 2001.

49. Wu, Y. J., Muldoon, L. L., Neuwelt, E. A. The chemoprotective agent *N*-acetylcysteine blocks cisplatin-induced apoptosis through caspase signaling pathway, *J Pharmacol Exp Ther*, 312(2), 424, 2005.

50. Ozyurt, H., Yildirim, Z., Kotuk, M., Yilmaz, H. R., Yagmurca, M., Iraz, M., Sogut, S., Gergerlioglu, S. Cisplatin-induced acute renal failure is ameliorated by erdosteine in a dose-dependent manner, *J Appl Toxicol*, 24(4), 269, 2004.

51. Satoh, M., Kashihara, N., Fujimoto, S., Horike, H., Tokura, T., Namikoshi, T., Sasaki, T., Makino, H. A novel free radical scavenger, edarabone, protects against cisplatin-induced acute renal damage *in vitro* and *in vivo*, *J Pharmacol Exp Ther*, 305(3), 1183, 2003.

52. Asna, N., Lewy, H., Ashkenazi, I. E., Deutsch, V., Peretz, H., Inbar, M., Ron, I. G. Time dependent protection of amifostine from renal and hematopoietic cisplatin induced toxicity, *Life Sci*, 76(16), 1825, 2005.

53. Yalcin, S., Muftuoglu, S., Cetin, E., Sarer, B., Yildirim, B. A., Zeybek, D., Orhan, B. Protection against cisplatin-induced nephrotoxicity by recombinant human erythropoietin, *Med Oncol*, 20(2), 169, 2003.

54. Francescato, H. D., Coimbra, T. M., Costa, R. S., Bianchi Mde, L. Protective effect of quercetin on the evolution of cisplatin-induced acute tubular necrosis, *Kidney Blood Press Res*, 27(3), 148, 2004.

55. Kadikoylu, G., Bolaman, Z., Demir, S., Balkaya, M., Akalin, N., Enli, Y. The effects of desferrioxamine on cisplatin-induced lipid peroxidation and the activities of antioxidant enzymes in rat kidneys, *Hum Exp Toxicol*, 23(1), 29, 2004.

56. Fujihara, C. K., Sena, C. R., Malheiros, D. M., Mattar, A. L., Zatz, R. Short-term nitric oxide inhibition induces progressive nephropathy after regression of initial renal injury, *Am J Physiol Renal Physiol*, 290(3), F632, 2006.

57. Srivastava, R. C., Farookh, A., Ahmad, N., Misra, M., Hasan, S. K., Husain, M. M. Evidence for the involvement of nitric oxide in cisplatin-induced toxicity in rats, *Biometals*, 9(2), 139, 1996.

58. Saad, S. Y., Najjar, T. A., Daba, M. H., Al-Rikabi, A. C. Inhibition of nitric oxide synthase aggravates cisplatin-induced nephrotoxicity: effect of 2-amino-4-methylpyridine, *Chemotherapy*, 48(6), 309, 2002.

59. Saleh, S., El-Demerdash, E. Protective effects of L-arginine against cisplatin-induced renal oxidative stress and toxicity: role of nitric oxide, *Basic Clin Pharmacol Toxicol*, 97(2), 91, 2005.

60. Cornelison, T. L., Reed, E. Nephrotoxicity and hydration management for cisplatin, carboplatin, and ormaplatin, *Gynecol Oncol*, 50(2), 147, 1993.

61. Hanigan, M. H., Deng, M., Zhang, L., Taylor, P. T., Jr., Lapus, M. G. Stress response inhibits the nephrotoxicity of cisplatin, *Am J Physiol Renal Physiol*, 288(1), F125, 2005.

62. Zhang, J. G., Lindup, W. E. Cisplatin-induced changes in adenine nucleotides in rat kidney slices: amelioration by tiopronin and procaine, *J Pharm Pharmacol*, 49(11), 1136, 1997.

63. Esposito, M., Vannozzi, M. O., Viale, M., Fulco, R. A., Collecchi, P., Merlo, F., De Cian, F., Zicca, A., Cadoni, A., Poirier, M. C. Para-aminobenzoic acid suppression of *cis*-diamminedichloroplatinum(II) nephrotoxicity, *Carcinogenesis*, 14(12), 2595, 1993.

64. Vassallo, R., Lipsky, J. J. Theophylline: recent advances in the understanding of its mode of action and uses in clinical practice, *Mayo Clin Proc*, 73(4), 346, 1998

65. Atessahin, A., Yilmaz, S., Karahan, I., Ceribasi, A. O., Karaoglu, A. Effects of lycopene against cisplatin-induced nephrotoxicity and oxidative stress in rats, *Toxicology*, 212(2–3), 116, 2005.

66. Kondo, Y., Himeno, S., Satoh, M., Naganuma, A., Nishimura, T., Imura, N. Citrate enhances the protective effect of orally administered bismuth subnitrate against the nephrotoxicity of *cis*-diamminedichloroplatinum, *Cancer Chemother Pharmacol*, 53(1), 33, 2004.

67. Kohda, Y., Matsunaga, Y., Yonogi, K., Kawai, Y., Awaya, A., Gemba, M. Protective effect of serum thymic factor, FTS, on cephaloridine-induced nephrotoxicity in rats, *Biol Pharm Bull*, 28(11), 2087, 2005.

68. Ramesh, G., Reeves, W. B. Salicylate reduces cisplatin nephrotoxicity by inhibition of tumor necrosis factor-alpha, *Kidney Int*, 65(2), 490, 2004.

69. Al-Majed, A. A., Abd-Allah, A. R., Al-Rikabi, A. C., Al-Shabanah, O. A., Mostafa, A. M. Effect of oral administration of Arabic gum on cisplatin-induced nephrotoxicity in rats, *J Biochem Mol Toxicol*, 17(3), 146, 2003.

70. Conklin, K. A. Cancer chemotherapy and antioxidants, *J Nutr*, 134(11), 3201S, 2004.

71. Ajith, T. A., Jose, N., Janardhanan, K. K. Amelioration of cisplatin induced nephrotoxicity in mice by ethyl acetate extract of a polypore fungus, Phellinus rimosus, *J Exp Clin Cancer Res*, 21(2), 213, 2002.

72. Annie, S., Rajagopal, P. L., Malini, S. Effect of *Cassia auriculata* Linn. root extract on cisplatin and gentamicin-induced renal injury, *Phytomedicine*, 12(8), 555, 2005.

73. Shirwaikar, A., Malini, S., Kumari, S. C. Protective effect of Pongamia pinnata flowers against cisplatin and gentamicin induced nephrotoxicity in rats, *Ind J Exp Biol*, 41(1), 58, 2003.

74. Shirwaikar, A., Issac, D., Malini, S. Effect of Aerva lanata on cisplatin and gentamicin models of acute renal failure, *J Ethnopharmacol*, 90(1), 81, 2004.

75. Shirwaikar, A., Setty, M., Bommu, P. Effect of lupeol isolated from Crataeva nurvala Buch.-Ham. stem bark extract against free radical induced nephrotoxicity in rats, *Ind J Exp Biol*, 42(7), 686, 2004.

76. Kim, S. H., Hong, K. O., Hwang, J. K., Park, K. K. Xanthorrhizol has a potential to attenuate the high dose cisplatin-induced nephrotoxicity in mice, *Food Chem Toxicol*, 43(1), 117, 2005.

77. Shimeda, Y., Hirotani, Y., Akimoto, Y., Shindou, K., Ijiri, Y., Nishihori, T., Tanaka, K. Protective effects of capsaicin against cisplatin-induced nephrotoxicity in rats, *Biol Pharm Bull*, 28(9), 1635, 2005.

78. Naidu, M. U., Shifow, A. A., Kumar, K. V., Ratnakar, K. S. Ginkgo biloba extract ameliorates gentamicin-induced nephrotoxicity in rats, *Phytomedicine*, 7(3), 191, 2000.

79. Disel, U., Paydas, S., Dogan, A., Gulfiliz, G., Yavuz, S. Effect of colchicine on cyclosporine nephrotoxicity, reduction of TGF-beta overexpression, apoptosis, and oxidative damage: an experimental animal study, *Transplant Proc*, 36(5), 1372, 2004.

80. Shi, S., Zheng, S., Jia, C., Zhu, Y., Xie, H. The effect of an antioxidant tea polyphenols on cell apoptosis in rat model of cyclosporine-induced chronic nephrotoxicity, *Zhonghua Wai Ke Za Zhi*, 40(9), 709, 2002.

81. Wang, C., Salahudeen, A. K. Cyclosporine nephrotoxicity: attenuation by an antioxidant-inhibitor of lipid peroxidation *in vitro* and *in vivo*, *Transplantation*, 58(8), 940, 1994.

82. Parra Cid, J. R., Garcia, C., Alvarez, C., De Arriba, G. Antioxidant nutrients protect against cyclosporine A nephrotoxicity, *Toxicology*, 189(1–2), 99, 2003.

83. Naidu, M. U., Kumar, K. V., Shifow, A. A., Prayag, A., Ratnakar, K. S. Lacidipine protects against cyclosporine-induced nephrotoxicity in rats, *Nephron*, 81(1), 60, 1999.

84. Shifow, A. A., Kumar, K. V., Naidu, M. U., Ratnakar, K. S. Melatonin, a pineal hormone with antioxidant property, protects against gentamicin-induced nephrotoxicity in rats, *Nephron*, 85(2), 167, 2000.

85. Kumar, K. V., Shifow, A. A., Naidu, M. U., Ratnakar, K. S. Carvedilol: a beta blocker with antioxidant property protects against gentamicin-induced nephrotoxicity in rats, *Life Sci*, 66(26), 2603, 2000.

86. Kumar, K. V., Naidu, M. U., Shifow, A. A., Ratnakar, K. S. Probucol protects against gentamycin-induced nephrotoxicity in rats, *Indian J Pharmacol*, 32, 108, 2000.

87. Khan, M., Shobha, J. C., Mohan, I. K., Naidu, M. U., Sundaram, C., Singh, S., Kuppusamy, P., Kutala, V. K. Protective effect of *Spirulina* against doxorubicin-induced cardiotoxicity, *Phytother Res*, 19(12), 1030, 2005.

88. Ciferri, O. *Spirulina*, the edible microorganism, *Microbiol Rev*, 47(4), 551, 1983

89. Sheshadri, C. V., Umesh, B. V. *Spirulina*—A nutrition food for the masses, *Invention Intelligence*, 28980, 253, 1992.

90. Johnson, P., Shubert, E. Availability of iron to rats from *spirulina*, a blue green alga, *Nutr Res*, 6, 85, 1986.

91. Delpeuch, F. E. A. Consumption as food and nutrition composition of blue-green algae among populations in the Kanem region of Chad, *Ann. Nutr. Aliment*, 29, 497, 1976.

92. Chamorro, G. A., Herrera, G., Salazar, M., Salazar, S., Ulloa, V. Subchronic toxicity study in rats fed *Spirulina*, *J Pharm Belg*, 43(1), 29, 1988.

93. Chamorro, G., Salazar, M., Favila, L., Bourges, H. Pharmacology and toxicology of *Spirulina* alga, *Rev Invest Clin*, 48(5), 389, 1996.

94. Tulliez, J., Bories, G., Boudene, C., Fevrier, C. Hydrocarbons of the spiruline algae: nature, metabolism of heptadecane by rats and swine, *Ann Nutr Aliment*, 29(6), 563, 1975.

95. Chamorro, G., Salazar, M. Teratogenic study of *spirulina* in mice, *Arch Latinoam Nutr*, 40(1), 86, 1990.

96. Fevrier, C., Seve, B. Incorporation of a spiruline (*Spirulina maxima*) in swine food, *Ann Nutr Aliment*, 29(6), 625, 1975.

97. Sautier, C., Tremolieres, J. Food value of the spiruline algae to man, *Ann Nutr Aliment*, 29(6), 517, 1975.

98. Schwartz, J., Shklar, G., Reid, S., Trickler, D. Prevention of experimental oral cancer by extracts of *Spirulina*-Dunaliella algae, *Nutr Cancer*, 11(2), 127, 1988.

99. Wang, Y., Chang, C. F., Chou, J., Chen, H. L., Deng, X., Harvey, B. K., Cadet, J. L., Bickford, P. C. Dietary supplementation with blueberries, spinach, or *spirulina* reduces ischemic brain damage, *Exp Neurol*, 193(1), 75, 2005.

100. Ayehunie, S., Belay, A., Baba, T. W., Ruprecht, R. M. Inhibition of HIV-1 replication by an aqueous extract of *Spirulina platensis* (*Arthrospira platensis*), *J Acquir Immune Defic Syndr Hum Retrovirol*, 18(1), 7, 1998.

101. Hayashi, K., Hayashi, T., Kojima, I. A natural sulfated polysaccharide, calcium spirulan, isolated from *Spirulina platensis*: *in vitro* and *ex vivo* evaluation of anti-herpes simplex virus and anti-human immunodeficiency virus activities, *AIDS Res Hum Retroviruses*, 12(15), 1463, 1996.

102. Gonzalez, R., Rodriguez, S., Romay, C., Gonzalez, A., Armesto, J., Remirez, D., Merino, N. Anti-inflammatory activity of phycocyanin extract in acetic acid-induced colitis in rats, *Pharmacol Res*, 39(1), 1055, 1999.

103. Remirez, D., Gonzalez, R., Merino, N., Rodriguez, S., Ancheta, O. Inhibitory effects of *Spirulina* in zymosan-induced arthritis in mice, *Mediators Inflamm*, 11(2), 75, 2002.

104. Miranda, M. S., Cintra, R. G., Barros, S. B., Mancini Filho, J. Antioxidant activity of the microalga *Spirulina maxima*, *Braz J Med Biol Res*, 31(8), 1075, 1998.

105. Premkumar, K., Pachiappan, A., Abraham, S. K., Santhiya, S. T., Gopinath, P. M., Ramesh, A. Effect of *Spirulina fusiformis* on cyclophosphamide and mitomycin-C induced genotoxicity and oxidative stress in mice, *Fitoterapia*, 72(8), 906, 2001.

106. Upasani, C. D., Balaraman, R. Protective effect of *Spirulina* on lead-induced deleterious changes in the lipid peroxidation and endogenous antioxidants in rats, *Phytother Res*, 17(4), 330, 2003.

107. Khan, M., Shobha, J. C., Mohan, I. K., Rao Naidu, M. U., Prayag, A., Kutala, V. K. *Spirulina* attenuates cyclosporine-induced nephrotoxicity in rats, *J Appl Toxicol*, 26(5), 444, 2006.

108. Sies, H. Relationship between free radicals and vitamins: an overview, *Int J Vitam Nutr Res Suppl*, 30, 215, 1989.

109. Coyle, J. T., Puttfarcken, P. Oxidative stress, glutamate, and neurodegenerative disorders, *Science*, 262(5134), 689, 1993.

110. Cuzzocrea, S., Riley, D. P., Caputi, A. P., Salvemini, D. Antioxidant therapy: a new pharmacological approach in shock, inflammation, and ischemia/reperfusion injury, *Pharmacol Rev*, 53(1), 135, 2001.

111. Surh, Y. J., Kundu, J. K., Na, H. K., Lee, J. S. Redox-sensitive transcription factors as prime targets for chemoprevention with anti-inflammatory and antioxidative phytochemicals, *J Nutr*, 135(12 Suppl), 2993S, 2005.

112. Soccio, M., Toniato, E., Evangelista, V., Carluccio, M., De Caterina, R. Oxidative stress and cardiovascular risk: the role of vascular NAD(P)H oxidase and its genetic variants, *Eur J Clin Invest*, 35(5), 305, 2005.

113. Demmig-Adams, B., Adams, W. W., 3rd. Antioxidants in photosynthesis and human nutrition, *Science*, 298(5601), 2149, 2002.

114. Vadiraja, B. B., Gaikwad, N. W., Madyastha, K. M. Hepatoprotective effect of C-phycocyanin: protection for carbon tetrachloride and R-(+)-pulegone-mediated hepatotoxicty in rats, *Biochem Biophys Res Commun*, 249(2), 428, 1998.

115. Yang, C. W., Lee, S. H., Lim, S. W., Jung, J. Y., Kim, W. Y., Kim, H. W., Choi, B. S., Li, C., Cha, J. H., Kim, Y. S., Kim, J., Bang, B. K. Cyclosporine or FK506 decrease mature epidermal growth factor protein expression and renal tubular regeneration in rat kidneys with ischemia/reperfusion injury, *Nephron*, 92(4), 914, 2002.

116. Bhat, V. B., Madyastha, K. M. C-phycocyanin: a potent peroxyl radical scavenger *in vivo* and *in vitro*, *Biochem Biophys Res Commun*, 275(1), 20, 2000.

117. Bhat, V. B., Madyastha, K. M. Scavenging of peroxynitrite by phycocyanin and phycocyanobilin from *Spirulina platensis*: protection against oxidative damage to DNA, *Biochem Biophys Res Commun*, 285(2), 262, 2001.

118. Romay, C., Armesto, J., Remirez, D., Gonzalez, R., Ledon, N., Garcia, I. Antioxidant and anti-inflammatory properties of C-phycocyanin from blue-green algae, *Inflamm Res*, 47(1), 36, 1998.

119. Romay, C., Ledon, N., Gonzalez, R. Effects of phycocyanin extract on prostaglandin E2 levels in mouse ear inflammation test, *Arzneimittelforschung*, 50(12), 1106, 2000.

120. Remirez, D., Fernandez, V., Tapia, G., Gonzalez, R., Videla, L. A. Influence of C-phycocyanin on hepatocellular parameters related to liver oxidative stress and Kupffer cell functioning, *Inflamm Res*, 51(7), 351, 2002.

121. Premkumar, K., Abraham, S. K., Santhiya, S. T., Ramesh, A. Protective effect of *Spirulina fusiformis* on chemical-induced genotoxicity in mice, *Fitoterapia*, 75(1), 24, 2004.

122. Farooq, S., Asokan, D., Kalaiselvi, P., Sakthivel, R., Varalakshmi, P. Prophylactic role of phycocyanin: a study of oxalate mediated renal cell injury, *Chem Biol Interact*, 149(1), 1, 2004.

123. Cummings, B. S., Schnellmann, R. G. Cisplatin-induced renal cell apoptosis: caspase 3-dependent and -independent pathways, *J Pharmacol Exp Ther*, 302(1), 8, 2002.

124. Lau, A. H. Apoptosis induced by cisplatin nephrotoxic injury, *Kidney Int*, 56(4), 1295, 1999.

125. Khan, M., Varadharaj, S., Shobha, J. C., Naidu, M. U., Parinandi, N. L., Kutala, V. K., Kuppusamy, P. C-phycocyanin ameliorates doxorubicin-induced oxidative stress and apoptosis in adult rat cardiomyocytes, *J Cardiovasc Pharmacol*, 47(1), 9, 2006.

126. Khan, M., Varadharaj, S., Ganesan, L. P., Shobha, J. C., Naidu, M. U., Parinandi, N. L., Tridandapani, S., Kutala, V. K., Kuppusamy, P. C-phycocyanin protects against ischemia-reperfusion injury of heart through involvement of p38 MAPK and ERK signaling, *Am J Physiol Heart Circ Physiol*, 290(5), H2136, 2006.

127. Sandau, K., Pfeilschifter, J., Brune, B. The balance between nitric oxide and superoxide determines apoptotic and necrotic death of rat mesangial cells, *J Immunol*, 158(10), 4938, 1997.

128. Hammes, M. S., Lieske, J. C., Pawar, S., Spargo, B. H., Toback, F. G. Calcium oxalate monohydrate crystals stimulate gene expression in renal epithelial cells, *Kidney Int*, 48(2), 501, 1995.

129. Farooq, S. M., Ebrahim, A. S., Subramhanya, K. H., Sakthivel, R., Rajesh, N. G., Varalakshmi, P. Oxalate mediated nephronal impairment and its inhibition by C-phycocyanin: a study on urolithic rats, *Mol Cell Biochem*, 284(1–2), 95, 2006.

130. Mazzon, E., Britti, D., De Sarro, A., Caputi, A. P., Cuzzocrea, S. Effect of *N*-acetylcysteine on gentamicin-mediated nephropathy in rats, *Eur J Pharmacol*, 424(1), 75, 2001.

131. Cuzzocrea, S., Mazzon, E., Dugo, L., Serraino, I., Di Paola, R., Britti, D., De Sarro, A., Pierpaoli, S., Caputi, A., Masini, E., Salvemini, D. A role for superoxide in gentamicin-mediated nephropathy in rats, *Eur J Pharmacol*, 450(1), 67, 2002.

132. Kuhad, A., Tirkey, N., Pilkhwal, S., Chopra, K. Renoprotective effect of *Spirulina fusiformis* on cisplatin-induced oxidative stress and renal dysfunction in rats, *Ren Fail*, 28(3), 247, 2006.

133. Kapoor, R., Mehta, U. Effect of supplementation of blue green alga (*Spirulina*) on outcome of pregnancy in rats, *Plant Foods Hum Nutr*, 43(1), 29, 1993.

134. Katusic, Z. S. Superoxide anion and endothelial regulation of arterial tone, *Free Radic Biol Med*, 20(3), 443, 1996.

135. Rivas-Cabanero, L., Rodriguez-Lopez, A. M., Martinez-Salgado, C., Saura, M., Lamas, S., Lopez-Novoa, J. M. Gentamicin treatment increases mesangial cell nitric oxide production, *Exp Nephrol*, 5(1), 23, 1997.

136. Balaraman, R., Gulati, O. D., Bhatt, J. D., Rathod, S. P., Hemavathi, K. G. Cadmium-induced hypertension in rats, *Pharmacology*, 38(4), 226, 1989.

137. Jeyaprakash, K., Chinnaswamy, P. Effect of *spirulina* and Liv-52 on cadmium induced toxicity in albino rats, *Ind J Exp Biol*, 43(9), 773, 2005.

8 *Spirulina* and Immunity

Andrea T. Borchers, Amha Belay, Carl L. Keen, and M. Eric Gershwin

CONTENTS

INTRODUCTION

The main function of the immune system in humans and animals is to detect and then neutralize or destroy invading pathogens, such as viruses, bacteria, fungi, and parasites. In addition, it is responsible for eliminating worn-out and abnormal self-cells. For these purposes, two types of immune responses have evolved, classified as innate and adaptive. Innate immune responses are also called nonspecific because they can be triggered by certain molecular patterns common to whole classes of pathogens and do not vary in subsequent encounters with the same antigen. The major mechanisms of innate immunity include phagocytosis, inflammation, complement activation, and induction of cell death. The main classes of phagocytes, that is, cells able to engulf entire bacteria or particulate matter, are neutrophils and macrophages. The chemical messengers they and some other cell types produce play an important role in the initiation of an inflammatory response. The killing of virus-infected cells and cancer cells through induction of programmed cell death or apoptosis is accomplished by natural killer (NK) cells.

Adaptive immune responses are highly specific for a particular antigen and become stronger and faster in subsequent encounters. They are the responsibility of B cells and T cells. The main function of B cells is to produce antibodies, which neutralize pathogens or stimulate their elimination by other cell types. There are five major classes (isotypes) of antibodies: immunoglobulin (Ig)A, IgD, IgE, IgG, and IgM, with IgA and IgG having 2 and 4 subclasses, respectively. Resting B cells express IgM and IgD on their cell surface as antigen receptors. Upon activation, B cells start to secrete IgM. It is only later in the immune response that they undergo a process called isotype switching and begin to produce other types of Ig. T cells are classified into helper T cells and cytotoxic T cells. One subclass of helper T cells provides help to macrophages in killing pathogenic microorganisms they have engulfed. The other subclass plays a vital role in inducing B cell antibody production. Cytotoxic T cells directly eliminate infected cells by initiating apoptosis.

All immune cells are ultimately derived from the same precursor or progenitor cells in the bone marrow, which eventually differentiate into myeloid (mono-cytes/macrophages, neutrophils, basophils, eosinophils, and mast cells) and lymphoid cells (B and T cells). Differentiation occurs under the influence of a variety of growth factors and cytokines. The differentiation of lymphoid progenitors into lymphocytes takes place in the central lymphoid organs, that is, bone marrow in the case of B cells and thymus in the case of T cells. After their maturation in these primary lymphoid organs, both types of lymphocytes migrate to the peripheral lymphoid tissues, that is, the lymph nodes, spleen, and lymphoid tissues associated with mucosa. It is in these peripheral lymphoid tissues that the reaction of B and T lymphocytes with foreign antigens takes place.

During immune responses, immune cells themselves and several other cell types start to produce a variety of messenger molecules, including chemokines and cytokines. Chemokines attract specific immune cells or subsets of them to the affected tissue(s). Cytokines are vital in shaping the exact nature of the response and in coordin-ating the functions of the various cell types involved. They do so in part by inducing the production of numerous proteins and the activity of certain enzymes, some of which produce further chemical messengers.

Spirulina is the designation commonly, but incorrectly, used for several types of cyanobacteria (blue-green algae) belonging to the Oscillatoriaceae family. The algae used for dietary supplements and animal feed belong to the genus *Arthrospira*. In order to avoid confusion, we will follow the common practice of calling them *Spirulina* rather than *Arthrospira*. Three species of these algae have been used in the experiments described here: *S. platensis*, *S. fusiformis*, and *S. maxima*.

Spirulina contains approximately 60% protein, a variety of polysaccharides, essential fatty acids, vitamins and minerals, and phenolic compounds. One of the major proteins in *Spirulina* (15%–20% of algal dry weight) is C-phycocyanin, which consists of the apoprotein and covalently attached phycocyanobilin chromophores, which are responsible for the blue coloring of these cyanobacteria. In addition to whole *Spirulina*, some of its polysaccharide fractions and C-phycocyanin have been investigated for their ability to influence immune functions.

SPIRULINA AND THE INNATE IMMUNE SYSTEM

MACROPHAGE PHAGOCYTOSIS

Spirulina has been reported to inhibit tumorigenesis in experimental animals and to induce the regression of existing tumors.[1–4] There are indications that one of the mechanisms involved in this protective effect is the stimulation of innate immune responses, in particular macrophage phagocytosis and production of chemokines and cytokines.

In vitro, addition of *Spirulina* to macrophages obtained from the lung of cats significantly raised the percentage of phagocytic macrophages without affecting the number of particles that each of these macrophages engulfed.[5] Similarly, in chicks that had received *Spirulina* as part of their diet (10–10,000 ppm) for 3 or 7 weeks, the proportion of phagocytic macrophages was significantly increased compared to unsupplemented controls.[6] The number of ingested particles per phagocytic macrophage was not significantly affected. In another study, however, dietary supplementation of chicks with 0.5%, 1.0%, or 2.0% *Spirulina* for 14, 35, or 42 days significantly enhanced not only the percentage of macrophages involved in phagocytosis but also the number of phagocytosed particles per macrophage.[7] These macrophages also exhibited significantly greater lipopolysaccharide (LPS)-induced production of nitrite than those obtained from unsupplemented animals.[7] Spontaneous nitrite production (in the absence of LPS or other stimuli) was also markedly higher in macrophages from many of the *Spirulina*-treated groups compared to controls, although the difference did not always reach statistical significance. Nitrite measures the synthesis of nitric oxide. This molecule, along with other reactive nitrogen and oxygen species, plays an important role in the killing of the pathogens that have been engulfed through phagocytosis.

The results of another study suggest that dietary *S. platensis* also significantly increases the phagocytic activity of peritoneal macrophages in mice.[8] Note that *Spirulina* constituted 10% or 20% of the diet in this experiment, and no adjustments were made for the high content of protein and other essential nutrients in *Spirulina*. Food intake and body weight gain were almost identical in the control group and the two groups who received different dietary levels of this alga. However, many of the individual nutrients of *Spirulina* are known to enhance immune functions. Therefore, it cannot be ruled out that the overall improvement in the nutrient composition of the diet rather than specific immunomodulatory substances in *Spirulina* were responsible for the observed effects, which included enhanced antibody production by B cells and increased proliferation of T cells (discussed below).

In contrast to whole *Spirulina*, perfusion of mouse liver with C-phycocyanin was associated with a concentration-dependent decrease in phagocytosis by Kupffer cells, the resident macrophages in the liver.[9] There has also been a report that phycocyanin inhibited the respiratory burst associated with neutrophil phagocytosis.[10] It is not clear, however, whether phycocyanin suppressed phagocytosis or rather neutralized the resulting reactive oxygen species through its ability to scavenge free radicals, which was demonstrated in this and other studies.[10,11] In addition, it has been reported that phycocyanin induced a murine macrophage cell line to undergo apoptosis.[12]

MACROPHAGE CHEMOKINE AND CYTOKINE PRODUCTION

Macrophages are the main source of several cytokines that promote the inflammatory response and, therefore, are collectively referred to as proinflammatory cytokines. Two of the main representatives of this group are tumor necrosis factor (TNF)-α and interleukin (IL)-1. *In vitro*, a hot water extract of *Spirulina*, containing 36% protein (compared to 60% in whole algae) and 10% polysaccharides, enhanced the IL-1 activity in mouse peritoneal macrophages.[8] When human peripheral blood mononuclear cells, that is, immune cells obtained from the circulation, were stimulated with the soluble fraction of a *Spirulina* dietary supplement, IL-1β production was increased twofold compared to incubation in medium alone.[13] The combination of the mitogen PHA with *Spirulina* resulted in even greater stimulation of IL-1β synthesis.

Injections of a mixture of *Spirulina* and Dunaliella algae into hamster buccal pouches with established tumors resulted in significant tumor regression, and this was associated with a marked increase in the number of TNF-α-producing cells in the affected pouches.[3] These cells were mostly macrophages and were located primarily adjacent to the regressing carcinomas.

In vitro, a high-molecular-weight polysaccharide fraction from *Spirulina*-induced transcription (mRNA production) of IL-1β and TNF-α in a human monocyte cell line.[14,15] It also increased mRNA levels of several chemokines, that is, small proteins involved in attracting specific subsets of immune cells to sites of inflammation.[15] However, the authors were unable to show changes in the protein concentrations of IL-1β, TNF-α and most of these chemokines with the exception of IL-8 and macrophage inflammatory protein 1β.[15]

In contrast to the results obtained with *Spirulina* and its polysaccharides, pretreatment of rats with an intraperitoneal (ip) injection of phycocyanin almost completely inhibited the 82-fold increase in serum TNF-α concentrations induced by treatment with thyroid hormone, a model of oxidative stress in the liver.[9] Similarly, in mice, oral administration of phycocyanin 1 h before injection of LPS, a bacterial cell wall component that is known to induce high levels of proinflammatory cytokines, dose-dependently and significantly reduced the LPS-induced increase in serum TNF-α levels, with significant inhibition occurring at doses ≥ 100 mg/kg.[16] Of note, phycocyanin alone did not markedly affect serum TNF-α concentrations.

Together these results suggest that whole *Spirulina* enhances macrophage functions, such as phagocytosis and production of chemokines and cytokines. This effect may be attributable at least partially to the polysaccharide fraction. In contrast, the available data suggest that C-phycocyanin down-regulates these macrophage activities.

INFLAMMATION

Inflammation is characterized by pain, redness, swelling, and heat. These symptoms result from the activities of cytokines and chemokines along with a variety of other vasoactive and inflammatory mediators such as histamine, prostaglandins, and leukotrienes, but also reactive oxygen and nitrogen species. They mainly target local blood vessels, where they enhance blood flow, induce vasodilation, and increase the permeability of vessel walls. These changes allow fluids and plasma proteins to leak into the affected tissue. Cytokines also induce the expression of molecules that make it possible for immune cells to pass between the cells lining the blood vessels and to enter the affected tissue. Together, these alterations result in the infiltration of immune cells into the site of inflammation.

Inflammatory responses have a vital role in the protection of an organism against invading pathogens. However, many of the substances released during inflammatory responses harm not only invading microbes but also surrounding host cells, and prolonged (chronic) inflammation is generally associated with major tissue damage. Therefore, it is desirable to have substances that can minimize or prevent chronic inflammatory processes as well as inappropriate inflammatory reactions, such as those resulting from allergies against innocuous substances.

Although *Spirulina* can stimulate the production of some of the major proinflammatory cytokines, TNF-α and IL-1, there have been several investigations of its ability to inhibit inflammatory reactions. Even more data are available on the anti-inflammatory activities of phycocyanin.

Prostaglandins and Leukotrienes

One important group of inflammatory mediators are the prostaglandins and leukotrienes. They are the products of enzymatic pathways involving cyclooxygenase (COX) and lipoxygenase (LOX), respectively. It is the inducible isoform COX-2, rather than the constitutively expressed COX-1 that is responsible for the production of prostaglandins during inflammatory reactions.

A high-molecular-weight polysaccharide fraction of *Spirulina* induced COX-2 mRNA expression in a monocyte cell line.[15] In contrast, phycocyanin was shown to selectively inhibit COX-2 activity *in vitro*,[17] and to reduce the LPS-induced production of prostaglandin E2 in a mouse macrophage cell line, without affecting LPS-induced COX-2 protein expression.[12] In addition, oral administration of phycocyanin dose dependently decreased the concentrations of leukotriene B4 and prostaglandin E2 in inflamed tissue in mouse models of inflammation.[18,19] Furthermore, phycocyanin administered orally 1 h before induction of inflammation inhibited several types of acute and subchronic inflammatory responses.[20] Consistent with the ability of phycocyanin to inhibit prostaglandin and leukotriene synthesis, inhibition was greatest in models where inflammation is thought to be mediated predominantly by products of the COX and LOX pathways. Studies of the anti-inflammatory activities of phycocyanin and *Spirulina* are summarized in Table 8.1.

Reactive Oxygen and Nitrogen Species

Inflammatory responses are accompanied by markedly increased production of reactive oxygen species. Oxidative stress, in turn, induces the transcription of numerous genes encoding proinflammatory mediators or the enzymes producing them. Both *Spirulina* and phycocyanin can scavenge peroxyl, hydroxyl, alkoxyl, and superoxide radicals and have been shown to act as antioxidants *in vivo* and to induce enzymes that participate in the defense against oxidative damage.[21]

TABLE 8.1
Studies on the Anti-Inflammatory Effects of Orally Administered *Spirulina* and Phycocyanin

Model	Compound	Doses(s) (mg/kg)	Dosing schedule	Animals	Results of *Spirulina*- or phycocyanin-treated group compared to controls	Reference
Mouse ear inflammation induced by arachidonic acid	Phycocyanin	50, 100, or 200	1 h before topical application of arachidonic acid	OF1 mice	Dose-dependent inhibition of ear edema (maximum inhibition ~70%); inhibition of prostaglandin E2 levels in the inflamed ear; inhibition of leukotriene B4 levels in the inflamed ear	20 18, 19
Mouse ear inflammation induced by TPA	Phycocyanin	100, 200, or 300	1 h before topical application of TPA	OF1 mice	Dose-dependent inhibition (maximum 46%) of ear edema; dose-dependent reduction (maximum 47%) of myeloperoxidase activity as a marker of neutrophil infiltration	20
Carrageenan-induced rat paw edema	Phycocyanin	50, 100, or 200	1 h before carrageenan injection	Sprague Dawley rats	No inhibition of edema (increase in paw thickness) at 50 mg/kg, but significant inhibition with 100 and 200 mg/kg (maximum 44%)	20
Cotton pellet granuloma	Phycocyanin	50, 100, or 200	Once daily for 7 days after implantation of cotton pellets	Sprague Dawley rats	No inhibition at 50 mg/kg, but 30% and 36% inhibition (reduction of granuloma weight) with 100 and 200 mg/kg, respectively	20

Condition	Compound	Dose	Animal	Effect	Ref.
Adjuvant-induced arthritis	*S. fusiformis*	800	Swiss albino mice	Decreased paw volume; lower lysosomal enzyme activities (as a marker of inflammation) in plasma, liver, and spleen; reduced protein-bound carbohydrates (as a measure of tissue damage)	24
Zymosan-induced arthritis	Spirulan®	100 or 400	OF1 mice	Once daily for 9 days (Days 4–12 after zymosan injection). Prevention of joint destruction or pannus formation and reduction in bone erosion; attenuated joint inflammation (infiltration); decreased β-glucuronidase activity in the synovial fluid	25
Zymosan-induced arthritis	Phycocyanin	25, 50, or 100	OF1 mice	Once daily for 8 days (Days 4–12 after zymosan injection). Prevention of joint destruction or pannus formation and pronounced reduction in bone erosion; attenuated joint inflammation (infiltration); dose-dependent inhibition of β-glucuronidase activity in the synovial fluid	26
Acetic acid-induced colitis	Phycocyanin	150, 200, or 300	Wistar rats	30 min before acetic acid enema. Inhibition of inflammatory cell infiltration of colonic tissue; decreased myeloperoxidase activity, indicating reduction of neutrophil infiltration; reduced damage score	27

Dosing column: Adjuvant-induced arthritis — Once daily for 8 days (days 11–18 after injection of Freund's adjuvant).

a TPA = 12-*O*-tetradecanoyl-phorbol-13-acetate.

Although nitric oxide produced during inflammatory responses by the inducible form of nitric oxide synthase (iNOS) plays a vital role in the killing of intracellular pathogens, excessive levels can have harmful effects, particularly in the systemic circulation. The effects of *Spirulina* and phycocyanin on systemic production of nitric oxide, measured as serum nitrite concentrations, contrast with those described above in macrophages.[7] *Spirulina* given orally to mice did not affect serum nitrite levels by itself, but inhibited the gentamycin-induced increase in serum nitrite concentrations in a dose-dependent manner.[22] Similar results were obtained in animals treated with cisplatin.[23] Oral administration of phycocyanin 1 h before intraperitoneal injection of LPS dose dependently and significantly reduced the LPS-induced rise in serum nitrite levels.[16] Similarly, intraperitoneal administration of phycocyanin significantly reversed the increase in serum nitrite concentrations resulting from the administration of thyroid hormone.[9] In addition, it inhibited the concomitant increase in liver iNOS activity to the levels seen in control animals.

Animal Models of Inflammatory Diseases

Rheumatoid arthritis is an autoimmune disease characterized by chronic inflammation of various joints, resulting in joint erosion. In an animal model of rheumatoid arthritis, oral administration of *S. fusiformis* (800 mg/kg per day) from Day 11 to Day 18 after arthritis induction resulted in significant suppression of inflammation[24] (see also Table 8.1). In a different model *Spirulina* given orally for 8 days, starting 4 days after induction of arthritis, also significantly reduced inflammation and joint destruction.[25] The higher dose (400 mg/kg) provided markedly better protection than the lower dose (100 mg/kg), but both were significantly less effective than the reference compound, triamcinolone. Orally administered phycocyanin at doses of 25, 50, or 100 mg/kg significantly inhibited inflammation and structural joint damage in the same model.[26] Note that four-fold higher doses of *Spirulina* were required to obtain similar anti-inflammatory effects as seen after treatment with phycocyanin. Since phycocyanin constitutes ~20% of *Spirulina* dry weight, these observations are consistent with the hypothesis that phycocyanin is mainly responsible for the anti-inflammatory activity of this alga in experimental arthritis. However, that still leaves the question of why the anti-inflammatory effects of phycocyanin in *Spirulina* predominate in this model whereas the proinflammatory activity of other constituents prevails in others.

Orally administered phycocyanin also showed anti-inflammatory activity in acetic acid-induced colitis, an animal model of inflammatory bowel disease.[27] Pretreatment with various doses of phycocyanin 30 min before the induction of colitis dose dependently inhibited both inflammation and histological damage. It also markedly reduced myeloperoxidase activity, a marker of neutrophil infiltration, which has been shown to correlate with the severity of the damage to the intestinal mucosa.

ALLERGIC INFLAMMATION

Allergic inflammation involves the same types of mediators as other inflammatory responses, but they are induced by IgE antibodies binding to mast cells and thereby triggering the release of preformed and newly synthesized inflammatory agents from these cells. Among these agents, the histamine plays a central role. Anaphylaxis is a severe and potentially life-threatening systemic allergic reaction caused by IgE-mediated release of mediators from mast cells and basophils. Like other allergic reactions, anaphylaxis requires previous sensitization to the triggering antigen.

Spirulina or phycocyanin supplementation does not enhance sensitization to allergens, as demonstrated by the findings that antigen-specific IgE levels do not differ significantly in different unsupplemented and supplemented animals sensitized to either shrimp extract or ovalbumin (OVA).[28,29] Prolonged supplementation with phycocyanin may even suppress antigen-specific IgE production.[29]

There is growing evidence that, once allergic sensitization has occurred, *Spirulina* and phycocyanin can reduce the inflammatory response to allergen exposure *in vitro* and in animals. *In vitro*, brief preincubation of rat peritoneal mast cells with *S. platensis* was shown to result in significant inhibition of histamine release and TNF-α production mediated by IgE or compound 48/80, a histamine-releasing agent.[30] At a concentration of 1 μg/mL, *Spirulina* yielded 80% and 60% inhibition of IgE-mediated and 48/80-induced histamine release, respectively. Methanolic extracts of the same *Spirulina* species also inhibited compound 48/80-induced histamine release in another study.[31] Interestingly, after size fractionation, most fractions exhibited significant inhibitory activity. This suggests that *Spirulina* contains diverse agents capable of suppressing mast cell histamine release. Other researchers showed that one of these constituents is phycocyanin, which dose dependently inhibited compound 48/80-induced histamine release from rat peritoneal mast cells.[32] Note that the concentration required to obtain ~60% inhibition was three orders of magnitude higher than the effective dose of whole *Spirulina* in the previously discussed study (3 mg/mL vs. 1 μg/mL).[30] This lends further support to the suggestion that *Spirulina* contains several constituents capable of inhibiting the release of histamine from mast cells, at least *in vitro*.

When *S. platensis* powder suspended in saline was injected intraperitoneally 1 h before the induction of systemic anaphylaxis with compound 48/80, it dose dependently reduced mortality in rats.[30,33] *Spirulina* products from two providers were used in these studies and exhibited different effectiveness, one providing complete protection at doses ≥500 mg/kg,[30] and the other preventing mortality at doses ≥100 mg/kg.[33] In one of these studies, prevention of anaphylaxis was associated with a significant and dose-dependent decrease in serum histamine concentrations,[33] suggesting that the inhibition of histamine release constituted a major antianaphylactic mechanism. In the same study, *Spirulina* inhibited passive cutaneous anaphylaxis induced by local injection of anti-DNP IgE and intravenous antigen challenge.

Oral pretreatment with phycocyanin significantly reduced the IgE-mediated inflammatory response (ear swelling) to intracutaneous challenge with OVA following intraperitoneal sensitization.[32] It also inhibited myeloperoxidase activity, a marker of neutrophil infiltration. This may have been due to the ability of phycocyanin to reduce the production of leukotriene B4,[18] a substance that attracts neutrophils to the site of inflammation. Note, however, that phycocyanin at doses of 100–300 mg/kg was a much weaker inhibitor than the reference compound triamcinolone at 10 mg/kg. In another experiment reported in the same paper, oral phycocyanin dampened the skin reactions resulting from injection of histamine or of the histamine-releasing compound 48/80. This suggests that prevention of histamine release is not the only mechanism by which phycocyanin, and possibly also *Spirulina*, protect from allergic inflammation.

The cytokine IL-4 is known to play a central role in the production of IgE antibodies by B cells and the activation of several other cell types involved in the processes that lead to allergic symptoms. When peripheral blood mononuclear cells from healthy volunteers were incubated with the soluble fraction of a *Spirulina* supplement, their IL-4 production was significantly increased compared to cells incubated in medium alone.[13] The mitogen PHA induced markedly higher levels of this cytokine, and these were further enhanced (by up to fourfold) in the presence of *Spirulina*. This suggested the possibility that this alga could enhance allergic reactions. However, incubation with *Spirulina* alone also resulted in a 13-fold increase in IFN-γ synthesis and in combination with PHA induced significantly greater production of this cytokine than seen with PHA alone. IFN-γ can antagonize many of the functions of IL-4, and it is the ratio between these two cytokines, rather than their absolute levels, that determines the nature of the immune response. Nevertheless, the increase in IFN-γ production, though pronounced, was not statistically significant owing to high variability in the responses of individual subjects. This suggests that, in some individuals, the ability of *Spirulina* to induce IFN-γ production might not be strong enough to counterbalance the rise in IL-4.

In a recent placebo-controlled trial, 36 patients with allergic rhinitis were assigned to one of three groups receiving 1000 mg/d or 2000 mg/d of a *Spirulina*-based dietary supplement or placebo, respectively.[34] Before and after 12 weeks of supplementation, the ability of peripheral blood mononuclear cells, to produce certain cytokines in response to stimulation (with PHA) was examined. The higher, but not the lower, dose of *Spirulina* was associated with a significant reduction in the secretion of IL-4 compared to the baseline values of this group. Two other cytokines that could oppose the production of IL-4, IL-2, and IFN-γ, were not significantly affected by consumption of *Spirulina*. It remains to be established whether the discrepancies between the *in vitro* and *in vivo* cytokine responses are due to differential effects of *Spirulina* in healthy and allergic subjects or to differences between *in vitro* and *in vivo* conditions.

NK Cells

Natural killer (NK) cells represent another arm of the innate immune system. One of their main functions is to kill virus-infected cells, and they also play an important role in the destruction of certain types of tumor cells. Newly hatched chicks whose diet was supplemented with *Spirulina* for 7 weeks exhibited significantly enhanced NK cell cytotoxic activity compared to unsupplemented controls.[6] Oral administration of a hot water extract of *Spirulina* to four human volunteers for 4 weeks markedly increased the cytolytic activity of NK cells in two of them, but did not further augment it in the two other subjects, who exhibited high NK activity at baseline.[35] NK cells are an important source of interferon (IFN)-γ, a cytokine that activates macrophages and induces other immune responses vital for the elimination of intracellular pathogens. *Spirulina* supplementation was associated with significant production of IFN-γ by NK cells after stimulation with IL-12 and with even higher responses to the combination of IL-12 and IL-18. Both are well known inducers of IFN-γ, but were unable to elicit detectable levels of this cytokine in NK cells obtained before supplementation with *Spirulina*.

SPIRULINA IN ADAPTIVE IMMUNE RESPONSES

ANTIBODY PRODUCTION BY B CELLS

There are several studies investigating the effect of *Spirulina* on the antibody production by B cells in response to immunization (primary immune response) and challenge (secondary immune response) with a specific antigen. In the earliest of these studies, mice were fed diets containing 10% or 20% of *S. platensis*, immunized with sheep red blood cells after 7 weeks, and challenged after 9 weeks.[8] *Spirulina* feeding significantly increased the number of IgM antibody-producing cells in the spleen during the primary immune response, but had little effect on the synthesis of IgG antibodies during the secondary immune response. As discussed previously, this study suffers from the lack of adjustment for the higher protein and essential nutrient content of the *Spirulina*-supplemented diets.

In contrast, another group of researchers reported that *Spirulina* enhanced antigen-specific antibody production during the secondary, but not the primary, immune response.[6] In their experiments, newly hatched chicks received diets containing between 10 and 10,000 ppm of *Spirulina* for 3 or 7 weeks. Significantly higher antigen-specific antibody production (IgM and IgG) was seen at all dose levels of *Spirulina* in the strain treated for 7 weeks. In another strain supplemented for only 3 weeks, there was a significant increase in antigen-specific IgG only at the highest dose level (10,000 ppm).

Another study examined whether a hot water extract of *S. platensis* could affect experimental food allergy.[28] Note that the previous data from these investigators suggest that hot water extracts contain less protein and possibly higher concentrations of polysaccharides compared to whole *Spirulina*.[8] One group of mice received *S. platensis* one of two concentrations of the extract in their drinking water before they were immunized with, and then orally exposed to, shrimp extract. Another group was given *Spirulina* extract concomitantly with immunization and antigen stimulation. Concurrent *Spirulina* treatment did not significantly affect total and antigen-specific IgE concentrations in serum, indicating that it did not enhance the allergic response to this food antigen.[28] At the higher dose, *Spirulina* treatment significantly enhanced total serum levels of IgG1, the most common subclass of IgG, whereas the increase in antigen-specific IgG1 did not reach statistical significance. It also resulted in significantly greater total, but not antigen-specific, IgA levels in the intestinal contents. IgA is the antibody associated with mucosal surfaces. Since these are the major entry sites for many bacteria and viruses, secretory IgA is of central importance in the protection against these pathogens by preventing their adherence to, and penetration of, the epithelium, neutralizing toxins, and preventing viral multiplication.

In mice that received *Spirulina* extract before immunization and stimulation with shrimp antigens, IgA and IgG1 antibody production was examined in various lymphoid tissues.[28] Animals supplemented with the higher dose of *Spirulina* exhibited a marked increase in total, but not antigen-specific, IgA in the spleen and mesenteric lymph nodes, whereas such an increase was not observed in Peyer's patches. Mesenteric lymph nodes are the lymphatics of the colon, while Peyer's patches are lymph nodes in the intestinal wall near the junction of the ileum and colon. In contrast, total and antigen-specific IgG1 production in spleen and mesenteric lymph nodes did not differ significantly between supplemented and unsupplemented animals. These findings further underscore the ability of *Spirulina* to enhance the production of protective IgA antibodies overall without increasing the antigen-specific IgA response.

When mice were fed with a crude polysaccharide fraction of *Spirulina* for at least 4 days, cultured Peyer's patch cells isolated from these animals secreted significantly higher levels of IgA, and these levels were further increased after an additional day of supplementation.[36] The synthesis of IL-6 was also markedly increased in these cultures and the time course paralleled that of IgA production. This is consistent with the known ability of this cytokine to induce IgA synthesis in B cells. These findings suggest that polysaccharides participate in the stimulation of nonantigen-specific IgA production.

The effects of phycocyanin on antibody production have also been examined. Six weeks of supplementation with phycocyanin in the drinking water, resulting in a daily intake of ~57.5 mg/kg, was associated with an eightfold increase of antigen-specific IgA in Peyer's patches in response to immunization and rechallenge with ovalbumin (OVA).[29] Antigen-specific IgA was not seen in mesenteric lymph nodes of immunized animals that did not receive phycocyanin, but was markedly induced in mesenteric lymph nodes of supplemented animals. In the intestinal mucosa, treatment with phycocyanin substantially increased both total and OVA-specific IgA, whereas only the enhancement of total IgA reached statistical significance in the spleen. Splenic antigen-specific, but not total, IgG1 synthesis was significantly augmented in phycocyanin-treated animals. As had been observed with the hot water extract of whole *Spirulina*, supplementation with phycocyanin for 6 weeks did not significantly alter the antigen-specific IgE and IgG1 levels. Interestingly, when another strain of mice was supplemented for 6 weeks, the same results were obtained. However, extending the treatment with phycocyanin over a period of 8 weeks resulted in marked reduction in serum concentrations of OVA-specific IgE and IgG1. The levels of total and antigen-specific IgA in the intestinal mucosa were not affected by extended treatment.

Together, these results suggest that neither *Spirulina* nor its polysaccharides nor phycocyanin significantly affect the induction of antigen-specific IgE, suggesting little potential to increase allergic sensitization. All three fractions are able to markedly enhance total, but not antigen-specific IgA levels. This is likely to provide increased protection from invading pathogens.

Effect on T Cells

In vitro, a hot-water extract of *S. platensis* dose dependently induced the proliferation of mouse spleen cells, but not thymus cells.[8] Together with the observation that the *Spirulina* extract enhanced macrophage functions, including phagocytosis and IL-1 production, these results suggested that *Spirulina* did not affect T cell function directly, but through activation of macrophages. In the same investigation, spleen cells from mice fed diets containing 10% or 20% *Spirulina* extract also exhibited significantly increased proliferation in response to T-cell mitogens, but not to a B-cell mitogen. Similarly, dietary supplementation of newly hatched chicks with *Spirulina* for 7 weeks significantly enhanced T lymphocyte proliferation at the highest dose provided (10,000 ppm), but not at 10 or 100 ppm.[6] No significant effect on lymphoproliferation was seen in another strain of chicks supplemented for 3 weeks only.

Dietary administration of a crude polysaccharide fraction of *Spirulina* significantly augmented the secretion of INF-γ by spleen cells starting 3 days after the beginning of supplementation, with further incremental increases seen after one and two additional days.[36] The cellular source was not determined but is likely to be T cells or NK cells.

Spirulina and the Generation of Immune Cells (Hematopoiesis)

It was recently shown that a hot water extract of *S. platensis*, phycocyanin, and a cell wall extract (presumably containing mostly polysaccharides) all induced proliferation in bone marrow cells.[37] When spleen or peritoneal-exudate cells were incubated with these extracts, the culture supernatants induced colony formation in bone marrow cells. Each colony represents the progeny of a single precursor or stem cell. This ability seemed to be at least partly attributable to the induction of granulocyte-macrophage colony-stimulating factor (GM-CSF) and IL-3. Serum and supernatant from cultures of lymphoid organs obtained from mice that had been orally treated with the different *Spirulina* extracts also induced significant colony formation in bone marrow cells. Even greater induction was obtained with serum from mice that had received the extracts intraperitoneally. Note, however, that serum from these mice reportedly did not contain detectable levels of GM-CSF or IL-3.

Absorption of *Spirulina* Constituents

Several different polysaccharide fractions have been isolated from *Spirulina*, some of them with molecular weights exceeding 10 million Da.[14,38] These polysaccharides were shown to exhibit biological activities, such as immunomodulation and enhancement of hematopoiesis, not only *in vitro* but also after oral administration.[36-38] This is consistent with the findings that oral administration of certain mushroom polysaccharides can enhance immune functions and inhibit carcinogenesis.[39] Other fungal polysaccharides, however, are ineffective when given orally, although they show significant biological activity after intravenous or intraperitoneal administration. Humans and many animals can digest certain types of polysaccharides into small fragments or even their individual sugar constituents and subsequently absorb these oligo- or monosaccharides. It seems highly unlikely that such small fragments retain any biological activity. Many other plant, fungal, and bacterial polysaccharides are indigestible for humans and many animals because of the lack of the enzymes capable of breaking the types of linkages between individual sugars within these macromolecules.

It had long been thought that the inability to digest polysaccharides would prevent their absorption completely and that they would simply be excreted. The question then arises as to how these polysaccharides exert their effects after oral administration. Several groups of researchers demonstrated that, following the oral intake of some indigestible polysaccharides, fragments as large as 20,000 Da, (approximately 150 monosaccharides) reach the circulation.[39] However, the biological activity of polysaccharides *in vitro* and *in vivo* frequently declines with decreasing molecular weight,[39] as has also been demonstrated for certain activities of a *Spirulina* polysaccharide fraction.[40] An alternative explanation could be that contact between polysaccharides and intestinal epithelial cells or cellular components of the gut-associated lymphoid tissue ultimately results in the priming or activation of other immune cells. These activated cells could subsequently migrate to other tissues and thereby exert systemic immunomodulatory effects.

It also remains to be established how phycocyanin exerts biological activities *in vivo* since proteins are generally broken down into individual amino acids or small oligopeptides before absorption. The phycocyanobilin chromophore, however, structurally resembles the bile pigment bilirubin, which can be absorbed from any part of the small or large intestine as long as it remains unconjugated. This would suggest that the phycocyanobilin part of phycocyanin is mainly responsible for the antioxidant and anti-inflammatory effects seen after oral administration of phycocyanin. This is supported by the observation that this chromophore accounts for much of the radical scavenging and antioxidant properties of phycocyanin and *Spirulina*.[41]

CONCLUDING REMARKS

The data discussed here indicate that, in animals, *Spirulina* is able to stimulate a variety of immune functions, including macrophage phagocytosis and production of cytokines, chemokines and other inflammatory mediators, NK cell activity, B cell antibody production, and T cell proliferation and possibly cytokine secretion. Despite its ability to induce proinflammatory cytokines, *Spirulina* has also been shown to significantly inhibit inflammatory responses in a variety of animal models, including models of rheumatoid arthritis, colitis, and IgE-mediated local and systemic allergic reactions. This may indicate that *Spirulina* possesses truly immunomodulatory activities, enhancing suboptimal immune responses, while dampening immune system hyperactivity. Acute and chronic toxicity studies in animals indicate that *Spirulina* does not pose a health risk,[21] and isolated reports of possible adverse effects in humans are not clearly attributable to the consumption of *Spirulina*.[42,43] The US Food and Drug Administration (FDA) granted dried biomass of *Arthrospira platensis* GRAS (generally regarded as safe) status in 2003.[44] Little information is available on the effects of *Spirulina* supplementation on the human immune system. The few existing data suggest that it may be able to modulate immune functions in both healthy and allergic subjects.

REFERENCES

1. Schwartz, J., Shklar, G., Reid, S., and Trickler, D. 1988. Prevention of experimental oral cancer by extracts of *Spirulina-Dunaliella* algae. *Nutr Cancer* 11:127–134.
2. Schwartz, J., and Shklar, G. 1987. Regression of experimental hamster cancer by beta carotene and algae extracts. *J Oral Maxillofac Surg* 45:510–515.
3. Shklar, G., and Schwartz, J. 1988. Tumor necrosis factor in experimental cancer regression with alphatocopherol, beta-carotene, canthaxanthin and algae extract. *Eur J Cancer Clin Oncol* 24:839–850.
4. Dasgupta, T., Banerjee, S., Yadav, P.K., and Rao, A.R. 2001. Chemomodulation of carcinogen metabolising enzymes, antioxidant profiles and skin and forestomach papillomagenesis by *Spirulina platensis*. *Mol Cell Biochem* 226:27–38.
5. Qureshi, M.A., and Ali, R.A. 1996. *Spirulina platensis* exposure enhances macrophage phagocytic function in cats. *Immunopharmacol Immunotoxicol* 18:457–463.
6. Qureshi, M.A., Garlich, J.D., and Kidd, M.T. 1996. Dietary *Spirulina platensis* enhances humoral and cell-mediated immune functions in chickens. *Immunopharmacol Immunotoxicol* 18:465–476.
7. Al-Batshan, H.A., Al-Mufarrej, S.I., Al-Homaidan, A.A., and Qureshi, M.A. 2001. Enhancement of chicken macrophage phagocytic function and nitrite production by dietary *Spirulina platensis*. *Immunopharmacol Immunotoxicol* 23:281–289.
8. Hayashi, O., Katoh, T., and Okuwaki, Y. 1994. Enhancement of antibody production in mice by dietary *Spirulina platensis*. *J Nutr Sci Vitaminol (Tokyo)* 40:431–441.
9. Remirez, D., Fernández, V., Tapia, G., González, R., and Videla, L.A. 2002. Influence of C-phycocyanin on hepatocellular parameters related to liver oxidative stress and Kupffer cell functioning. *Inflamm Res* 5:351–356.
10. Romay, C., Armesto, J., Remirez, D., González, R., Ledon, N., and García, I. 1998. Antioxidant and anti-inflammatory properties of C-phycocyanin from blue-green algae. *Inflamm Res* 47:36–41.
11. Bhat, V.B., and Madyastha, K.M. 2000. C-phycocyanin: a potent peroxyl radical scavenger *in vivo* and *in vitro*. *Biochem Biophys Res Commun* 275:20–25.
12. Reddy, M.C., Subhashini, J., Mahipal, S.V., Bhat, V.B., Srinivas Reddy, P., Kiranmai, G., Madyastha, K.M., and Reddanna, P. 2003. C-Phycocyanin, a selective cyclooxygenase-2 inhibitor, induces apoptosis in lipopolysaccharide-stimulated RAW 264.7 macrophages. *Biochem Biophys Res Commun* 304:385–392.
13. Mao, T.K., Van de Water, J., and Gershwin, M.E. 2000. Effect of *Spirulina* on the secretion of cytokines from peripheral blood mononuclear cells. *J Med Food* 3:135–140.
14. Pugh, N., Ross, S.A., ElSohly, H.N., ElSohly, M.A., and Pasco, D.S. 2001. Isolation of three high molecular weight polysaccharide preparations with potent immunostimulatory activity from *Spirulina platensis*, *Aphanizomenon flos-aquae* and *Chlorella pyrenoidosa*. *Planta Med* 67:737–742.
15. Grzanna, R., Polotsky, A., Phan, P.V., Pugh, N., Pasco, D., and Frondoza, C.G. 2006. Immolina, a high-molecular-weight polysaccharide fraction of *Spirulina*, enhances chemokine expression in human monocytic THP-1 cells. *J Altern Complement Med* 12:429–435.
16. Romay, C., Delgado, R., Remirez, D., Gonzalez, R., and Rojas, A. 2001. Effects of phycocyanin extract on tumor necrosis factor-a and nitrite levels in serum of mice treated with endotoxin. *Arzneimittelforschung* 51:733–736.

17. Reddy, C.M., Bhat, V.B., Kiranmai, G., Reddy, M.N., Reddanna, P., and Mady-astha, K.M. 2000. Selective inhibition of cyclooxygenase-2 by C-phycocyanin, a biliprotein from *Spirulina platensis*. *Biochem Biophys Res Commun* 277:599–603.

18. Romay, C., Ledon, N., and Gonzalez, R. 1999. Phycocyanin extract reduces leuko-triene B4 levels in arachidonic acid-induced mouse-ear inflammation test. *J Pharm Pharmacol* 51:641–642.

19. Romay, C., Ledon, N., and Gonzalez, R. 2000. Effects of phycocyanin extract on prostaglandin E2 levels in mouse ear inflammation test. *Arzneimittelforschung* 50:1106–1109.

20. Romay, C., Ledon, N., and Gonzalez, R. 1998. Further studies on anti-inflammatory activity of phycocyanin in some animal models of inflammation. *Inflamm Res* 47:334–338.

21. Belay, A. 2002. The potential application of *Spirulina* (*Arthrospira*) as a nutritional and therapeutic supplement in health management. *JANA* (*Journal of the American Nutraceutical Association*) 5:27–48.

22. Kuhad, A., Tirkey, N., Pilkhwal, S., and Chopra, K. 2006. Effect of *Spirulina*, a blue-green algae, on gentamicin-induced oxidative stress and renal dysfunction in rats. *Fundam Clin Pharmacol* 20:121–128.

23. Kuhad, A., Tirkey, N., Pilkhwal, S., and Chopra, K. 2006. Renoprotective effect of *Spirulina fusiformis* on cisplatin-induced oxidative stress and renal dysfunction in rats. *Ren Fail* 28:247–254.

24. Rasool, M., Sabina, E.P., and Lavanya, B. 2006. Anti-inflammatory effect of *Spirulina fusiformis* on adjuvant-induced arthritis in mice. *Biol Pharm Bull* 29:2483–2487.

25. Remirez, D., González, R., Merino, N., Rodríguez, S., and Ancheta, O. 2002. Inhib-itory effects of *Spirulina* in zymosan-induced arthritis in mice. *Mediators Inflamm* 11:75–79.

26. Remirez, D., González, A., Merino, N., González, R., Ancheta, O., Romay, C., and Rodríguez, S. 1999. Effect of phycocyanin in zymosan-induced arthritis in mice— phycocyanin as an antiarthritic compound. *Drug Dev Res* 48:70–75.

27. González, R., Rodríguez, S., Romay, C., Ancheta, O., González, A., Armesto, J., Remirez, D., and Merino, N. 1999. Anti-inflammatory activity of phycocyanin extract in acetic acid-induced colitis in rats. *Pharmacol Res* 39:55–59.

28. Hayashi, O., Hirahashi, T., Katoh, T., Miyajima, H., Hirano, T., and Okuwaki, Y. 1998. Class specific influence of dietary *Spirulina platensis* on antibody production in mice. *J Nutr Sci Vitaminol* (*Tokyo*) 44:841–851.

29. Nemoto-Kawamura, C., Hirahashi, T., Nagai, T., Yamada, H., Katoh, T., and Hayashi, O. 2004. Phycocyanin enhances secretary IgA antibody response and suppresses aller-gic IgE antibody response in mice immunized with antigen-entrapped biodegradable microparticles. *J Nutr Sci Vitaminol* (*Tokyo*) 50:129–136.

30. Yang, H.N., Lee, E.H., and Kim, H.M. 1997. *Spirulina platensis* inhibits anaphylactic reaction. *Life Sci* 61:1237–1244.

31. Price, J.A., III, Sanny, C., and Shevlin, D. 2002. Inhibition of mast cells by algae. *J Med Food* 5:205–210.

32. Remirez, D., Ledón, N., and González, R. 2002. Role of histamine in the inhibitory effects of phycocyanin in experimental models of allergic inflammatory response. *Mediators Inflamm* 11:81–85.

33. Kim, H.M., Lee, E.H., Cho, H.H., and Moon, Y.H. 1998. Inhibitory effect of mast cell-mediated immediate-type allergic reactions in rats by spirulina. *Biochem Pharmacol* 55:1071–1076.

34. Mao, T.K., Van de Water, J., and Gershwin, M.E. 2005. Effects of a *Spirulina*-based dietary supplement on cytokine production from allergic rhinitis patients. *J Med Food* 8:27–30.

35. Hirahashi, T., Matsumoto, M., Hazeki, K., Saeki, Y., Ui, M., and Seya, T. 2002. Activation of the human innate immune system by *Spirulina*: augmentation of interferon production and NK cytotoxicity by oral administration of hot water extract of *Spirulina platensis*. *Int Immunopharmacol* 2:423–434.

36. Balachandran, P., Pugh, N.D., Ma, G., and Pasco, D.S. 2006. Toll-like receptor 2-dependent activation of monocytes by *Spirulina* polysaccharide and its immune enhancing action in mice. *Int Immunopharmacol* 6:1808–1814.

37. Hayashi, O., Ono, S., Ishii, K., Shi, Y., Hirahashi, T., and Katoh, T. 2006. Enhancement of proliferation and differentiation in bone marrow hematopoietic cells by *Spirulina* (*Arthrospira*) *platensis* in mice. *J Appl Phycol* 18:47–56.

38. Zhang, H.Q., Lin, A.P., Sun, Y., and Deng, Y.M. 2001. Chemo- and radio-protective effects of polysaccharide of *Spirulina platensis* on hemopoietic system of mice and dogs. *Acta Pharmacol Sin* 22:1121–1124.

39. Borchers, A.T., Stern, J.S., Hackman, R.M., Keen, C.L., and Gershwin, M.E. 1999. Mushrooms, tumors, and immunity. *Proc Soc Exp Biol Med* 221:281–293.

40. Lee, J.B., Srisomporn, P., Hayashi, K., Tanaka, T., Sankawa, U., and Hayashi, T. 2001. Effects of structural modification of calcium spirulan, a sulfated polysaccharide from *Spirulina platensis*, on antiviral activity. *Chem Pharm Bull* (*Tokyo*) 49:108–110.

41. Hirata, T., Tanaka, M., Ooike, M., Tsunomura, T., and Sakaguchi, M. 2000. Antioxidant activities of phycocyanobilin prepared from *Spirulina platensis*. *J Appl Phycol* 12:435–439.

42. Iwasa, M., Yamamoto, M., Tanaka, Y., Kaito, M., and Adachi, Y. 2002. *Spirulina*-associated hepatotoxicity. *Am J Gastroenterol* 97:3212–3213.

43. Lee, A.N., and Werth, V.P. 2004. Activation of autoimmunity following use of immunostimulatory herbal supplements. *Arch Dermatol* 140:723–727.

44. U.S. Food and Drug Administration. 2003. *www.cfsan.fda.gov/~rdb/opa-gras.html* accessed February 21, 2007.

9 NK Activation Induced by *Spirulina*

*Tsukasa Seya, Takashi Ebihara, Ken Kodama,
Kaoru Hazeki, and Misako Matsumoto*

CONTENTS

INTRODUCTION

Detection of microbial products depends on a sophisticated network of germline-encoded pattern-recognition receptors that recognize microbe-specific patterns, nucleic acids, and metabolic products.[1] These receptors trigger signaling leading to activation of transcription factors, which induce cytokines/interferons to orchestrate host defense. We have a variety of foods that may contain something similar to microbial patterns. Since epithelial cells in the intestine and colon express pattern-recognition receptors,[2] it is not surprising that these pattern-like molecules regulate the immune system through response to the pattern-recognition receptors in the colon epithelial cells.

The cyanobacterium, *Spirulina platensis*, has been taken as a health drink or pills for more than 15 years without any undesirable effect on humans.[3] Its safety for human consumption has also been confirmed through numerous toxicological studies. *Spirulina* is a filamentous cyanobacterium containing constituents with various host immune potential. High NK activation is induced in humans having *Spirulina*.[4] Ab production and NK activation are also observed in chicken having small amounts (~10,000 ppm) of *Spirulina*.[5] The sugar and lipid moieties of *Spirulina* are involved in raising host immune responses, although the exact molecules responsible for NK activation have not been identified. The mechanism of NK activation by *Spirulina* is currently thought to be mediated by two pathways (Figures 9.1 and 9.2): direct

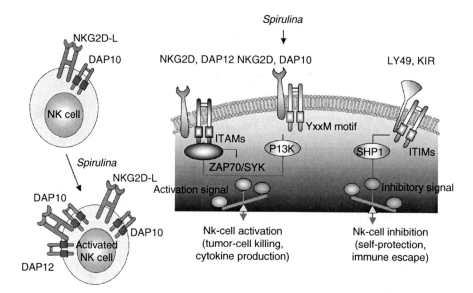

FIGURE 9.1 *Spirulina* extract induces up-regulation of the S-form of NKG2D receptor in NK cells. *Spirulina* directly acts on NK cells through lectin-like receptors and up-regulates the S-form of NKG2D (left panel). This form can activate DAP10 and DAP12, and PI3-kinase-mediated NK activation is accelerated (right panel).

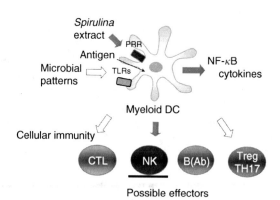

FIGURE 9.2 *Spirulina* extract induces maturation of myeloid dendritic cells through pattern recognition receptors (PRR). *Spirulina* contains a ligand that activates a putative PRR on dendritic cells. The PRR drives the dendritic cells to activate NK cells (gray arrows). Thus, NK cells are indirectly activated by another constituent of *Spirulina*. If a TLR ligand is simultaneously provided for dendritic cell maturation, the TLR is activated to confer CTL inducing abilities on the dendritic cells (white arrows). TLR ligands also induces IL-6, which activates TH17 cells.

activation of NK by *Spirulina* and indirect ways mainly through *Spirulina*-mediated dendritic cell activation.[6]

A hot water extract of *Spirulina* has been orally administered to patients as an anticancer and antiviral agent. Several reports supported the efficiency of oral administration of *Spirulina* for retardation of tumor progression in mice with tumor burden.[7] Tumor regressed in parallel with NK activation in mice.[6] In this review, we focus on the function of *Spirulina* as an NK-activating agent and introduce its potential for clinical application.

SPIRULINA NK ACTIVATION REVISITED

The experimental immunomodulatory function of *Spirulina* was first reported in mice in 1994.[8] This report introduced some evidence that *Spirulina* taken into mice facilitated antibody production, increased the ratio of activated peritoneal macrophages, and induced spleen cells to grow better in response to Con A.[8] In spleen cells in culture, addition of the hot water extract of *Spirulina* leads to enhanced interleukin-1 (IL-1) and then antibody production.[9] These results suggested that the initial target cells for *Spirulina* could be macrophages.

In 2002, human study on *Spirulina* was reported, where healthy male volunteers were given *Spirulina* orally every day for several weeks to be analyzed for the activity of their NK cells withdrawn at weekly or monthly intervals.[4] The cells in the collected blood were incubated with IL-12 alone or together with IL-18 to observe the release of interferon (IFN)-gamma there in response to these cytokines. The NK activities, measured as the IFN-gamma production in response to IL-12/IL-18 and NK target killing activity, were much higher for the cells taken 2 months after the inset of the *Spirulina* administration than for the cells taken from the same volunteers before the administration. The results reflect the reported findings that NK reciprocally activates dendritic cells[10] and IL-12/IL-18 may augment the NK cell activation.[11]

Successive studies suggested that *Spirulina* induces IFN-gamma and tumor cytotoxicity in part dependent on NK activity. *Spirulina* appears to directly act on a certain lectin-like receptor on NK cells to induce NK-activating receptors,[6] occurring independent of toll-like receptor (TLR). Unique points in this study are that (1) marked tumor regression is observed in mice with administration of *Spirulina*, suggesting that the NK cells actually participate in retardation of tumor growth, (2) Rae-1-positive tumor cells are selectively eliminated in *Spirulina*-fed mice, and (3) the S-form of NKG2D are induced in NK cells by *Spirulina*. Actually, PI3-kinase is activated secondary to the S-form of NKG2D and DAP10 in response to *Spirulina* extract in NK cells (Figure 9.1). It is also possible that unidentified pattern-recognition receptors (other than TLR) on dendritic cells participate in recognition of *Spirulina* extracts and make dendritic cells activate NK cells[12] (Figure 9.2). These receptors are not TLRs but others that recognize pattern molecules in *Spirulina*.[6] A major histocompatibility complex (MHC) low population of the tumor is selectively regressed by administration of *Spirulina*. Thus, the possible interpretation is that *Spirulina* extract activates mouse NK and the NK-mediated tumor cytotoxicity directs to the MHC-low population leading to retardation of tumor growth in the B16 syngeneic mouse model.

Structural investigation of *Spirulina* indicated that it contains glycolipids, such as *O*-β-D-galactosyl-(1-1′)-2′,3′-di-*O*-acyl-D-glycerol, which possess fatty acid moieties, palmitic acid, and linoleic or linolenic acids.[13] It is currently accepted that lipid moieties of microbes often serve as ligands of pattern-recognition receptors.[14,15] Thus, it is not surprising that *Spirulina* glycolipids serve as ligands for pattern-recognition receptors. Inducing IFN-gamma supports this possibility since T cells as well as NK cells are main producers of IFN-gamma.[4]

IMMUNE ACTIVATION BY *SPIRULINA*

There have been a number of reports relating to the functions of *Spirulina* in rodents. Zhang et al.[16] reported that the hot water extract of *Spirulina* showed significant hydroxy radical scavenging activity in mice. In another study, the methanolic extract of *Spirulina* showed weak antioxidant activity in rats.[17] Several papers suggested that the relevant substance is phycocyanin in *Spirulina*.[17,18] Using an experimental squamous cell cancer model of hamsters, administration of *Spirulina* extract has been reported to result in total tumor regression in 30% of animals.[19] Intraperitoneal injection of a polysaccharide extract of *Spirulina* was shown to inhibit proliferation of ascitic hepatoma cells in mice.[20] Calcium Spirulan, a polysaccharide isolated from *S. platensis*, inhibited lung metastasis of mouse B16 melanoma cells by intravenous administration.[21] Hence, phycocyanin and water-soluble components, presumably polysaccharides, may be responsible for antioxidant and anticancer effects in rodents.

In humans, rough *Spirulina* was reported to alleviate oral leukoplakia in pan tobacco chewers.[22] Water-soluble *Spirulina* components also inhibited the replication of human viruses, herpes simplex, cytomegalo, measles, mumps, and influenza A viruses.[23] The water extract also inhibited HIV replication in human T cells, T cell lines, and Langerhans cells.[24] Again, water-soluble polysaccharides appear to participate in the antioxidant, anticancer, and antiviral effects of *Spirulina*. These reports, together with our finding of modulation of pattern receptor signaling by the water extract in concert with immune modulation,[25] imply that the target of *Spirulina*-mediated immune activation is the innate immune system.

Nevertheless, it remains to be tested what kinds of cell wall components are readily extractable in the hot water-soluble fraction.[9] Only such extractable components can serve as receptor ligands. Absorption efficacy of the relevant components in the hot water extract of *Spirulina* has not been determined.

OTHER AGENTS

Chlorella,[26] mushrooms,[27,28] and agarics[29] are also categorized as plants and have been suggested to have immune potentiating abilities similar to *Spirulina*. Although there is little scientific background or results of physicochemical analyses to support these activities, it is becoming clear that animal cells, particularly those of the myeloid lineage, are equipped with a repertoire of microbe-recognizing receptors.[30] It is likely that some components of these materials can stimulate certain microbe receptors. Immune potentiation is representative of the anticancer and antiviral effects of these agents. In fact, several reports suggested that partially purified preparations of these agents provoke NF-kappaB and MAPK in human and mouse macrophages.[25] Clarification of the mechanism of immune potentiation by these materials and *Spirulina* would help to complete the outline of the primary or ancient host defense system and to understand its significance with regard to maintenance of health in humans.

BCG-*SPIRULINA* COMBINATION FOR CANCER IMMUNE THERAPY

A post operative immune therapy for cancer has been conducted using the cell-wall skeleton of BCG (BCG-CWS) in patients with lung cancer after surgical resection in the hospital of Osaka Medical Center for Cancer for > 10 years. In a typical study of patients with lung cancer, significant high 5-year survival with good QOL was observed compared to a historical control in the same hospital.[31,32] BCG-CWS acts as a potent adjuvant for induction of tumor-specific cytotoxic T lymphocytes (CTL), a potent effector for tumor cells. Thus, the mechanism of this adjuvant for induction of antitumor immunity has been investigated in our research group.

In C57BL/6 mouse B-16 melanoma implanting model, preadministration of the B16 melanoma antigenic peptide and BCG-CWS resulted in suppression of tumor growth.[33] Specific CTL against B16 melanoma was induced in parallel with tumor regression.[33] The CTL induction as well as retardation of tumor growth was completely diminished in MyD88-deficient mice.[33] Hence, the mechanism whereby BCG-CWS and tumor antigen contribute to regression of implanted tumor can be explained as follows: BCG acts as an adjuvant to activate TLR followed by the MyD88 adapter in antigen-presenting dendritic cells leading to up-regulation of antigen-presenting capacity and the levels of co-stimulators. This was true in *in vitro* dendritic cell stimulation with BCG-CWS both in mouse[33] and human.[34]

Simple subcutaneous administration of BCG-CWS would be effective if the patients are reserving tumor antigen.[31] However, in many cases, tumor turned MHC class I-negative and grew again in patients, irrespective of continuous BCG-CWS treatment. This finding is consistent with the fact that BCG-CWS lacks the ability to activate NK cells,[4,35] another effector for cancer. Administration of an NK-activating agent additionally to BCG-CWS adjuvant is expected to establish a powerful immune therapy for postoperative patients.

We developed a strategy of tumor immune therapy using BCG-CWS and *Spirulina*, which is now found to be a strong NK activator.[4,6] In transplanted tumor-bearing mice, effective tumor regression was observed if BCG-CWS and *Spirulina* were simultaneously administered.[6] Nearly complete remission could be introduced in about 80% of tumor-bearing mice through oral administration of *Spirulina* and subcutaneous injection of tumor debris conjugated with BCG-CWS.

The authors mentioned the mechanism whereby tumor was regressed by this combination therapy. According to their previous reports, microbial component acts as a maturation inducer of dendritic cells,[30] which play a major role in induction of tumor-specific CTL. CTL targets for high MHC-expressing tumor cell populations.

However, CTL fails to attack low MHC-expressing cells, which can be eliminated by NK cells. Since *Spirulina* is an efficient NK activator, MHC-negative tumor cells circumventing CTL attack to survive will be killed by *Spirulina*-mediated NK cells. Hence, this therapy should be adaptable to a variety of tumors. More extensive studies on the tumor-eliminating mechanism by the effector cells are in progress and part of them were presented in the meeting of Princess Takamatsu Cancer Research Meeting held on November 11–13, 2003 in Tokyo.[36] In the future, this combined adjuvant immune therapy will be adaptable to human patients with postoperative cancer.

FURTHER STUDIES

Bacteria, viruses, fungi, and cyanobacteria were known to potentiate host immunity for undefined mechanisms. It is so far accepted that certain components of microbial origin serve as ligands for TLRs and cytoplasmic NOD-like receptors in host macrophages/dendritic cells, which are nidus for activation cascades of the host immune system. Many factors including cytokines (IL-12, IL-6, TNF and IL-18), costimulators (CD80, CD86), and nitrogen oxide are up-regulated through Toll and cytoplasmic signaling, resulting in induction of cellular immunity.[37–39] However, the routes for induction of mature dendritic cells that commit NK activation or CTL induction have not been identified.

The point is why *Spirulina* is chosen for this case. *Spirulina* has been used as a healthy drink or pills for 10 years without any problem. We tested the effect of *Spirulina* on NK activity and IFN gamma-inducing activity in volunteers more than 40 years old.[4] The immune potentiating ability of *Spirulina* was revealed in this *in vivo* experiment. NK activation and IFN gamma production are enhanced after taking *Spirulina* and are continued for 12–24 weeks after stopping administration. This suggests the involvement of mucosal immunity in the Gut in *Spirulina*-mediated immune response.[40] *In vitro* experiment using preparations of human dendritic cells and blood cells, the *Spirulina* NK activation is attributable to water-extractable factors that directly interact with NK cells.[6] In addition, whole cell lysate of *Spirulina* contains factors that facilitate maturation of dendritic cells.[25] The relevant molecules responsible for this immune potentiating ability should be identified to substantiate the immune therapy involving *Spirulina*.

ACKNOWLEDGMENT

The authors are grateful to Drs Takagaki, Aoki and Abe (Dainippon Ink Co. Ltd) for supporting this work. This work was supported in part by the Osaka Community Foundation, Mitsubishi Foundation, and Takeda Foundation. Thanks are also due to our laboratory members for critical discussions.

REFERENCES

1. Medzhitov R, and Janeway CA. 1997. Innate immunity: the virtues of a nonclonal system of recognition. *Cell* 91: 295–8. Review.

2. Abreu MT, Fukata M, and Arditi M. 2005. TLR signaling in the gut in health and disease. *J. Immunol.* 174: 4453–60. Review.

3. Kay RA. 1991. Microalgae as food and supplement. *Crit. Rev. Food Sci. Nutr.* 30: 555–73.

4. Hirahashi T, Matsumoto M, Hazeki K, Saeki Y, Ui M, and Seya T. 2002. Activation of the human innate immune system by *Spirulina*: augmentation of interferon production and NK cytotoxicity by oral administration of hot water extract of *Spirulina platensis*. *Int. Immunopharmacol.* 2: 423–34.

5. Qureshi MA, Garlich JD, and Kidd MT. 1996. Dietary *Spirulina platensis* enhances humoral and cell-mediated immune functions in chickens. *Immunopharmacol. Immunotoxicol.* 18: 465–76.

6. Masuda H, Akazawa T, Ebihara T, Hazeki K, Hazeki O, Matsumoto M, and Seya T. 2007. Anti-tumor natural killer cell activation induced by *spirulina* extract. *Int. Immunopharmacol.* (submitted).

7. Mishima T, Murata J, Toyoshima M, Fujii H, Nakajima M, Hayashi T, Kato T, and Saiki I. 1998. Inhibition of tumor invasion and metastasis by calcium spirulan (Ca-SP), a novel sulfated polysaccharide derived from a blue-green alga, *Spirulina platensis*. *Clin. Exp. Metastasis.* 16: 541–50.

8. Cheng-Wu Z. 1994. Effect of polysaccharide and phycocyanin from *spirulina* on peripheral blood and hematopoietic system of bone marrow in mice. *Proc. of Second Asia Pacific Conf. on Algal Biotech.* (Abstr).

9. Hayashi O, Katoh T, and Okuwaki Y. 1994. Enhancement of antibody production in mice by dietary *spirulina*. *J. Nutr. Science Vitaminol (Tokyo)* 40: 431–41.

10. Gerosa F, Baldani-Guerra B, Nisii C, Marchesini V, Carra G, and Trinchieri G. 2002. Reciprocal activating interaction between natural killer cells and dendritic cells. *J. Exp. Med.* 195: 327–33.

11. Tanaka F, Hashimoto W, Okamura H, Robbins PD, Lotze MT, and Tahara H. 2000. Rapid generation of potent and tumor-specific cytotoxic T lymphocytes by interleukin 18 using dendritic cells and natural killer cells. *Cancer Res.* 60: 4838–44.

12. Matsuo-Tanabe M, Kawamoto T, Tanida S, Matsumoto M, and Seya T. 2004. Toll-like receptor 2 agonists with unique properties synthesized with reference to a product of *Streptosporangium*. *Immunology* 235–41.

13. Kataoka T, and Misaki A. 1983. Glycolipids isolated from *Spirulina maxima*: structure and fatty acid composition. *Agric. Biol. Chem.* 47: 2349–55.

14. Means TK, Golenbock DT, and Fenton MJ. 2000. Structure and function of Toll-like receptor proteins. *Life Sci.* 68: 241–58. Review.

15. Uehori, J, Fukase K, Akazawa T, Uematsu T, Akira S, Funami S, Shingai K, Matsumoto I, Azuma M, Toyoshima K, Kusumoto S, and Seya T. 2005. Dendritic cell maturation induced by muramyl dipeptide (MDP) derivatives: monoacylated MDP confers TLR2/TLR4 activation. *J. Immunol.* 174: 7096–103.

16. Zhang S, Xie J, Zhang J, Zhao J, and Jiang L. 1999. Electron spin resonance studies on photosensitized formation of hydroxyl radical by C-phycocyanin from *Spirulina platensis*. *Biochim. Biophys. Acta* 1426: 205–11.

17. Miranda MS, Cintra RG, Barros SB, and Filho J. 1998. Antioxidant activity of the microalga *Spirulina maxima*. *Braz. J. Med. Biol. Res.* 31: 1075–9.

18. Romay C, Ledon N, and Gonzalez R. 1999. Phycocyanin extract reduces leukotriene B4 levels in arachidonic acid-induced mouse-ear inflammation test. *J. Pharm. Pharmacol.* 51: 641–2.

19. Schwartz JL, Shklar G, Reid S, and Tricker D. 1988. Prevention of experimental oral cancer by extracts of *Spirulina*-Dunaliella algae. *Nutr. Cancer* 11: 127–34.

20. Li ZY, Li YG, Guo SY, Li L, and Zhang SL. 2000. Study of the factors of Cr(III) bioaccumulation on *Spirulina platensis. Sheng. Wu. Gong. Cheng. Xue. Bao.* 16: 108–12.

21. Seya T, Akazawa T, Matsumoto M, Begum NA, Azuma I, and Toyoshima K. 2003. Innate immune therapy for cancer: application of BCG-CWS and *spirulina* to patients with lung cancer. *Anticancer Res.* 23: 4369–76. Review.

22. Mathew B, Sankaranarayanan R, Nair PP, Varghese C, Somanathan T, Amma BP, Amma NS, and Nair MK. 1995. Evaluation of chemoprevention of oral cancer with *Spirulina fusiformis. Nutr. Cancer* 24: 197–202.

23. Hayashi K, Hayashi T, and Kojima I. 1996. A natural sulfated polysaccharide, calcium spirulan, isolated from *Spirulina platensis: in vitro* and *ex vivo* evaluation of anti-herpes simplex virus and anti-human immunodeficiency virus activities. *AIDS Res. Hum. Retroviruses* 12: 1463–71.

24. Ayehunie S, Belay A, Baba TW, and Ruprecht RM. 1998. Inhibition of HIV-1 replication by an aqueous extract of *Spirulina platensis* (*Arthrospira platensis*). *J. Acquir. Immune. Defic. Syndr. Hum. Retrovirol.* 18: 7–12.

25. Hazeki K, Hazeki O, Matsumoto M, and Seya T. 2003. Toll signaling induced by *Spirulina* extract in human myeloid dendritic cells. *Jpn Soc. Immunol.* (Proceedings). 33: 127 (Abstr).

26. Tanaka K, Tomita Y, Tsuruta M, Konishi F, Okuda M, Himeno K, and Nomoto K. 1990. Oral administration of *Chlorella vulgaris* augments concomitant antitumor immunity. *Immunopharmacol. Immunotoxicol.* 12: 277–91.

27. Borchers AT, Stern JS, Hackman RM, Keen CL, and Gershwin ME. 1999. Mushrooms, tumors, and immunity. *Proc. Soc. Exp. Biol. Med.* 221: 281–93.

28. Chang R. 1996. Functional properties of edible mushrooms. *Nutr. Rev.* 54: S91–3.

29. Ebina T, and Fujimiya Y. 1998. Antitumor effect of a peptide-glucan preparation extracted from Agaricus blazei in a double-grafted tumor system in mice. *Biotherapy* 11: 259–65.

30. Iwasaki A, and Medzhitov R. 2004. Toll-like receptor control of the adaptive immune responses. *Nat. Immunol.* 5: 987–95. Review.

31. Hayashi A, Doi O, Azuma I, and Toyoshima K. 1998. Immunofriendly use of BCG-cell wall skeleton remarkably improves the survival rate of various cancer patients. *Proc. Jpn. Acad.* 74(B): 50–8.

32. Seya T, Matsumoto M, Akazawa T, and Kodama K. 2006. Advance of adjuvant-augmented immunetherapy for cancer. *65th Annual meeting Jpn Cancer Assoc.* (Proceedings). 249 (Abstr).

33. Akazawa T, Masuda H, Saeki Y, Matsumoto M, Takeda K, Akira S, Azuma I, Toyoshima K, and Seya T. 2004. Adjuvant-mediated tumor regression and tumor-specific CTL induction are impaired in MyD88-deficient mice. *Cancer Res.* 64: 757–64.

34. Uehori J, Tsuji S, Matsumoto M, Kawata C, Takeuchi T, Akira S, Azuma I, Toyoshima K, and Seya T. 2003. Simultaneous blocking of human Toll-like receptor 2 and 4 suppresses myeloid dendritic cell maturation induced by *Mycobacterium bovis* bacillus Calmette-Guérin (BCG)-peptidoglycan (PGN). *Infect. Immun.* 71: 4238–49.

35. Matsumoto M, Seya T, Kikkawa S, Tsuji S, Shida K, Nomura M, Kurita-Taniguchi M, Ohigashi H, Yokouchi H, Takami H, Hayashi A, Azuma I, Masaoka T, Kodama K, and Toyoshima K. 2001. IFNγ-producing ability in blood of patients with lung cancer: production of IL-12 p40 and IL-18 in response to BCG-CWS. *Int. Immunopharmacol.* 1: 1559–69.

36. Akazawa T, Okuno M, Okuda Y, Tsujimura K, Takahashi T, Ikawa M, Okabe M, Ebihara T, Shingai M, Inoue N, Tanaka-Okamoto M, Ishizaki H, Miyoshi J, Matsumoto M, and Seya T. 2006. Antitumor NK activation induced by the Toll-like receptor3-TICAM-1 (TRIF) pathway in myeloid dendritic cells. *Proc. Natl. Acad. Sci. USA.* 104: 252–7.

37. Tsuji S, Matsumoto M, Takeuchi O, Akira S, Azuma I, Hayashi A, Toyoshima K, Seya T. 2000. Maturation of human dendritic cells by cell-wall skeleton of *Mycobacterium bovis* Bacillus Calmette-Guerin: involvement of Toll-like receptors. *Infect. Immun.* 68: 6883–90.

38. Seya T, Akazawa T, Matsumoto M, Begum NA, Azuma I, and Toyoshima K. 2003. Innate immune therapy for cancer: application of BCG-CWS and *spirulina* to patients with lung cancer. *Anticancer Res.* 23: 4369–76. Review.

39. Seya T, Akazawa T, Tsujita T, and Matsumoto M. 2006. Application of Toll-like receptor agonists to vaccine adjuvant therapy. *ECAM* 3: 31–8. Review.

40. Abreu MT, Fukata M, and Arditi M. 2005. TLR signaling in the gut in health and disease. *J. Immunol.* 174: 4453–60. Review.

10 Spirulina and Antibody Production

Osamu Hayashi, Kyoko Ishii, and Toshimitsu Kato

CONTENTS

INTRODUCTION

Immune responses are mediated by a variety of cells and soluble molecules or cytokines that are involved in signaling between cells during immune responses in an autocrine or paracrine manner. Macrophages and T and B lymphocytes play a central role in all immune responses, but other cells in the tissues also participate by signaling to the lymphocytes and by responding to the cytokines such as interleukins (ILs) and interferon γ (IFNγ) (Figure 10.1). Cell-mediated immunity, originally described as localized reactions to organisms such as intracellular pathogens, is mediated by phagocytes and lymphocytes. Humoral immunity, on the contrary, is mediated by antibodies in the circulating blood and lymph. It is not possible entirely, however, to consider cell-mediated and antibody-mediated responses separately. Although the environment surrounding us contains a great variety of infectious agents as antigens, most infections in normal individuals are short-lived and leave little permanent damage. This is due to the immune system, which combats infectious agents.[1,2]

Spirulina (*Arthrospira*)*platensis*, which is a helicoidal filamentous blue-green alga or cyanobacterium, has a history of being used as food for more than a 1000 years.[3,4] It has been commercially produced for almost 30 years as a human food

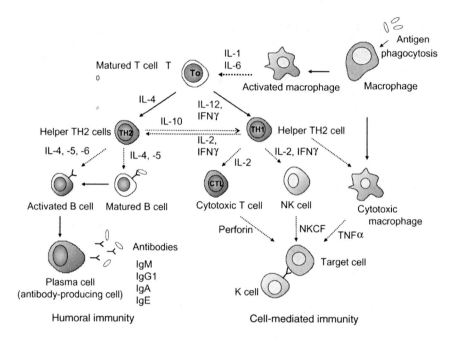

FIGURE 10.1   Immune systems and cytokines.

supplement, based on the advantages of mass cultivation and easy harvest of the micro alga.[5] Nutritional studies have demonstrated that it contains high-quality protein and other nutritional components such as vitamins; minerals; essential fatty acids, including γ-linolenic acid, and β-carotene.[6-8] More attention has been given to the study of the therapeutic effects of *Spirulina*. In addition to reports concerning its effectiveness in reducing hyperlipidemia, diabetes, and high blood pressure in man and animals, an antiviral effect against Herpes simplex has also been reported,[9] and some reports have also shown that *S. platensis* may be beneficial in treating some forms of atopic bronchial asthma and cancer involving immune functions.[10] It is therefore of interest from the nutritional and medical points of view to investigate whether *S. platensis* affects immunological indices.

In this chapter, we focused on the effects of *Spirulina* and its extracts, for example phycocyanin, on immune functions, especially on antibody responses in humans and experimental animals in *in-vivo* and *in-vitro* studies.

PRIMARY ANTIBODY RESPONSE AND MACROPHAGE FUNCTION IN MICE FED *SPIRULINA*

Some studies have shown that feeding *Spirulina* to fish and poultry resulted in increased disease resistance, improved survival, and growth rates, which was attributed to an improvement of immune functions.[7,11] Antitumor effect of *Spirulina* in hamster through stimulation of the immune response, involving T cell activation, has been also reported.[10]

TABLE 10.1
Immune Responses to SRBC in Mice Fed *Spirulina*

	Groups Control	SP-10	SP-20
Primary response to SRBC			
PFC ($\times 10^2/10^6$ cells)	13.7 ± 3.6	18.2 ± 3.9*	19.5 ± 4.1**
HA titers (2n)	7.3 ± 0.4	7.6 ± 0.5	7.6 ± 0.4
Secondary response to SRBC			
IgG-PFC ($\times 10^2/10^6$ cells)	19.3 ± 7.6	19.8 ± 8.1	14.1 ± 7.6
with 2-ME treatment	11.9 ± 0.2	12.3 ± 0.6	11.7 ± 0.8
without 2-ME treatment	11.9 ± 0.2	12.5 ± 0.6*	12.0 ± 1.0

Means ± SD of 10 mice *$p < .05$, **$p < .01$ compared to Control
Source: Hayashi, O., J. *Nutr. Sci. Vitaminol.*, 40, 435, 1994. With permission.

TABLE 10.2
Percentage of Peritoneal Phagocytic Cells Ingesting Latex Particles From Mice Fed *Spirulina*

Groups	Splenic PFC ($\times 10^6$ cells/mouse)	Phagocytic cell (%)
Control	13.7 ± 3.6	91.3 ± 6.1
SP-10	18.2 ± 3.95*	95.9 ± 2.4*
SP-20	19.5 ± 4.1**	93.9 ± 5.3

Means ± SD of 10 mice *$p < .05$, **$p < .01$ compared to Control.
Source: Hayashi, O., J. *Nutr. Sci. Vitaminol.*, 40, 435, 1994. With permission.

At the beginning of the study we used *in-vivo* and *in-vitro* systems to investigate whether *S. platensis* and its extracts enhance the immune response through primary response and macrophage function in mice. BALB/cAnNCrj mice used in the study were fed laboratory chow containing 10 or 20% (w/w) dried *Spirulina*. The mice gained body weight normally and consumed an equivalent amount of food and water compared to control mice during the experiment period of 7 weeks. The mice fed on *Spirulina* diet showed increased numbers of splenic antibody-producing cells, that is, plaque-forming cells (PFC) in the primary immune responses to sheep red blood cells (SRBC) (Table 10.1).[12] Immunoglobulin G (IgG)-antibody producing cells (IgG-PFC) in the secondary immune response, however, was hardly affected except for hemagglutination (HA) titer without 2-mercaptoethanol (2-ME) treatment, suggesting that *Spirulina* affects immunoglobulin M (IgM) antibody synthesis in the initial phase of the immune response. Phagocytic activity of peritoneal-exuded macrophages from the mice was significantly enhanced (Table 10.2). Proliferations of spleen cells by T-cell mitogens, concanavalin A (Con A), and phytohemagglutinin (PHA) were

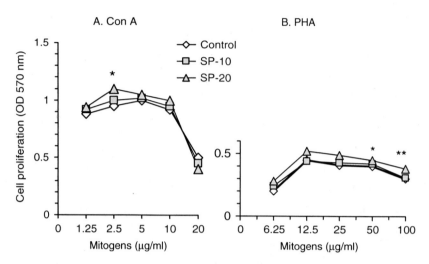

FIGURE 10.2 Mitogen-induced proliferation of spleen cells from mice fed *Spirulina* (Adapted from Hayashi, O., *J. Nutr. Sci. Vitaminol.*, 40, 436, 1994. With permission.) Means ± SD of 10 mice.
*$p < .05$, **$p < .01$ compared to Control.

also enhanced (Figure 10.2), whereas the mitogenic activity with LPS, a B-cell mitogen, was not affected. Adding either a hot-water extract of *Spirulina* (SpHW) or a culture supernatant of macrophages stimulated with SpHW to spleen cells in culture increased numbers of PFCs in *in-vitro* experiment. The culture supernatant of macrophages stimulated with SpHW contained significantly increased levels of both interleukin-1 (IL-1) activity (Figure 10.3) and TNFα. These results suggested that *Spirulina* enhanced the immune response in mice, particularly the primary response, by stimulating macrophage functions.

Lee et al.[13] reported that feeding prawns, *Penaeus merguiensis*, with *S. platensis* (0.3% w/w feed) enhanced phagocytic activity of the hemocytes from hemolymph against some bacteria such as *Vibrio harveyi*, *Escherichia coli*, *Salmonella typhimurium* used. They suggested that lipopolysaccharides and peptidoglycan in *Spirulina* might nonspecifically activate phagocytic hemocytes of the prawns. Liu et al.[14] reported that intraperitoneally injected polysaccharides of *Spirulina* increased the percentage of phagocytic cells in peritoneal macrophages in addition to increasing the hemolysin content in the blood of mice. Macrophages from chickens exposed to water-soluble extract of *Spirulina* also showed increased percentage of phagocytic cells as well as increased numbers of internalized unopsonized SRBC per phagocytic cell.[15] Pugh et al.[16] demonstrated that water-soluble polysaccharide preparations from food-grade *S. platensis* (a polysaccharide named "Immunlina") and from *Chlorella pyrenoidosa* (a polysaccharide named "Immurella") had immunostimulatory activity detected by a transcription bioassay for nuclear factor kappa B (NF-κB) in THP-1 human monocytes/macrophages, and substantially increased mRNA levels of interleukin 1β (IL-1β) and tumor necrosis factor-α (TNFα). Recently, Wu et al.[17] showed that both water extracts from *Chlorella* (*C. vulgaris*) and *Spirulina* (*S. maxima*) had potential activities of treatment of liver fibrosis inhibiting hepatic stellate cell (HSC)

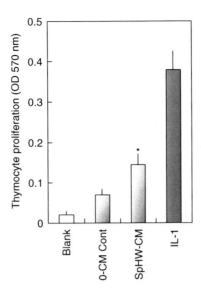

FIGURE 10.3 IL-1 activity in culture supernatant of peritoneal macrophages stimulated with SpHW (From Hayashi, O., *J. Nutr. Sci. Vitaminol.*, 40, 437, 1994. With permission.)
IL-1 activity in each culture supernatant of peritoneal macrophage, 0-CM and SpHW-CM, was measured by thymocyte-proliferation assay in the presence of phytohemagglutinin PHA. IL-1 is positive control.
Data represent means ± SD of three wells.
*$p < .05$ compared to Blank.

proliferation, which was due to their antioxidant activity. They also showed that the total amount of phenol contributing to antioxidant activity in *Spirulina* was almost five times greater than that of chlorella. Either SpHW or hot-water extract from *Chlorella vulgaris* (CHW) significantly increased the mitogenicity of spleen cells and/or the number of PFC in *in-vitro* spleen-cell culture.[18] Although major differences were not observed in these activities, some extracts from *Spirulina*, for example, dialysed substance of SpHW and cell wall substance of *Spirulina*, increased IL-1 activity in the culture of peritoneal macrophages, whereas induction of IL-1 activity by *Chlorella* extracts was not significant.[18]

Listeria monocytogenes is a facultative intracellular bacterium, capable of surviving and multiplying in macrophage-rich organs such as liver and spleen. We expected bactericidal activity in murine macrophages, which were stimulated with *Spirulina* in *in-vivo* experiment or in *in-vitro* culture. In spite of significant induction of IL-1 activity, however, SpHW did not enhance bactericidal activity against *L. monocytogenes* in the macrophages.[19]

MUCOSAL IgA RESPONSE IN MICE TREATED WITH *SPIRULINA*

Secretory immunoglobulin A (IgA) antibodies work as the predominant isotype in most secretory tissues or mucosal surfaces and exhibit various biological properties

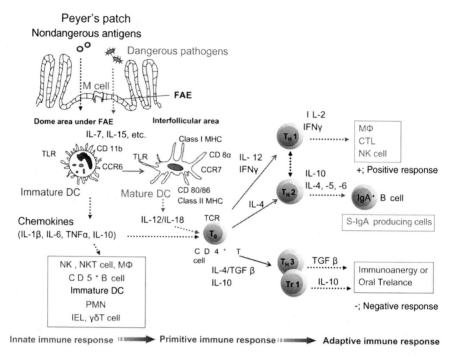

FIGURE 10.4 Innate and adaptive responses in mucosal immunity
FAE; Follicle-associated epitherium, DC; Dendritic cell, TLR; Toll-like receptor,
CCR; Chemokine receptor

as the first line of immune defense, for example agglutination of micro-organisms; neutralization of bacterial enzymes, toxins, and viruses; immune exclusion; blocking adherence of bacteria to the epithelium; and reduction of antigens or allergen absorption.[20] The intestine is the largest single immune organ; it consists of more than 200 m² of mucosal surface available for antigen uptake and contains more than 70% of an organism's plasma cells. An organism produces more IgA than the organism's production of IgG.[20,21]

The mucosal immune system evolves mechanisms that can discriminate between harmless antigens, commensal microorganisms, and dangerous pathogens. The ability of the system to distinguish between "dangerous" and "nondangerous" agents is essential for mounting protective immune responses.[22] The lymphoid follicles associated with mucosa house two types of dendritic cells; a subpopulation of immature dendritic cells located in close contact with the follicles-associated epithelium (FAE) and a subpopulation of mature, differentiated dendritic cells present in the interfollicular region associated with T cells (Figure 10.4). Following the antigen processing, primitive or early immune response is induced within several hours after infection in association with NK, $\gamma\delta$T, CD5$^+$B cells and others, and then antigen-specific adaptive immune response is induced several days later. Dendritic cells process the antigen and present it to T cells in the form of peptides bound to the expressed major histocompatibility complex (MHC) molecules. ILs-7 and -15 secreted from epithelial cells work as cytokines that enhance the proliferation and differentiation of intraepithelial lymphocytes (IELs) and other cells such as dendritic cells for innate and primitive immune responses. "Nondangerous" or harmless antigens like food are presented to T cells by immature dendritic cells that express costimulatory molecules in low levels. Production of IL-10 and TGFβ leads to activation of regulatory Tr-1 or Th3 cells, which in turn inhibits the immune response and induces "oral mucosal tolerance." "Dangerous" antigens like pathogenic microorganisms, on the other hand, induce the maturation of dendritic cells, which express the surface costimulatory molecules such as CD80/86 antigens and produce IL-12 for activation of Th1 cells followed by acquired positive response.

We then investigated antibody responses of IgA and other classes, such as IgE and IgG1, as possible evidence of the protective effects of *Spirulina* toward food allergy and microbial infection.[23] In this study, antibody productions were monitored in mice treated with a hot-water extract of *Spirulina*, SpHW concurrently or protectively ingested with oral administration of crude shrimp extract as an antigen. Soy- and shrimp- extract antigens had been known to induce IgE antibody response significantly following serial oral injection in C3H/HeJ mice.[24] In a primary experiment, ingestion of *Spirulina* extracts alone did not increase the basal of IgE antibody up to 5 weeks.

EFFECT OF CONCURRENTLY INGESTED SpHW WITH ANTIGEN ADMINISTRATION

We first observed antibody levels in the blood and intestinal contents of the mice treated with SpHW concurrently ingested with antigen administration of shrimp (Figure 10.5). Concentrated and diluted SpHW (SPC and SPD) solutions were prepared by dilution of SpHW to 15- and 60-fold, respectively, and were given to Ag-SPC and Ag-SPD groups aseptically. Ag group was given sterilized water. The groups were immunized intraperitoneally with a mixture of crude shrimp extract and inactivated *Bordetella pertussis* adjuvant as primary immunization followed by oral administration of crude shrimp extract twice a week through an animal feeding catheter for 5 weeks.

Total IgA level in the intestine of Ag group that was orally immunized with antigen alone was almost the same as that of normal nonimmunized animals. IgA antibody levels in the intestine of the Ag-SPD group that concurrently ingested SPD with antigen administration were significantly higher than that of Ag group (Figure 10.6A). Antigen-specific IgE level that was increased in the Ag group, however, was not further enhanced by *Spirulina* concurrently ingested with antigen, as shown in the Ag-SPC and Ag-SPD groups in Figure 10.6B. *Spirulina* seemed to neither induce nor enhance allergic reaction such as food allergy dependent on an IgE. IgG1 antibody increased by oral administration of shrimp antigen, on the other hand, was further enhanced by the treatment of *Spirulina* extract in Ag-SPD group (Data not shown).

EFFECT OF PROTECTIVELY INGESTED SpHW BEFORE ANTIGEN ADMINISTRATION

The enhancement of IgA antibody production in the intestine by *Spirulina* extract was further confirmed. In this experiment, SPD was protectively given to both SPD and SPD-Ag groups for 4 weeks before and for 1 week after primary immunization

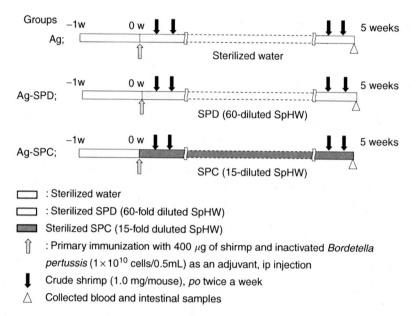

FIGURE 10.5 Concurrent ingestion of *Spirulina* extract, SPC and SPD, with crude shrimp antigen administration
Five mice per group were used in the experiment.

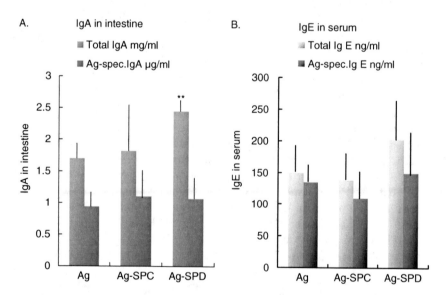

FIGURE 10.6 IgA (A) IgE (B) antibody productions in mice treated with SpHW concurrently ingested with antigen stimulation
Means ± SD of six mice
**$p < .01$ compared to Ag group

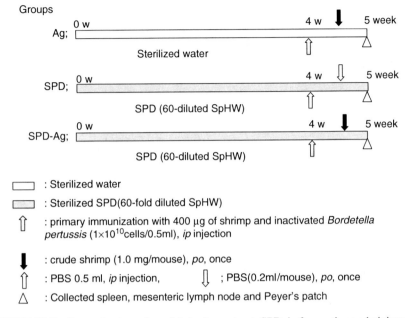

Groups

: Sterilized water

: Sterilized SPD(60-fold diluted SpHW)

⇑ : primary immunization with 400 µg of shrimp and inactivated *Bordetella pertussis* (1×10^{10}cells/0.5ml), *ip* injection

⬇ : crude shrimp (1.0 mg/mouse), *po*, once

⇑ : PBS 0.5 ml, *ip* injection,   ⇓ ; PBS(0.2ml/mouse), *po*, once

△ : Collected spleen, mesenteric lymph node and Peyer's patch

FIGURE 10.7   Protective ingestion of *Spirulina* extract, SPD, before antigen administration Five mice per group were used in the experiments.

(Figure 10.7). Crude shrimp extract antigen with *Bordetella* adjuvant was intraperitoneally injected as described in the former experiment and crude shrimp extract was orally administered once after the primary immunization. IgA antibody production in culture cells of some lymphoid organs from mice treated with *Spirulina* extract was examined.

IgA antibody levels in the culture supernatant of cells of lymphoid organs, especially in the spleen and mesenteric lymph node of the SPD-Ag group was significantly enhanced in comparison with Ag groups as shown in Figure 10.8, whereas neither antigen stimulation alone in Ag group nor administration of SPD alone in SPD group increased the IgA antibody in any lymphoid organ.

In conclusion, these results from the experiments in both concurrent and protective ingestion of *Spirulina* showed that *Spirulina* at least neither induced nor enhanced allergic reaction like food allergy dependent on IgE antibody, and that *Spirulina* ingested both concurrently with antigen and before antigen administration significantly enhanced IgA antibody production to protectively affect against infection or allergic reaction.

Secretory IgA antibodies exhibit synergistic interaction with antibacterial substances such as lysozyme and lactoferrin.[20] Cholera toxin, bacterial lipopolysaccharides or lipid A, muramyl dipeptide, and a synthetic or nonbacterial lipoidal amine, are known as mucosal adjuvants and have been found to potentiate secretory immune response to stimulate the production of IgA antibody.[25] It has also been known that orally ingested lactic acid bacteria—*Bifidobacterium longum*, *B. breve*, and *Lactobacillus casei*—increased mucosal IgA response to antigen in *in vitro* or *in vivo* studies

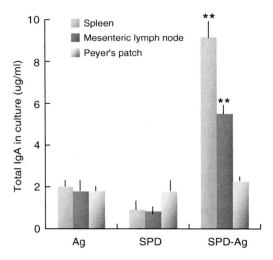

FIGURE 10.8   Total IgA antibody in cell-culture supernatant of lymphoid organs from mice protectively ingested with *Spirulina* extract before antigen stimulation as shown in Figure 10.7 (Adapted from Hayashi, O., *J. Nutr. Sci. Vitaminol.*, 44, 848, 1998. With permission.)
Means ± SD of five mice
**p < .01 compared to Ag group

in animals and in humans.[26,27] The role of cytokines in orchestrating the mucosal immune response has been greatly investigated for the potential of therapeutic applications to improve mucosal responses and to control systemic autoimmunity.[28] Further experiments concerning the mechanisms of stimulating local immune response by *Spirulina*, in regard to cytokine production, are necessary, in addition to investigations of the enhancing effect of *Spirulina* on IgA production in humans.

DISTINCT EFFECTS OF PHYCOCYANIN INGESTION ON SECRETORY IgA AND ALLERGIC IgE ANTIBODY RESPONSES IN MICE

Spirulina contains phycocyanin, a blue, 270-kDa photosynthetic pigment protein, which accounts for approximately 15% of the dry weight of *Spirulina*.[3] Previously we investigated the effect of phycocyanin ingestion on the immune response of the intestinal mucosa, and found that ingestion of phycocyanin promoted IgA antibody production in mice immunized with aqueous solution of ovalbumin (OVA) as an antigen.[29] In Peyer's patches that are contained in the peripheral lymphoid tissues, production of total IgA antibody was also promoted by phycocyanin. However, the antigen-specific IgA antibodies in both Peyer's patches and mesenteric lymph nodes were undetected, probably because OVA, used as an antigen, was an aqueous solution. Aqueous antigen could be too easily degraded in the digestive tract to retain functional antigenicity. In order to solve this problem, we prepared OVA antigen-entrapped biodegradable microparticles made of poly (DL-lactide-co-glycolide), and

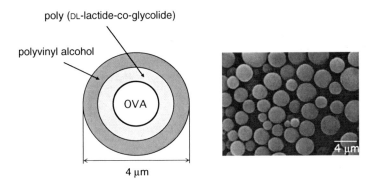

FIGURE 10.9 (Water-in-oil)-in-water emulsion (left) and Scanning electron micrograph (right) of OVA microparticles (Adapted from Nemoto-Kawamura, C., *J. Nutr. Sci. Vitaminol.*, 50, 132, 2004. With permission.)
Scale bar: 4 μm.
Average diameter was 4 μm.

used as a stimulating antigen for local antibody response in the mucous. Antigen that has been entrapped in biodegradable microparticles may circumvent the problem of antigen degradation.[30–32] We focused on the study of immune responses in the intestinal mucosa, mesenteric lymph nodes, and Peyer's patches in mice that had ingested phycocyanin. The effect of phycocyanin on type I allergy was also studied by measuring serum IgE levels and its relation to inflammation.

OVA-entrapped biodegradable microparticles (OVA microparticles) were prepared using the (water-in-oil)-in-water (w/o/w) emulsion solvent evaporation technique.[33] A mixture of OVA aqueous solution and poly (DL-lactide-co-glycolide) in dichloromethane (DCM) was homogenized at 8000 rpm for 10 s in a micro homogenizer followed by addition of polyvinyl alcohol aqueous solution. Sediment of a (water-in-oil)-in-water (w/o/w) emulsion obtained by secondary homogenization similar to the first step was washed three times with sterile distilled water by centrifugation, and lyophilized to recover the resulted microparticles. To determine the shape of the microparticles and to determine the average value of diameter, more than 400 microparticles in each batch were observed by scanning electron microscopy (Figure 10.9). Average diameter of the microparticles was 4 μm. Protein contents of the microparticles were found to be 15% as a standard of bovine serum albumin, measured by using a bicinchoninic acid kit.

Antigen-entrapped microparticles may be a useful tool to study the mucosal immune responses. Some investigators have shown that microparticles of 3–4 μm diameters activated both mucosal and systemic immunity [32] and resulted in the greatest increase in serum antigen-specific IgG1 antibody levels in mice.[34] We reported as a preliminary experiment that microparticles having a diameter of approximately 4 μm also exhibited strong adhesion to Peyer's patches.[35] These data were consistent with the idea that there was an appropriate particle size that renders the microparticles effective. As a result of using antigen-entrapped microparticles with 4 μm average diameters, OVA-specific IgA antibody was successfully induced. In addition to

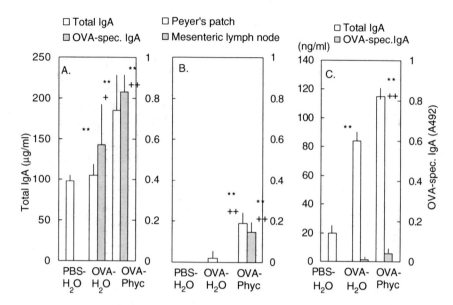

FIGURE 10.10 Total and OVA-specific IgA antibodies in intestinal mucosa (A) and in cell-culture supernatants of Peyer's patch and mesenteric lymph node (B), and of spleen (C) from mice treated with phycocyanin for 6 weeks

Values of each antibody level are expressed as means $\pm$ SD of 5 mice.

$*p < .05$, $**p < .01$ compared to each PBS-H_2O control, and $+; p < .05$, $++; p < .01$ compared to each OVA-H_2O.

enhancement of the mucosal response, OVA microparticles increased both total and antigen-specific IgA and IgG1 antibody in the spleen and the serum, suggesting that microparticles antigen enhanced systemic immune response as well as local immune response in mucous.

In the mice that ingested 0.05% phycocyanin solution for 6 weeks, a marked increase in the antigen-specific IgA antibody level as well as the total IgA antibody was observed in the intestinal mucosa (Figure 10.10A), the Peyer's patches, and mesenteric lymph nodes (Figure 10.10B), which comprise a major part of the gut-associated lymphoid tissues (GALT), and also in the spleen cells (Figure 10.10C), whereas neither IgG1 nor IgE was affected (Figure 10.11A). Phycocyanin ingestion for 8 weeks, on the other hand, suppressed the production of antigen-specific IgG1 and IgE antibody in the serum (Figure 10.11B). Tokuyama et al.[36] reported that mice treated simultaneously with retinoic acid and interleukin-5 (IL-5) enhanced IgA antibody production as a result of enhancing the class switch of B cells to IgA-antibody-producing precursor cells, while IgG1 antibody was strongly inhibited. This antagonistic antibody behavior produced by phycocyanin suggests that phycocyanin exerts its inhibitory effects against allergy through at least two ways: amplification of IgA production in the mucosal immunity to defend against the invasion of allergens, and suppression of IgE and IgG1 production in the systemic immunity to minimize excessive responses to allergens. IL-6 and IL-10 are also known to be involved in

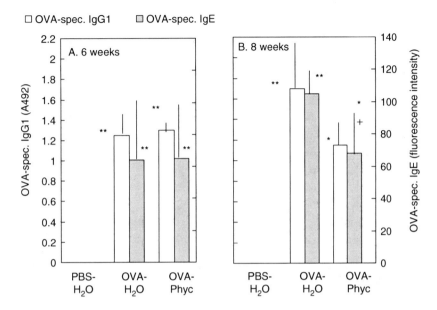

FIGURE 10.11 OVA-specific IgG1 and IgE antibody levels in serum of BALB/cA mice treated with phycocyanin for 6 (A) or 8 weeks (B).
Values of each antibody level are expressed as mean $\pm$ SD ($n = 6$).
**$p < .01$ compared to PBS-H_2O and $^+p < .05$, $^{++}p < .01$ compared to OVA-H_2O

the class switching to IgA-antibody-producing precursor cells.[22] The isotype class switching to IgA antibody is mediated by TGF-β, while switching to IgG1 and IgE antibodies is induced by IL-4.[22] These cytokines may also be involved in the promotion of IgA antibody production and the inhibition of IgG1 and IgE antibody production by phycocyanin ingestion.

As shown in Figure 10.11A and other papers,[23,29] serum OVA-specific IgE antibody, as well as IgG1, were not affected by 5–6 week treatment with phycocyanin. Further prolongation of phycocyanin treatment up to 8 weeks may contribute to the significant suppression of OVA-specific IgE antibody response, that is, suppression of Th2 function and/or enhancement of suppressor T cell or Th1 function. In contrast, significant reduction of intestinal vascular permeability in mice by Evans blue-leaking method was observed following 6-week treatment with phycocyanin (Figure 10.12). It was noted that the reduction of permeability preceded by 2 weeks the suppression of antigen-specific IgE level in the course of 8 weeks of phycocyanin ingestion. Remirez et al.[37] reported that phycocyanin itself prevented allergic dermatitis in rats by inhibiting the release of histamine caused by compound 48/80. They also reported that oral administration of phycocyanin (50–200 mg/kg) 1 h before application of arachidonic acid prevented inflammatory edema in rat ears by reducing productions of prostaglandin E_2 (PGE_2) and leukotriene B_4 (LTB_4) through inhibiting the activity of cyclooxygenase (COX-2), a prostaglandin-synthesizing enzyme.[38] Phycocyanin possibly alleviated the inflammation independent of IgE antibody. *Spirulina* products

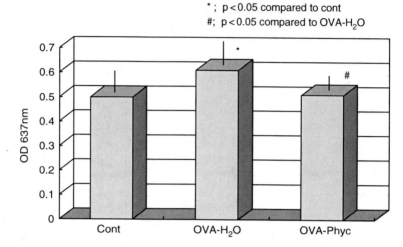

FIGURE 10.12   Intestinal vascular permeability in mice treated with phycocyanin for 6 weeks (Adapted from Nemoto-Kawamura, C., *J. Nutr. Sci. Vitaminol.*, 50, 134, 2004. With permission.)
Vascular permeability was determined by Evans blue-leakage method.
Optical density measured at 637 nm is expressed as means ± SD of 5 mice.
*$p < .05$ compared to Cont and #$p < .05$ compared to OVA-H_2O

containing phycocyanin not only are useful dietary supplements but also strengthen the defense mechanisms against infectious diseases and also strengthen the protective mechanisms against food allergy and other inflammatory diseases.

INCREASE OF IgA ANTIBODY LEVELS IN HUMANS CUSTOMARILY INGESTING *SPIRULINA*

We now are gaining an understanding of the possibility of enhancement of mucosal and/or systemic antibody responses, especially in regard to production of IgA antibody in the intestine by continuous ingestion of *Spirulina* or its extracts involving phycocyanin as shown in Figures 10.8 and 10.10 in animal studies. We then investigated salivary IgA antibody levels in the subjects who ingested commercial *Spirulina* tablets as a health food in various periods of usage in their daily life. We detected a correlation between the salivary IgA level and the amount of *Spirulina* ingested. Salivary glands have been recognized as a part of the common mucosal immune system, and saliva has been used by researchers for studies of the influence of various parameters on the human mucosal immune system.[39]

One hundred and thirty four employees of a manufacturing company, average age; 43.2 ± 12.1 years old (from 20 to 62 years old), were enrolled in the study and asked to offer saliva as specimens and to answer some questionnaires about duration and experience of *Spirulina* ingestion.[40] About 127 saliva specimens from 91 men and 36 women were collected after having obtained consent from each subject. Secreted

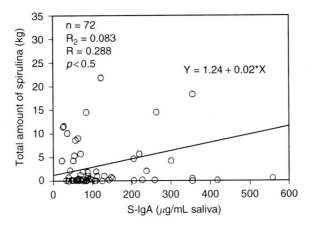

FIGURE 10.13 Correlation between total S-IgA levels in saliva of subjects and total amount of *Spirulina* ingested by subjects (From Ishii, K., *J. Kagawa Nutr. Univ.*, 30, 30, 1999. With permission.)

saliva from each subject was collected in dental roller cotton being kept in the mouth for 3 min, and saliva specimens were obtained as supernatant after centrifugation. Secretory-IgA (S-IgA) antibody level in saliva was determined by ELISA. Total S-IgA level of the group ingesting *Spirulina* (SP) continuously (Continuous group, $n = 33$) in men was significantly higher ($p < .05$) than that of the group ingesting SP discontinuously (Discontinuous group, $n = 22$). Total S-IgA level of the group ingesting SP for more than 1 year was significantly increased ($p < .01$) in comparison to the group ingesting SP for less than half a year. Further, S-IgA levels in the saliva from the 72 subjects of men and women, who ingested *Spirulina* continuously ($n = 43$) and discontinuously ($n = 29$), were positively correlated to total amount of *Spirulina* ingested by the subjects (Figure 10.13). Correlation coefficient R was 0.288 and was statistically significant ($p < .05$).

ENHANCEMENT OF PROLIFERATION AND DIFFERENTIATION OF IMMUNE COMPETENT CELLS BY *SPIRULINA*

Phycocyanin has been known to promote the growth of a human myeloid cell line, RPMI 8226.[41,42] Recently, Liu et al.[39] reported that phycocyanin inhibited growth of human leukemia K562 cells and enhanced the arrest of the cell growth at G1 phase, suggesting enhancement of differentiation of the cells. To evaluate whether *Spirulina* has potentials to enhance or sustain immune functions as a consequence of promoting proliferation or differentiation of immune competent-cells, we investigated effects of *Spirulina* and its extracts, SpHW, phycocyanin (Pc), and SpCW, on proliferation of bone marrow cells and induction of colony-forming activity.

Results were as follows: in addition to the enhancement of proliferation of bone-marrow cells, culture supernatants of the spleen cells stimulated with *Spirulina*

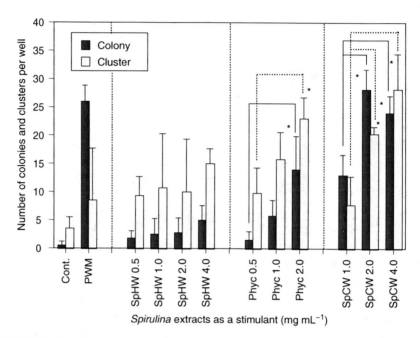

FIGURE 10.14 Colony and cluster formation of bone marrow-cells in soft agar assay cultured with supernatant of spleen cells stimulated with *Spirulina* extracts (From Hayashi, O., *J. Appl. Phycol.*, 18, 52, 2006. With permission.)
Spleen cells were stimulated with 0.5, 1.0, 2.0 and 4.0 mg/ml of *Spirulina* extract. Peritoneal-exudes cells were stimulated with 2.0 mg/ml *Spirulina* extract. Values are means ± SD of three samples.

extracts, especially Pc or SpCW, increased colony-formation of bone marrow cells (Figure 10.14). High amount of granulocyte macrophage colony-stimulating factor (GM-CSF) or IL-3 as a colony-forming activity was detected in the culture supernatants of the spleen cells as well as in peritoneal-exudes cells stimulated with the *Spirulina* extracts, especially with SpCW (Table 10.3). Multipotent colony-stimulating factors such as G- and GM-CSF and IL-3, which have been known to be produced by a variety of cells including monocytes and lymphocytes, can support proliferation of immature hematopoietic cells.[43] Valtieri et al.[44] reported that in *in vitro* system using the IL-3-dependent granulocytic lineage 32D clone 3 (Cl3) cells derived from normal murine bone marrow, G-CSF stimulated terminal differentiation of the cells into neutrophilic granulocytes. *Spirulina* and its components such as phycocyanin can affect enhancing proliferation or differentiation of immune competent-cells in lymphoid organs including bone marrow cell, which may cause normally sustaining or enhancing immune functions.

Colony-forming activity was also significantly induced in the blood, spleen, and Peyer's patch cells in mice that ingested *Spirulina* extracts, SpHW, Phyc or SpCW, orally for 5 weeks in *in vivo* study (Figure 10.15). Ratios of neutrophils and lymphocytes of the mice fed with SpHW and SpCW were, in fact, consequently increased in the peripheral blood (Figure 10.16). In addition, ratios of reticulocytes by SpHW and

TABLE 10.3

GM-CSF and IL-3 Contents in Culture Supernatants (CS) of Spleen Cells Stimulated with *Spirulina* Extracts

Stimulated with	Colonies/well	GM-CSF pg/ml of CS	IL-3 pg/ml of CS
Control	0.5 ± 0.7	<4	47.3 ± 4.0
SpHW	2.8 ± 2.6	<4	76.7 ± 8.0
Phycocyanin	14.0 ± 5.9	9.2 ± 0.7	94.7 ± 10.8
SpCW	28.2 ± 5.5	1206 ± 333	481.7 ± 144.4

Values are means $\pm$ SD of 3 samples.

Source: Hayashi, O., *J. Appl. Phycol.*, 18, 50, 2006. With permission.

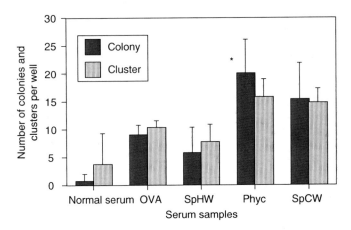

FIGURE 10.15 Colony and cluster formation of bone marrow-cells in soft agar assay cultured with serum from mice fed with *Spirulina* extracts for five consecutive days (From Hayashi, O., *J. Appl. Phycol.*, 18, 52, 2006. With permission.)

Values are means $\pm$ SD of three samples.

lymphocytes by Phyc were increased in the bone marrow of the mice. Zhang et al.[45] found that c-phycocyanin and polysaccharide isolated from *Spirulina* increased leukocyte and bone marrow nucleated cell counts as well as the number of colony-forming unit-granulocyte and macrophage (CFU-GM) in the gamma-ray irradiated mice. They also found that c-phycocyanin possessed high erythropoietin activity. These findings support our results.

Much evidence for clinical applications of hematopoietic growth factors such as GM-CSF and IL-3 to bone marrow failure patients has been accumulated to date. These cytokines as well as erythropoietin are effectively used to decrease cytopenias associated with high-dose chemotherapy, bone marrow transplantation, and leukemia patients,[46] and a phase I study of aerosolized GM-CSF recently demonstrated tolerance and possible efficacy in patients with malignant metastases to the lungs,

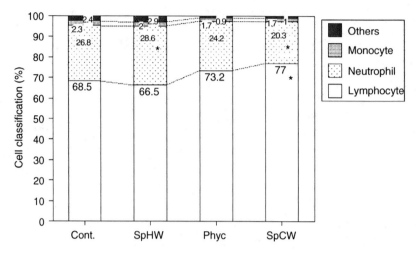

FIGURE 10.16 Classification of peripheral blood cells of mice fed with *Spirulina* extracts for 5 weeks (From Hayashi, O., *J. Appl. Phycol.*, 18, 54, 2006. With permission.) Values are means of six mice.

possibly through upregulation of antigen-specific cytotoxic T-cells.[47] It is known that various food compounds and the metabolites involving phycocyanin in *Spirulina* can influence the processes in cellular differentiation, apoptosis, and proliferative potential, and there is considerable evidence that vitamins and micronutrients are able to regulate gene expression of cancer cells, resulting in influence on the carcinogenic process.[48]

Nondialyzable extracts of some vegetables such as spinach induced the differentiation of other myeloid leukemia and promyelocytic cell lines U937 and HL-60 cells, respectively.[49] All-*trans*-retinoic acid and vitamin D3 are known as being among the physiologic agents that can modulate the proliferation and differentiation of hematopoietic cells.[50] Vitamin plus IFNγ treatment and enrichment with polyunsaturated fatty acids such as arachidonic acid, eicosapentaenoic acid or docosahexaenoic acid also significantly enhanced the expression of monocytic surface antigens CD11b and CD14 on human premonocytic U937 cells and resulted in enhancement of immunoregulatory effects.[51] In addition to our present results, it can be suggested that *Spirulina* is useful in providing complementary nutrients for modulating or maintaining the immune system and that it also may have potential therapeutic benefits for improvement of weakened immune functions caused by, for example, the use of anti-cancer and anti-infectious drugs or HIV-related diseases.

CONCLUSION AND OUTLOOK

At present, very few epidemiologic intervention studies have been done with humans concerning the use of *Spirulina* for health benefits. Hirahashi et al.[52] reported on the molecular mechanism of the human immune potentiating capacity of *Spirulina*. NK-mediated cytolysis and IFN γ production of NK cells collected from 12 healthy volunteers (age 40–65 years) who continued daily drinking of 50 ml of a hot-water extract of *Spirulina* were assayed. Enhancements of NK-mediated cytolysis and IFN γ production were observed in more than 50% subjects 2 months after the beginning of administration. In a study in India,[53] an experiment for assessment of *S. fusiformis* as a source of vitamin A was performed using six healthy preschool children aged 3–5 years as subjects. After stabilization by an almost carotene-free diet taken for 7 days, a single dose of *Spirulina* powder containing 1.2 mg of vitamin A fed along with each morning meal for 1 month improved serum retinol levels significantly, from 21.4 ± 6.23 to 30.3 ± 6.88 of retinol μg/dl. Average absorption rate of total carotene was 72.3%, which was almost the same as that observed in a vitamin A-directly supplemented group, suggesting the potential use of *Spirulina* as a dietary source of provitamin A. Nakaya et al.[54] reported a cholesterol lowering effect of *Spirulina* in studies of 30 healthy Japanese male volunteers as subjects who had mild hyperlipidemia or mild hypertension. Total serum cholesterol level and low-density lipoprotein (LDL) cholesterol were significantly reduced, while neither high-density lipoprotein (HDL)-cholesterol nor triglyceride was changed by 4.2 g of *Spirulina* administration per day for 4 or 8 weeks. Another intervention study was carried out to assess the effect of *Spirulina* on lipid metabolism, antioxidant capacity, and immune function in elderly Koreans.[55] About 6 male and 6 female subjects between the ages of 65–70 were given 7.5 g of *Spirulina* per day for 6 months. Concentrations of triglycerides, and total- and LDL-cholesterol in plasma decreased 4 weeks after the beginning of supplementation. Antioxidant capacity improved, and peripheral blood lymphocyte proliferation rate and plasma C3 levels detected as immune functions were also increased. Recently, Mao et al.[56] found that daily feeding of *Spirulina* 1000 mg or 2000 mg as dietary supplement for 12 weeks in allergic individuals of 36 patients reduced IL-4 production in peripheral blood lymphocytes, while it seemed to be ineffective for the secretion of Th1 cytokines, IFNγ and IL-2, indicating suppression of the differentiation of Th2 cells mediated, in part, by inhibiting the production of IL-4.

Nourishment should be taken essentially by diet. However, reflecting busy life styles of people today and their preferences in healthcare, especially in current aging society, eating habits have changed in developed nations in particular, and opportunities for using so-called health food supplements have increased. Through many studies using experimental animals and in some human studies, we have demonstrated the potential application of *Spirulina* (*Arthrospira*) as a nutritional and therapeutic supplement. We now expect *Spirulina* not only to be utilized effectively for people recovering from illness or for those in an unhealthy state but also for sustaining a healthy state among the general public, including the elderly. It is necessary to accumulate further data and evaluate it scientifically, from the viewpoints of evidence-based nutrition (EBN) and evidence-based healthcare (EBH), in order to assure the proper assessment and utilization of health foods.

REFERENCES

1. Male, D. and Roitt, I., Introduction to the immune system, in *Immunology*, Fifth edition, Roitt, I., Brostoff, J., and Male, D., Eds., Mosby, London, 1998, pp. 1–11.
2. Rook, G. and Balkwill, F., Cell-mediated immune reactions, in *Immunology*, Fifth edition, Roitt, I., Brostoff, J., and Male, D., Eds., Mosby, London, 1998, pp. 121–35.

3. Ciferri, O., *Spirulina*, the edible microorganisms, *Microbiol. Rev.*, 47, 551–78, 1983.

4. Vonshak, A., *Spirulina platensis (Arthrospira): Physiology, Cell-Biology and Biotechnology*, Taylor & Francis Ltd., UK, 1997.

5. Kay, R. A., Microalgae as food and supplement, *Crit. Rev. Food Sci. Nutr.*, 30, 555–73., 1991.

6. Belay, A., The potential application of *Spirulina (Arthorspira)* as a nutritional and therapeutic supplement in health management, *J. Am. Nutraceut. Ass.*, 5, 27–48, 2002.

7. Belay, A. et al., Current knowledge on potential health benefits of *Spirulina, J. Appl. Phycol.*, 5, 235–41, 1993.

8. Khan, Z., Bhadouria, P., and Bisen, P. S., Nutritional and therapeutic potential of *Spirulina, Curr. Pharm. Biotechnol.*, 6 (5), 373–9, 2005.

9. Hayashi, K., Hayashi, T., and Maeda, M., Calcium spirulan, an inhibitor of enveloped virus replication, from a blue-green alga *Spirulina platensis, J. Nat. Prod.*, 59, 83–87, 1996.

10. Schwarz, J. et al., Prevention of experimental oral cancer by extracts of *Spirulina-Dunaliela* algae, *Nutr. Cancer*, 11, 127–34, 1988.

11. Belay, A., Katoh, T., and Ota, Y., *Spirulina (Arthrospira)*: potential application as an animal feed supplement, in *International Association of Applied Algology 7th International Conference*, 1996, p. 23.

12. Hayashi, O., Katoh, T., and Okuwaki, Y., Enhancement of antibody production in mice by dietary *Spirulina platensis, J. Nutr. Sci. Vitaminol. (Tokyo)*.40 (5), 431–41, 1994.

13. Lee, Y.-K. et al., Enhancing phagocytic activity of hemocytes and disease resistance in the prawn *Penaeus merguiensis* by feeding *Spirulina platensis, J. Appl. Phycol.*, 15, 279–87, 2003.

14. Liu, L. et al., Study on effect and mechanism of polysaccharides on *Spirulina platensis* on body immune functions improvement, *Marine Science*, 6, 44–49, 1991.

15. Quresh, M. A., Kidd, M. T., and Ali, R. A., *Spirulina platensis* extract enhances chicken macrophages functions after *in vitro* exposure, *J. Nutr. Immunol.*, 3, 35–44, 1995.

16. Pugh, N. et al., Isolation of three high molecular weight polysaccharide preparations with potent immunostimulatory activity from *Spirulina platensis, Aphanizomenon flos-aquae* and *Chlorella pyrenoidosa, Planta Med.*, 67 (8), 737–42, 2001.

17. Wu, L. C. et al., Antioxidant and antiproliferative activities of *spirulina* and chlorella water extracts, *J. Agric. Food Chem.*, 53 (10), 4207–12, 2005.

18. Hayashi, O. et al., Effects of the extracts from *Spirulina* and *Chlorella* on the immune function of mice in culture, *Ann. Inst. Nutr. Sci. Kagawa Nutr. Univ.*, 13, 71–77, 1994.

19. Isobe, K. et al., Bactericidal activity of mouse macrophages stimulated with *Spirulina* extracts, *J. Kagawa Nutr. Univ.*, 26, 61–66, 1995.

20. Kilian, M. and Russell, M. W., Function of mucosal immunoglobulins, in *Handbook of Mucosa Immunology*, Orga, P. L., Mestecky, J., Lamm, M. E. et al., Eds., Academic Press, New York, 1994.

21. Schmucker, D. L. et al., Basis for the age-related decline in intestinal mucosal immunity, *Clin. Dev. Immunol.*, 10 (2–4), 167–72, 2003.

22. Tlaskalova-Hogenova, H. et al., Mucosal immunity: Its role in defense and allergy, *Int. Arch. Allergy Immunol.*, 128, 77–89, 2002.

23. Hayashi, O. et al., Class specific influence of dietary *Spirulina platensis* on antibody production in mice, *J. Nutr. Sci. Vitaminol. (Tokyo)*, 44, 841–51, 1998.

24. Bozelka, B. E. et al., Soy- and shrimp-specific IgE responses in orally and intraperitoneally immunized mice, *Int. Archs. Allergy appl. Immun.*, 83, 271–77, 1987.

25. Elson, C. O. and Dertzbaugh, M., Mucosal adjuvants, in *Handbook of Mucosal Immunology*, Orga, P. L., Mestecky, J., Lamm, M. E. et al., Eds., Academic Press, New York, 1994, pp. 391–402.

26. O'Hara, A. M. et al., Functional modulation of human intestinal epithelial cell responses by *Bifidobacterium infantis* and *Lactobacillus salivarius*, *Immunology*, 118 (2), 202–15, 2006.

27. Takahashi, T. et al., Effects or orally ingested *Bifidobacterium longum* on mucosal IgA response of mice to dietary antigens, *Biosci. Biotechnol. Biochem.*, 62, 10–15, 1998.

28. Lee, A. N. and Werth, V. P., Activation of autoimmunity following use of immunostimulatory herbal supplements, *Arch. Dermatol.*, 140 (6), 723–7, 2004.

29. Nemoto-Kawamura, C. et al., Effects of *Spirulina* phycocyanin ingestion on the mucosal antibody responses in mice, *J. Phys. Fit. Nutr. Immunol.*, 13, 102–11, 2003.

30. Eldridge, J. H. et al., Controlled vaccine release in the gut-associated lymphoid tissues I. Orally administered biodegradable microspheres target the Peyer's patches, *J. Controlled Release*, 11, 205–14, 1990.

31. Challacombe, S. J. et al., Enhanced secretory IgA and systemic IgG1 antibody responses after oral immunization with biodegradable microparticles containing antigen, *Immunology*, 76, 164–68, 1992.

32. Challacombe, S. J., Rahman, D., and O'Hagan, D. T., Salivary, gut, vaginal and nasal antibody responses after oral immunization with biodegradable microparticles, *Vaccine*, 15, 169–75, 1997.

33. Jeffery, H., Davis, S. S., and O'Hagan, D. T., The Preparation and characterization of poly(lactide-co-glycolide) microparticles. II. The entrapment of a model protein using a (water-in-oil)-in-water emulsion solvent evaporation technique, *Pharm. Res.*, 10, 362–68, 1993.

34. Uchida, T. and Goto, S., Oral delivery of poly(lactide-co-glycolide) microspheres containing ovalbumin as vaccine formulation: Particle size study, *Biol. Pharm. Bull.*, 17, 1272–76, 1994.

35. Ning, Y. et al., Age-related change of mouse Peyer's patch in scanning electron-microscopic observation and its relation to mucosal immune response, *J. Phys. Fit. Nutr. Immunol.*, 13, 90–101, 2003.

36. Tokuyama, H. and Tokuyama, Y., The regulatory effects of all-trans-retinoic acid on isotypes switching: Retinoic acid induces IgA switch rearrangement in cooperation with IL-5 and inhibits IgG1 switching, *Cell. Immunol.*, 192, 41–47, 1999.

37. Remirez, D., Ledon, N., and Gonzalez, R., Role of histamine in inhibitory effects of phycocyanin in experimental models of allergic inflammatory response, *Mediators Inflamm.*, 11, 81–85, 2002.

38. Romay, C., Ledon, N., and Gonzalez, R., Effects of phycocyanin extract on prostaglandin E_2 levels in mouse ear inflammation test, *Arzneimittel-Forschung/Drug Research*, 50 (II), 1106–09, 2000.

39. Gleeson, M., Cripps, A. W., and Clancy, R., Modifiers of the human mucosal immune system, *Immunol. Cell Biol.*, 73, 397–404, 1995.

40. Ishii, K. et al., Influence of dietary *Spirulina platensis* on IgA level in human saliva, *J. Kagawa Nutr. Univ.*, 30, 27–33, 1999.

41. Shinohara, K. et al., Algal phycocyanins promote growth of human cells in culture, *In Vitro Cell. Dev. Biol.*, 2, 1057–60, 1988.

42. Liu, Y. et al., Inhibitory effect of phycocyanin from *Spirulina platensis* on the growth of human leukemia K562 cells., *J. Appl. Phycol.*, 12, 125–30, 2000.

43. Ihle, J. N., Interleukin-3 and hematopoiesis, *Chem. Immunol.*, 51, 65–106, 1992.

44. Valtieri, M. et al., Cytokine-dependent granulocytic differentiation. Regulation of proliferative and differentiative responses in a murine progenitor cell line, *J. Immunol.*, 138, 3829–35, 1987.

45. Zhang, C.-W., Effect of polysaccharide and phycocyanin from *Spirulina* on peripheral blood and hematopoietic system of bone marrow in mice, *Proceeding of 2nd Asia Pacific Conference on Algal Biotechnology, China*, 58, 1994.

46. Vose, J. M. and Armitage, J. O., Clinical applications of hematopoietic growth factors, *J. Clin. Oncol.*, 13 (4), 1023–35, 1995.

47. Rao, R. D. et al., Aerosolized granulocyte macrophage colony-stimulating factor (GM-CSF) therapy in metastatic cancer, *Am. J. Clin. Oncol.*, 26 (5), 493–98, 2003.

48. Sacha, T. et al., The effect of beta-carotene and its derivatives on cytotoxicity, differentiation, proliferative potential and apoptosis on the three human acute leukemia cell lines: U-937, HL-60 and TF-1, *Biochim. Biophys. Acta*, 1740, 206–14, 2005.

49. Kobori, M. et al., Effect of non-dialyzable extracts of vegetables on the differentiation of U-937 human myeloid leukemia cell line, *Nippon Shokuhin Kagaku Kogaku Kaishi*, 42 (1), 61–68, 1995.

50. Collins, S. J., The role of retinoids and retinoic acid receptors in normal hematopoiesis, *Leukemia*, 16, 1905–86, 2002.

51. Obermeier, H., Hrboticky, N., and Sellmayer, A., Differential effects of polyunsaturated fatty acids on cell growth and differentiation of premonocytic U937 cells, *Biochim. Biophys. Acta*, 1266, 179–85, 1995.

52. Hirahashi, T. et al., Activation of the human innate immune system by *Spirulina*: augmentation of interferon production and NK cytotoxicity by oral administration of hot water extract of *Spirulina platensis*, *Int Immunopharmacol*, 2 (4), 423–34, 2002.

53. Annapurna, V. et al., Bioavailability of *Spirulina* carotenes in preschool children, *J. Clin. Biochem. Nutr.*, 10, 145–51, 1991.

54. Nakaya, N., Homma, Y., and Goto, Y., Cholesterol lowering effect of *Spirulina*, *Nutrition Reports International*, 1329–37, 1988.

55. Kim, W. H. and Park, J. Y., The effect of *Spirulina* on lipid metabolism, antioxidant capacity and immune function in Korean elderlies, *Korean J. Nutr.*, 36 (3), 287–97, 2003.

56. Mao, T. K., Water, V., and Gershwin, M. E., Effect of a *Spirulina*-based dietary supplement on cytokine production from allergic rhinitis patients, *J. Med. Food*, 8 (1), 27–30, 2005.

11 *Spirulina* as an Antiviral Agent

*Blanca Lilia Barrón, J. Martín Torres-Valencia,
Germán Chamorro-Cevallos, and Armida
Zúñiga-Estrada*

CONTENTS

INTRODUCTION

Spirulina now named *Arthrospira* is a cyanobacteria that belongs to kingdom Monera and division Cyanophyta. Cyanobacterias also know as blue-green alga, have been consumed as a food for many centuries. Traditionally it was used by Mexicans during the Aztec civilization, and it is currently used by the natives in the Lake Chad area.[1,2] The most commonly used species of *Spirulina* for nutritional supplements are *Spirulina platensis* and *Spirulina maxima*. They are produced commercially and sold as food supplement in health food stores around the world. Early interest in *Spirulina* was focused mainly on its potential as a source of protein, vitamins, especially vitamin B12 and provitamin A (β-carotene), and essential fatty acids like γ-linolenic acid (GLA). Recently more attention has been given to the study of its therapeutic effects, which include reduction of cholesterol and nephrotoxicity by heavy metals, anticancer properties, protection against radiation, and enhancement of the immune system.[3] *Spirulina* also possesses other biological functions such as antiviral, antibacterial, antifungal, and antiparasite activities.[4–6,1]

Actinomycetes have been the most prolific producers of new bioactive metabolites, and at the present time, yield known compounds at a rate in excess of 95% of all active leads discovery in primary screening. Therefore, the interest in identifying naturally occurring molecules with antiviral properties has been largely intensified, mainly searching for new sources of cultivable microorganisms. A high priority has been given for new antiviral drugs against human immunodeficiency virus type 1 (HIV-1), which has caused the most important pandemic disease, the acquired immunodeficiency syndrome (AIDS), since 1981.

Cyanophytes or cyanobacterias are widely distributed in nature, and relatively little systematic screening for antiviral activity had been done. In 1987 Patterson et al., started the screening of extracts of cultured cyanophytes for antiviral activity. Their goal was to examine the distribution of antiviral compounds among blue-green alga and determine whether particular geographic or physical sites are especially likely to yield active leads. They analyzed lipophilic and hydrophilic extracts from 694 strains of cultured cyanophytes, representing 334 species. The extracts were evaluated for antiviral activity against three human pathogenic viruses: herpes simplex type 2 (HSV-2), as representative of double stranded DNA viruses with a nuclear cell cycle; the respiratory syncytial virus (RSV) as representative of single-stranded RNA viruses, with a cellular cytoplasm cycle; and HIV-1, as representative of retroviruses. Approximately 10% of the extracts exhibited antiviral activity against HSV-2 and HIV-1, whereas 2% had activity against RSV. The antiviral activity was more commonly associated with lipophilic extracts than hydrophilic extracts. This survey of blue-green alga for the presence of antiviral activities showed that this biological activity is widely distributed among cyanophytes, and the order Chroococcales proved to be the most prolific producer of antiviral compounds. The substratum from which the organisms were collected showed little correlation with the presence of antiviral compounds. And there was not any relation among the conditions of cultivation of the organisms and the presence of antiviral activity.[7]

Another study published by Gustafson et al., 1989, showed that after the screening of extracts from cultured cyanobacterias (blue-green alga) by using a tetrazolium-based microculture many of these were remarkably active against HIV-1. The microculture assay used to guide the fractionation and purification process revealed a new class of HIV-1 inhibitory compounds, the sulfonic acid-containing glycolipids. These pure compounds were active against HIV-1 in different human lymphoblastoid cells.[8]

In another primary screening of aqueous extracts from terrestrial plants, cyanobacteria, marine invertebrates, and alga, approximately 15% of them showed anti-HIV activity, and this activity was found to be associated to anionic polysaccharides.[9]

Specific screening for inhibitors of reverse transcriptase (RT) from two retroviruses: avian myeloblastosis virus (AMV) and HIV-1, using the lipophilic and hydrophilic extracts of approximately 900 strains of cultured blue-green alga showed that 2% of the aqueous extracts have an anti-RT activity for both viruses. This inhibitory activity could not be attributed entirely to the degradation of transcript DNA, template RNA, or enzyme protein in the reaction mixture. The inhibition of the RT was associated to sulfolipids extracted from cyanobacterias.[10]

These studies on cyanobacterias clearly show the enormous potential of these organisms to produce antiviral compounds which have new targets in the viral replication cycles.

SPIRULINA ANTIVIRAL STUDIES *IN VITRO*

The first report studying the antiviral properties from the blue-green alga *Spirulina* was published by Hayashi et al. in 1993. *In vitro*, they demonstrated that a hot water soluble extract prepared from *S. platensis* inhibited the replication of herpes simplex virus type 1 (HSV-1) in HeLa cells, in a dose-dependent concentration, from 0.08 to 50 mg/mL. The extract did not have a virucidal effect, and the viral inhibition was due to an interference with the penetration event.[11]

After this report, a new antiviral research era started. Hayashi and Hayashi, 1996, by a bioactivity-directed fractionation of the hot water extract from *S. platensis*, isolated a novel sulfated polysaccharide chelating calcium ion, termed calcium spirulan (Ca–SP) as an antiviral principle. Ca–SP was obtained by gel filtration on Sepharose 6B of the hot water extract of *Spirulina* treated with 10% trichloroacetic acid, and a further purification step was done by DEAE cellulose chromatography. Ca–SP did not show antiviral effect against noneveloped viruses such as poliovirus and coxsackievirus. But it showed to be a very effective antiviral agent against enveloped viruses such as HSV-1, human cytomegalovirus (HCMV), measlesvirus, mumpsvirus, influenza A virus and HIV-1, with high therapeutic index (IC50/EC50, concentration required to reduce cell growth by 50% /concentration required to reduce virus replication by 50%) of 8,587, 578, 371, 274, 574, and 1,261, respectively. The antiviral activity of Ca–SP is due to a selective inhibition of the penetration event of HSV-1 into the host cell, effect previously observed with the aqueous extract of *Spirulina*.[12]

Ca–SP besides its antiviral activity, has shown an antitumor effect. It has successfully inhibited experimental lung metastasis. This effect is probably associated to its binding properties, especially to rhamnose receptors located on the cellular surface. It has been demonstrated that rhamnose is a major component in Ca–SP, and lung-metastasizing tumor cells from different types of primary tumor sites, present specific receptors for rhamnose.[13]

Other papers have confirmed and extended the studies about the antiviral properties of *S. platensis* on HIV-1 replication. Ayehunie et al., 1996, by using an aqueous extract of *S. platensis* and different human cells, T cell lines, and peripheral blood mononuclear cells (PMBC) infected with HIV-1, found that the extract at a concentration of 5–10 μg/mL reduced viral production and syncytium formation by 50%.

Same result was found for Rausher murine leukemia virus (RLV) at a concentration of 9–30 μg/mL. The inhibitory effect of the *Spirulina* extract was associated directly to an inactivation of HIV-1 virions.[14] A further study with this extract and HIV-1 on T cell lines, PMBC, and Langerhans cells showed that the extract inhibited 50% of the viral infection at concentrations of 0.3–1.2 μg/mL, and the therapeutic indices ranged between 200 and 6000. It was also confirmed that the inactivation of HIV-1 was a result of a direct virus inactivation. The antiviral activity was associated to the polysaccharide fraction and also to a fraction depleted of polysaccharides and tannins.[15]

It is known that *Spirulina* contains 2–5% of sulfolipids.[16] Sulfolipids from *S. platensis* have proved to be effective against HIV. Sulfolipids inhibit efficiently and selectively only the DNA polymerase activity of the HIV-RT, requiring a concentration of 24 nM for a 50% inhibition. Both the sulfonic acid moiety and the fatty acid ester side chain have a substantial effect in potentiating the extent of inhibition.[17]

A protein-bound pigment allophycocyanin purified from *S. platensis*, has shown an antiviral activity against enterovirus 71, in both rhabdomyosarcoma cells and African green monkey kidney cells. The allophycocianin inhibit 50% of enterovirus 71-induced cytophtic effect, viral plaque formation, and viral-induced apoptosis at concentrations of 0.056–0.101 μM. It has been shown to be more effective in preventing enterovirus infection when it was added to the cells before viral infection, than after, suggesting that it may interfere with a very early stage of viral replication such as virus adsorption and penetration.[18]

Several polysaccharide fractions isolated from *S. platensis* have showed a broad–spectrum antiviral activity, characterized by a strong inhibition *in vitro* of human viruses such as: HCMV, HSV-1, HHV-6 and HIV-1. The ongoing biochemical analysis of these preparations (intracellular and extracellular polysaccharides) indicates the presence of spirulan-like substances, in addition to a small group of other uncharacterized polysaccharides and possibly protein components. The highest inhibition was observed with the extracellular fractions, which presented a therapeutic index of 209.2 for HCMV. The extracellular fraction was isolated from culture supernatant by centrifugation of culture broth, liophylization and dialysis against deionized and ultrapure water. Apparently, this is the first description of antiviral activity of substances isolated from the extracellular fraction of *Spirulina*.[19]

These findings demonstrate that *Spirulina* besides the Ca–SP contains other compounds with antiviral properties.

Other *Spirulina* species, such as *S. maxima* has also shown antiviral activity against human and animal herpesviruses such as: HSV-2, HCMV, and suid herpesvirus 1 or pseudorabies virus (SuHV-1). However, this antiviral activity was not observed against other enveloped viruses such as: two measles strains (Edmonston-Zagreb vaccine strain and subacute sclerosing panencephalitis Halle strain) and vesicular stomatitis virus (VSV). Similarly to *S. platensis* the *S. maxima* extract does not have a virucidal effect on herpesvirus, both extracts inhibit herpesvirus infection by blocking the adsorption and penetration events of t7he viral replication cycle. According to the antiviral results obtained with the extracts from *S. maxima* using solvents with different polarity, the antiviral effect is related to the presence of highly polar compounds.[20]

Table 11.1 presents a summary of the *in vitro* antiviral studies of *Spirulina*.

TABLE 11.1
Studies on *Spirulina* Antiviral Activity *In Vitro*

Cellular system	Virus	*Spirulina*	Inhibitory concentrations	Reference
HeLa	HSV-1	Aqueous extract from S. platensis	0.08–50 mg/mL	Hayashi, et al., 1993[11]
		Sulfated polysaccharide	EC$_{50}$ (μg/mL)	Hayashi et al.,
HeLa	HSV-1	(Ca-SP) isolated from	0.92	1996[12]
HEL	HCMV	the *S. platensis*	8.30	
Vero	Measlesvirus	aqueous extract	17.00	
Vero	Mumpsvirus		23.00	
MDCK	Influenza A virus		9.40	
MT4	HIV-1		2.30	
T cell lines	HIV-1	Aqueous extract from	EC$_{50}$ (μg/mL)	Ayehunie et al.,
PMBC	RVL	*S. platensis*	5–10	1996[14]
			9–30	
T cell lines	HIV-1	Aqueous extract from	EC$_{50}$ (μg/mL)	Ayehunie et al.,
PMBC		*S. platensis*	0.3–1.2	1998[15]
Langerhans cells		Polysaccharide fraction Fraction depleted of polysaccharides and tannins		
UN	HIV	*S. platensis* sulfolipids	UN	Blinkova et al., 2001[42]
Rhabdomyosarcoma cells	Enterovirus 71	Allophycocyanin purified from	0.045 μM	Shih et al., 2003[18]
African green monkey kidney cells		*S. platensis*	0.056–0.101 μM	
HFF	HCMV HSV-1 HHV-6	Spirulan-like polysaccharides from *S. platensis*		Rechter et al, 2006[19]
	Influenza A virus HIV-1	intracellular and extracellular fractions	31–93 μg/mL 0.8–94 μg/mL	
		Aqueous extract from	EC$_{50}$	Hernandez-Corona
Vero	HSV-2	*S. maxima*	0.069 mg/mL	et al., 2002[20]
MDBK	SuHV-1		0.103	
MRC-5	HCMV		0.142	
Vero	HSV-1		0.333	

EC$_{50}$, concentration required to reduce virus replication by 50%; HeLa, human cervical cancer cell line; HEL, human embryonic lung cells; Vero, African Green monkey kidney cell line; MDCK, Madin-Darby canine kidney cell line; MT4, human T cell line; PBMC, Peripheral blood mononuclear cells; HFF, primary human foreskin fibroblasts; MDBK, Madin-Darby bovine kidney cells; MRC-5, human embryo lung fibroblasts. HSV-1, herpes simplex virus type 1; HCMV, human cytomegalovirus; HIV-1, human immunodeficiency virus type 1; RLV, Rauscher murine leukemia virus; SuHV-1, suid herpesvirus 1 (pseudorabies virus); UN, unknown.

SPIRULINA ANTIVIRAL STUDIES *IN VIVO*

The therapeutic efficacy of the *Spirulina* hot water soluble extract has been evaluated against HSV-1 corneal infection in hamsters. Hamsters fed with the extract at a dose of 100 or 500 mg/Kg body weight per day, for 7 days before the HSV-1 infection, have shown longer mean survival times, while all the animals of the control group died 8 days after the infection; about 15–30% of the animals treated with the extract remained alive. No evidence of toxicity was detected in the hamsters fed with food containing the *Spirulina* extract. These results suggest that the consumption of *Spirulina* in the diet may prevent herpetic encephalitis.[11]

The aqueous extract of *S. maxima* has also been tested using the zosteriform HSV-2 infection in mice. These animals received a topical application of the extract immediately before the viral infection, and after that, twice a day, for 5 days. The extract was used at a concentration of 3 mg/Kg body weight per day. HSV-2 could be recovered from a site of viral inoculation on the third day after infection, and on the next 5 days. There were no differences on the viral isolation from the zosteriform infection in the viral infected-control group, and in the *Spirulina*-treated infected group. However, 5 days after the viral infection, 7 out of 12 (58%) animals from the control-infected group developed signs of encephalitis, in comparison to 1 out of 12 (8.3%) from the *Spirulina*-treated infected group. The infected group showed severe signs of encephalitis like, kyphosis, piloerection, and rear limb ataxia, as well as a reduction on the body weight gain. The *Spirulina*-treated infected group showed a similar rate of body weight gain than the control groups: the *Spirulina*-treated mock infected and the noninfected groups. The virus was recovered from the central nervous system of the infected control group, but not from the *Spirulina*-treated infected group. These results suggest that *S. maxima* extract does not prevent the initial infection on the skin, but may successfully interfere with the neuroninvasiveness property of herpes simplex virus.[21]

When zosteriform infected mice received orally the *Spirulina* aqueous extract at the same concentration used for topical application, there were no differences on the rate of infection or development of encephalitis, between the infected-untreated group and the infected *Spirulina*-treated group. These findings were probably due to a low dose of the extract. None of the *Spirulina*-treated animals showed signs of toxicity, neither by topical application or oral ingestion. Therefore, it would be important to test higher concentrations or even better, to fractionate the extract and use higher concentration of the fractions with antiviral activity.[21]

In agreement with the idea that *Spirulina* contains different compounds with antiviral properties, an antiviral protein with molecular weight of 29 kDa has been identified from *S. plantensis*. This protein is active against the viral diseases produced by the nuclear polyhedrosis virus in the silkworm larvae *Bombyx mori*. The mechanism for this antiviral activity is still unknown and it could be similar to other antiviral proteins with carbohydrate-binding properties like cyanovirin.[22]

Proteins with antiviral properties have been found in other cyanobacteria like *Nostoc ellipsosporum*. From these cyanobacteria, an antiviral 11-kDa protein named cyanovirin (CV-N) has been isolated and purified. This protein belongs to the group of carbohydrate-binding proteins (CBP) which have been found in many species including cyanobacterias, sea corals, alga, plants, invertebrates, and vertebrates. CBPs have shown a potent anti-HIV activity, presumably acting by direct binding to the glycans that are abundantly present on the HIV-1 gP120 envelope. CN-V has shown to inhibit HIV infections in a vaginal transmission model in *Macaca fascicularis* infected with a pathogenic recombinant chimeric SIV/HIV.[23]

The antiviral effect observed in experiments *in vivo* with *Spirulina* or its extracts can not only be explained on the basis of a direct antiviral activity against the virus, because *Spirulina* has also immunomodulatory properties. In human volunteers who have received an oral dose of a hot water extract of *Spirulina*, more than 50% of them showed an enhancement of NK functions (IFN gamma production and cytolysis). The INF gamma was produced in an IL-12/IL18 dependent-pathway. It has been suggested that *Spirulina* may be involved in the signaling response through Toll in blood cells. *In vitro* stimulation of blood cells with Bacillus Calmette-Guérin (BCG) was more potent in volunteers who received the *Spirulina*. These results indicate that in humans *Spirulina* acts directly on myeloid lineages either directly or indirectly on NK cells.[24]

Patients with chronic viral hepatitis treated for 1 month with *Spirulina* did not show any improvement in the aminotransferases levels or in their general state.[25] This result could be explained because until now, there is not any *in vitro* study showing that *Spirulina* has an antiviral effect on hepatitis B or C viruses, which are the viruses involved in chronic hepatitis. On the other hand, even though *Spirulina* could enhance the immune response of the patients, it is known that viral chronic hepatitis are related to alterations on the immune response induced by the viral infections.

Negative results with *Spirulina* either in patients or experimental animals could be the result of an insufficient concentration of the antiviral principle in the anatomical site where the virus is being replicated, or that the virus tested is not sensitive to the antiviral principles produced by *Spirulina*. For example *S. platensis* extracts have shown no antiviral activity against viruses like poliovirus and coxsackievirus.[12] A similar situation has been found with *S. maxima* which has no antiviral activity against human adenovirus, poliovirus, rotavirus SA-11, measles vaccine virus, SSPE, and VSV.

Teas et al., 2004, have pointed out an intriguing epidemiological finding about HIV/AIDS rates. There is an enormous difference in the rate of HIV/AIDS incidence and prevalence found in Eastern Asia, 1/10,000 adults in Japan and Korea, compared to Africa, 1/10 adults, and such differences can be explained not only on the basis of intravenous drug use but also on the basis of sexual behavior. Even in Africa the HIV/AIDS rates vary, Chad reported low rates (2–4/100). These epidemiological data have been analyzed together with the alga consumption. People in Japan and Korea eat seaweed daily, and the Kanamemba, one of the major tribal group in Chad eat *Spirulina*, daily. The every day average consumption of alga in Asia and Africa ranges from 1 to 2 tablespoons (3–13 g). According to this general analysis, they have proposed the hypotheses that some of the differences in HIV/AIDS rates could be related to a regular consumption of dietary alga, which could prevent HIV infection and reduce the viral load among those infected. This hypothesis sounds interesting but it requires a deeper analysis of all the possible variables in order to determine if

TABLE 11.2

Studies on *Spirulina* Antiviral Activity *In Vivo*

Animal model	*Spirulina*	Dose	Reference
HSV-1 corneal infection of hamsters	Aqueous extract from *S. platensis*. Absorbed to solid food	100–500 mg/kg body weight, per day. For 7 days before viral infection	Hayashi, et al., 1993[11]
Zosteriform HSV-2 infection in mice	Aqueous extract from *S. maxima*. Topical application	3 mg/kg body weight, twice per day. Immediately before infection and for 5 days after infection	Barron et al. (unpublished results)[21]
Zosteriform HSV-2 infection in mice	Aqueous extract from *S. maxima*. Orally administered	3 mg/kg body weight, twice per day. Immediately before infection and for 5 days after infection	Barron et al. (unpublished results)[21]
Polyhedrosis virus infection in the silkworm larvae *Bombyx mori*	*S. platensis* by leaf dip method as a fed supplement. The resistance to viral infection was associated to a 29 kDa protein	At a concentration of 2–20%	Babu et al., 2005[22]
Human patients with viral chronic hepatitis	*S. platensis* as a food supplement for 1 month	Unknown	Baicus and Tanasescu, 2002[25]

HSV-1, herpes simplex virus type 1; HSV-2, herpes simplex virus type 2.

alga consumption has any beneficial effect either on AIDS symptoms or on preventing HIV infection.[26]

Table 11.2 presents a summary of the *Spirulina* studies *in vivo*.

SPIRULINA CHEMICAL COMPOSITION

The chemical composition of *Spirulina* has been analyzed since 1970, showing high protein concentration, 60–70% of its dry weight, whose nutritive value is related to the quality of amino acid. *Spirulina* contains essential amino acids, including leucine, isoleucine and valine. It also contains a relative high concentration of provitamin A, vitamin B_{12} and β-carotene. *Spirulina* have 4–7% lipids, essential fatty acids as linolenic and γ-linolenic acid,[27] and ω-3 and ω-6 polyunsaturated fatty acids.[28] Cyanobacteria and algae possess a wide range of colored compounds, including carotenoids, chlorophyll, and phycobiliproteins. C-phycocyanin is the principal phycobiliprotein.[29] A selenium-containing phycocyanin has been isolated from *S. platensis*.[30] *S. platensis* contains about 13.5% carbohydrates, the

o-rhamnosyl-acofriose: –o-Rha–o-Aco–   o-rhamnosyl-rhamnose: –o-UA–o-Rha–

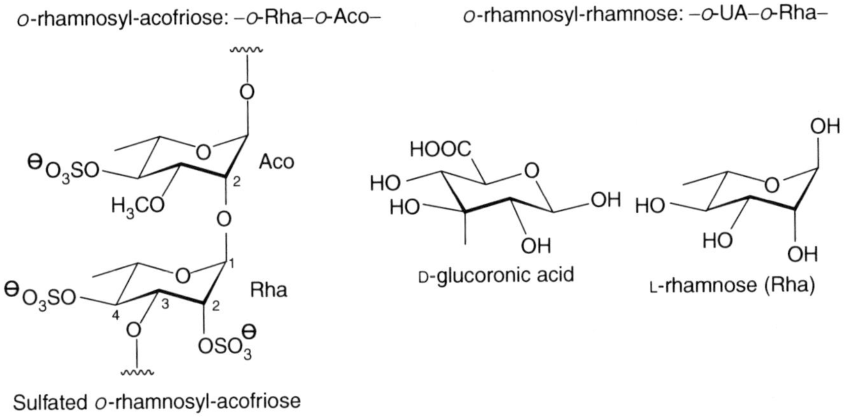

Sulfated o-rhamnosyl-acofriose

FIGURE 11.1   Two types of disaccharide repeating units of Ca–SP.

sugar composition is mainly composed of glucose, along with rhamnose, mannose, xylose, galactose, and two unusual sugars: 2-O-mehtyl-L-rhamnose and 3-O-methyl-L-rhamnose (acofriose).[31] (Figure 11.1). Nowadays the antiviral activity of *Spirulina* has been attributed to three groups of substances: sulfated polysaccharides, sulfoglycolipids, and a protein-bound pigment, the allophycocianin. It is interesting to emphasize that two of these groups of substances possess the sulfate moiety.

SPIRULINA ANTIVIRAL CHEMICAL STRUCTURES AND THEIR ANTIVIRAL MECHANISMS

ANTIVIRAL POLYSACCHARIDES

Calcium Spirulan

The sulfated polysaccharide named calcium spirulan (Ca–SP) isolated by bioassay-guide separation of the hot water extract from *S. platensis*, is a polymerized carbohydrate molecule unique to *Spirulina* containing both sulfur and calcium, which has a molecular weight of 250,000 to 300,000 Da.[12] Detailed structural analyses of their oligosaccharide derivatives performed by electroscopy ionization mass spectrometry (ESI-MS) and collision-induced dissociation tandem mass spectroscopy, showed that Ca–SP is composed of two types of disaccharide repeating units, O-rhamnosyl-acofriose and O-hexuronosyl-rhamnose (aldobiuronic acid)[32] (Figure 11.1). It was suggested that in the first disaccharide repeating unit the link is → 3)-α-L-Rha-(1 → 2)-α-L-Aco-(1 →. Until now, the link in aldobiuronic acid repeating unit is not clear. The sulfated groups were indicated to be substituted at the C-2 or C-4 position of 1,3-linked rhamnose, and at the C-4 position of acofriose. The sulfated units of →3)-α-L-Rha-(1 → 2)-α-L-Aco-(1 → might be essential for the Ca–SP activity.[32,33]

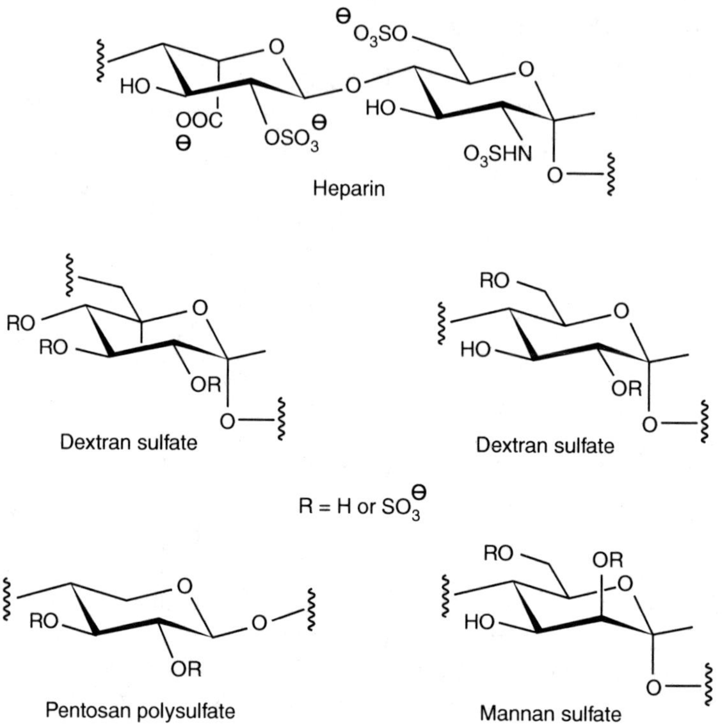

FIGURE 11.2   Structures of anti-HIV sulfated polysaccharides.

Sulfated polysaccharides are well-known as potent inhibitors of HIV-1 and -2 replications *in vitro*. It has been demonstrated that sulfated homopolysaccharides are more potent than heteropolysaccharides, and the sulfate group is necessary for anti-HIV activity.[34] The most interesting ones include heparin, dextran sulfate, dextrin sulfate, pentosan polysulfate, and mannan sulfate (Figure 11.2), which are responsible for the inhibition of virus-cell binding.[35] These compounds are also effective against other enveloped viruses, such as HSV, and HCMV, which usually cause opportunistic infections in immunocompromised patients. The polysulfates have shown a differential inhibitory activity against different HIV strains, suggesting that the target molecules for polysulfates are not the same. Experiments with dextran sulfate have shown that the antiviral activity is enhanced by increasing the molecular weight and degree of sulfation. Moreover, Ca–SP at low concentration does not produce an enhancement of virus-induced syncytium, as is observed in dextran sulfate cultures. Ca–SP has a low anticoagulant activity and a longer half-life in the blood of mice, compared to sulfate dextran. Calcium molecule of Ca–SP was shown to be essential for the inhibition of the viral infection,[36] however; calcium ion can be replaced by sodium or potassium ions preserving its antiviral activity against HSV-1 infection. While divalent or trivalent metal cations reduce its activity, it is noteworthy that substitution by Pb^{2+} ion increases the antiviral activity more than Mg^{2+} ion.

Despolymerization of sodium-spirulan with hydrogen peroxide reduce the antiviral activity as its molecular weight is decreased.[37]

Sulfated polysaccharides exert their anti-HIV activity by shielding off the positively charged amino acids in the V3 loop of the viral envelope glycoprotein gp120. The V3 loop is necessary for virus attachment to cell surface heparan sulfate, a primary binding site, before a more specific binding occurs to the CD4 receptor of CD4[+] T-cells.[38,35]

Spirulan-like

Several polysaccharides isolated from extracelullar fractions of *S. platensis* have showed a broad-spectrum antiviral activity, characterized by a strong inhibition *in vitro* of human viruses such as: HCMV, HSV-1, HHV-6, and HIV-1. These extracellular extracts are composed of 41% of carbohydrates and 57% proteins. Fractionation of one of these extracts by ion exchange chromatography revealed that the antiviral activity was basically in the anionic polysaccharide (spirulan-like substances), but not in proteins fractions. A detailed study in HCMV showed that the spirulan-like substances inhibit HCMV by interfering with both the adsorption and penetration stages of the viral infection. The early inhibition in HCMV replication cycle is similar to the one observed with HSV-1, but it is different for HHV-6, which is inhibited by these substances after the infection step, indicating that there are difference in the mode of action between HCMV and HHV-6. In addition, a second inhibitory effect is observed latter, during intracellular steps of HCMV replication.

To explain these effects, it has been suggested that besides the antiviral activity displayed by negatively charged polysaccharides, which may initially bind to the virus itself or to cellular surfaces, more effective antiviral activity might result from the binding of the polysaccharides to cellular surfaces. Thereby, polysaccharides might interfere with viral entry, but also induce regulatory stimuli giving way to intracellular antiviral effects. One of these intracellular antiviral mechanisms could be IFN induction; however, it has been demonstrated that none of spirulan-like molecules induce significant levels of IFN-α, β.

Therefore, the intracellular anti-HCMV must be related to other mechanisms rather than to IFN activity.[19] It has been proposed that it is unlikely that spirulan-like molecules could effectively penetrate into the cells. But by confocal laser scanning microscopic (CLSM) analysis, sodium-spirulan (Na-SP), a modified spirulan molecule in which the calcium ion was replaced by sodium, has demonstrated to be internalized in HSV-1 infected cells[37]; therefore they might interfere with the viral replication events.

Immulina

Immulina is another polysaccharide isolated from *S. platensis*, which showed potent immunostimulatory activity and does not contain sulfur or calcium. This substance is structurally complex, with an estimated molecular weight above ten million Daltons, is highly water soluble and comprise between 0.5% and 2.0% of microalgal weight.[39]

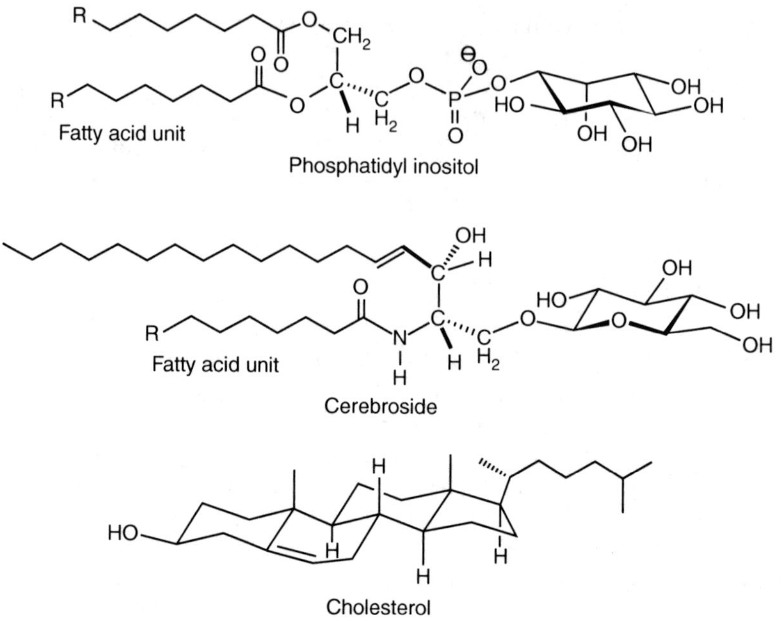

FIGURE 11.3 Structures of phosphatidyl inositol, cerebroside, and cholesterol.

The antiviral activity of water soluble extracts of *Spirulina* can also be explained by the combined action of Ca–SP and Immulina.

SULFOGLYCOLIPIDS

The three main kinds of membrane lipids are phospholipids (like phosphatidyl inositol), glycolipids (like cerebroside), and cholesterol (Figure 11.3). Cholesterol is present in all animal membranes, but absent in prokaryotes. Sulfoglycolipids, as the name implies, consist of three distinct moieties: a backbone lipid, a carbohydrate, and a sulfate moiety. An example of a sulfoglycolipid is presented by 2-palmitoyl-3-hydroxyphthioceranoyl-2′-sulfate-$\alpha - \alpha'$-D-trealose (Ac$_2$SGL) (Figure 11.4), which was isolated as mycobacterial antigen from *Mycobacterium tuberculosis*.[40] *In vitro* studies have revealed that sulfoglycolipids isolated from *Spirulina* exhibit strong antiviral properties. Helper T-cells exposed to sulfoglycolipids isolated from blue-green algae were protected from HIV infection.[8] The chemical structure of the sulfoglycolipids from *Spirulina* remains unknown.

ANTIVIRAL PROTEINS

Allophycocianin

The allophycocyanin is a red fluorescent protein, isolated from *S. platensis*. This antiviral-protein is a member of the phycobiliprotein family, and can be found in blue-green alga, red alga, and cryptomonadas. It has a molecular weight of 104,000 Da

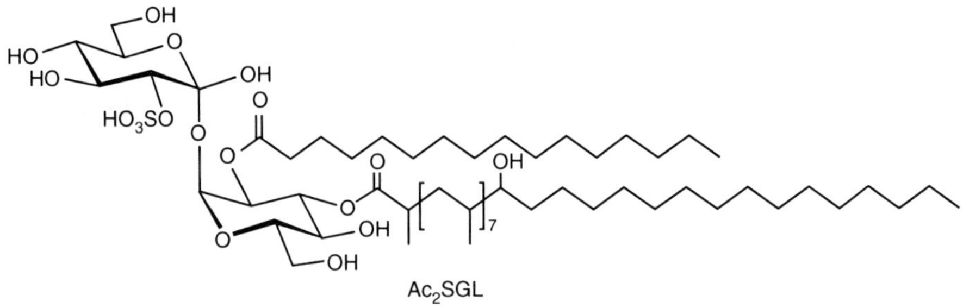

FIGURE 11.4 Structure of 2-palmitoyl-3-hydroxyphthioceranoyl-2′-sulfate-$\alpha - \alpha'$-D-trealose (Ac$_2$SGL).

and consists of two distinguishable protein subunits, which contain at least three covalently attached bilin chromophores, open chain tetrapyrroles with no metal complexes.[41] The antiviral mechanism for this alga-protein remains to be elucidated, but it has shown to abate the apoptotic activity in enterovirus 71-infected cells. It is known that enterovirus 71 infection induces apoptosis and apoptosis may help to spread viral progeny, but also contribute to the viral-induced pathology, especially if it occurs in nonreplicating cells such as neurons. During the last outbreak of enterovirus 71 infection in Taiwan, the postmortem studies clearly showed that enterovirus 71 infected the central nervous system, therefore it can be speculated that a molecule like the allophycocianin could be very helpful to reduce the severe consequences associated with the enterovirus 71 Infection.[18] Allophycocianin could also be useful as a therapeutic treatment for other diseases in which the apoptotic activity is increased and related to the pathology of the disease.

Carbohydrate-Binding Proteins (CBP)

An antiviral protein with molecular weight of 29 kDa has been identified from *S plantensis*.[22] This protein belongs to the group of carbohydrate-binding proteins (CBP) which have been found in many species including cyanobacteria, sea corals, alga, plants, invertebrates, and vertebrates. CBPs have shown a potent anti-HIV activity, presumably acting by direct binding to the glycans that are abundantly present on the HIV-1 gP120 envelope. The cyanovirin (CV-N) protein is a CBP isolated from the cyanobacteria *Nostoc ellipsosporum*. It is an antiviral 11-kDa protein, which has been successfully expressed as a recombinant protein in *Streptococcus gordonii*. This bacteria produces two forms of the CV-N, one is attached to the bacterial surface and the other, is secreted in soluble form in the supernatant of liquid bacterial cultures. The secreted form of CV-N can tightly bind to HIV-1 gp120, whereas CV-N displayed on the bacterial cell wall surface is able to efficiently capture HIV virions. Also, it has been expressed in *Lactobacillus jensenii*.[23] These bacterial systems could be very useful to express and delivery these antiviral proteins in mucosal tissues, and protect the sites from infection of viruses like HV-1, which are highly inhibited by this type of proteins.[23]

SPIRULINA PATENT

The only antiviral compound from *Spirulina* that has been patented is the antiviral polysaccharide purified from *S. platensis* by Hayashi et al. 1996[12]. The US Patent 5585365 was issued on December 17, 1996, and claims that this polysaccharide has a molecular weight of 250,000–300,000 Da, contains rhamnose, glucose, fructose, ribose, galactose, xylose, mannose, glucuronic acid, and galacturonic acid, which can be used as a method for prophylactic or therapeutic treatment of viral diseases, produced by HIV, HSV, HCMV, measles virus, mumps virus, and influenza virus.

The *Spirulina* polysaccharide can be used as an ingredient of antiviral pharmaceutical compositions (liquid, powders, capsules), in foods or drinks like chocolate, tea, biscuits, hamburgers, and others alike. It is recommended to administrate orally the polysaccharide for humans, and animals such as domestic animals: cattles, pigs, sheeps, goats, and pets like dogs, cats, at a dose of about 5–200 mg/kg weight per day, depending on general conditions, severity of the diseases among other factors.

It is worth to say that until now, there are not any published results about human or animal trials showing the antiviral prophylactic or therapeutic efficacy of this polysaccharide.

CONCLUSIONS

It has been clearly demonstrated that *Spirulina* contains several biological active molecules, some of them per se, have shown antiviral activities. The successful ability of viruses to infect specific cell types is due in part to the property of these viruses to bind to particular structures or receptors on the surface of cells. This interaction is highly specific and involves both, viral proteins known as viral attachment proteins (VAP) and cellular receptors. Therefore, any interference affecting the binding between both molecules will impair the virus infection. According to these observations, it is reasonable that Ca–SP, spirulan-like polysaccharides and sulfoglycolipids, and CBPs from *Spirulina* present strong and wide antiviral activity due at least to their interaction with the specialized binding proteins either from the virus or cells receptors. Therefore, *Spirulina*'s antiviral principles are good candidates for antiviral therapeutical use in patients with AIDS, who usually suffer several herpesvirus opportunistic infections. Besides the wide antiviral effect, sulfated-polysaccharides from *Spirulina* have shown to target more than one step in the viral replication cycle, property that is very advantageous for therapeutic use, because it reduces the occurrence of drug-resistant viruses.

Finally, the antiviral molecules produced by *Spirulina* could be specifically modified to obtain more useful and efficient drugs for antiviral therapy, either for topical or systemic use. The study of *Spirulina* antiviral properties has a long way to go.

REFERENCES

1. Ciferri, O. and Tiboni, O., The biochemistry and industrial potential of *Spirulina*, *Ann. Rev. Microbiol.*, 39, 503, 1985.

2. Belay, A., The potential application of *Spirulina* (*Arthrospira*) as a nutritional and therapeutic supplement in health management, *J. A.N.A.,* 5, 27, 2002

3. Belay, A., et al., Current knowledge on potential health benefits of *Spirulina, J. Apl. Phycol.*, 5, 235, 1993.

4. Khan, Z., Bhadouria, P., and Bisen, P.S., Nutritional and theraeutic potential of *Spirulina, Curr. Pharm. Biotechnol.*, 6, 373, 2005.

5. Lee, A.N. and Werth, V.P., Activation of autoimmunity following use of immunostimulatory herbal supplements, *Arch. Dermatol.*, 140, 723, 2004.

6. Chamorro, G., et al., Update on the pharmacology of *Spirulina* (*Arthrospira*), an unconventional food, *Arch. Latinoam. Nutr.*, 52, 232, 2002.

7. Patterson G.M.L., et al., Antiviral activity of cultured blue-green algae (cyanophyta), *J. Phycol.*, 28, 125, 1993.

8. Gustafson, K.R. et al., AIDS-Antiviral sulfolipids from cyanobacteria (blue-green algae), *J. Natl. Cancer Inst.*, 81, 1254, 1989.

9. Cardellina, J.H.2nd., et al., A chemical screening strategy for the dereplication and prioritization of HIV-inhibitory aqueous natural products extracts, *J. Nat. Prod.*, 56, 1123, 1993.

10. Lau, A.F., et al., Inhibition of reverse transcriptase activity by extracts of cultured blue-green algae (cyanophyta), *Planta Med.*, 59, 148, 1993.

11. Hayashi, K., Hayashi, T., and Morita, M., An extract from *Spirulina* platenses is a selective inhibitor of herpes simplex virus type 1 penetration into HeLa cells, *Phytoter. Res.* 7, 76, 1993.

12. Hayashi, T. et al., Calcium spirulan, an inhibitor of enveloped virus replication, from a blue-green alga *Spirulina platensis, J. Nat. Prod.*, 59, 83, 1996.

13. Mishima, T., et al., Inhibition of tumor invasion and metastasis by calcium spirulan (Ca-SP), a novel sulfated polysaccharide derived from a blue-green alga, *Spirulinaplatensis, Clin. Exp. Metastasis.*, 16, 541, 1998.

14. Ayehunie, S., et al., Inhibition of HIV-1 replication by an aqueous extract of *Spirulina* (*Arthrospira platensis*), 7th IAAA Conference, Knysna, South Africa April 17, 1996.

15. Ayehunie, S., et al., Inhibition of HIV-1 replication by an aqueous extract of *Spirulina platensis* (*Arthrospira platensis*), *J. AIDS Hum. Retrovirol.*, 18, 7, 1998.

16. Babadzhanov, A.S. et al., Chemical composition of *Spirulina platensis* cultivated in Uzbekistan, *Chem. Nat. Compounds*, 40, 276, 2004.

17. Loya, S., et al., The inhibition of the reverse transcriptase of HIV-1 by the natural sulfoglycolipids from cyanobacteria: contribution of different moieties to their high potency, *J. Nat. Prod.*, 61, 891, 1998.

18. Shih, S.R., et al., Inhibition of enterovirus 71-induced apoptosis by allophycocyanin isolated from a blue-green alga *Spirulina platensis, J. Med. Virol.*, 70, 119, 2003.

19. Rechter, S., et al., Antiviral activity of *Arthrospira*-derived spirulan-like substances, *Antiviral Res.*, 72, 197, 2006.

20. Hernandez-Corona, et al., Antiviral activity of *Spirulina* maxima against herpes simplex virus type 2, *Antiviral Res.*, 56, 279, 2002.

21. Barron, B.L., et al., Antiviral activity of a hot water extract from *Spirulina* maxima on the herpes zosteriform infection of mice. (unpublished)

22. Babu, S.M., Gopalaswamy, G., and Chandramohan N., Identification of an antiviral principle in *Spirulina platensis* against Bombyx mori Nuclear Polyhedrosis Virus (BmNPV), *Indian J. Biotechno.*, 4, 384, 2005.

23. Balzarini, J., Inhibition of HIV entry by carbohydrate-binding proteins, *Antiviral Res.*, 71, 237, 2006.

24. Hirahashi, T., et al., Activation of the human innate immune system by *Spirulina*: augmentation of interferon production and NK cytotoxicity by oral administration of hot water extract of *Spirulina platensis, Int. Immunopharmacol.*, 2, 423, 2002.

25. Baicus, C. and Tanasescu, C., Chronic viral hepatitis, the treatment with spiruline for one month has no effect on the aminotransferases, *Rom J. Intern. Med.*, 40, 89, 2002.

26. Teas, J., et al., Algae a poor man's HAART?, *Med. Hypotheses.*, 62, 507, 2004.

27. Sánchez, M. et al., *Spirulina* (*Arthrospira*): An edible microorganism. A review, http://www.javeriana.edu.co/universitas_scientiarum/vol8n1/J_bernal.htm, 2007.

28. Wu, L.-C. et al., Antioxidant and antiproliferative activities of *Spirulina* and *Chlorella* water extracts, *J. Agric. Food Chem.*, 53, 4207, 2005.

29. Hsiao, G. et al., C-Phycocyanin, a very potent and novel platelet aggregation inhibitor from *Spirulina platensis, J. Agric. Food Chem.*, 53, 7734, 2005.

30. Huang, Z. et al., Characterization and antioxidant activity of selenium-containing phycocyanin isolated from *Spirulina platensis, Food Chem.*, 100, 1137, 2007.

31. Shekharam, K.M., Venkataraman, L.V., and Salimath, P.V., Carbohydrate composition and characterization of two unusual sugars from the blue green alga *Spirulina platensis, Phytochemistry*, 26, 2267, 1987.

32. Lee, J.B. et al., Structural analysis of calcium spirulan (Ca-SP)-derived oligosaccharides using electrospray ionization mass spectrometry, *J. Nat. Prod.*, 63, 136, 2000.

33. Lee, J.B., et al., Further purification and structural analysis of calcium spirulan from *Spirulina platensis, J. Nat. Prod.*, 61, 110, 1998.

34. Schaeffer, D.J. and Krylov, V.S., Anti-HIV activity of extracts and compounds from algae and cyanobacteria, *Ecotoxicol Environ Saf.*, 45, 208, 2000.

35. Cos, P. et al., Plant substances as anti-HIV agents selected according to their putative mechanism of action, *J. Nat. Prod.*, 67, 284, 2004.

36. Hayashi, K., Hayashi, T., and Kojima, I., A natural sulfated polysaccharide, calcium spirulan, isolated from *Spirulina platensis*: *in vitro* and *ex vivo* evaluation of anti-herpes simplex virus and anti-human immunodeficiency virus activities, *AIDS Res. Hum. Retroviruses*, 12, 1463, 1996.

37. Lee, J.B., et al., Effects of structural modification of calcium spirulan, a sulfated polysaccharide from *Spirulina* platensis, on antiviral activity, *Chem. Pharm. Bull. (Tokyo).*, 49, 108, 2001.

38. Witvrouw, M., and De Clercq, E., Sulfated polysaccharides extracted from sea algae as potential antiviral drugs, *Gen. Pharmacol.*, 29, 497, 1997.

39. Pugh, N. et al., Isolation of three high molecular weight polysaccharide preparation with potent immunostimulatory activity from *Spirulina platensis, Aphanizomenon flos-aquae* and *Chlorella pyrenoidosa, Planta Med.*, 67, 737, 2001.

40. Gilleron, M. et al., Diacylated sulfoglycolipids are novel mycobacterial antigens stimulating CD1-restricted T cells during infection with *Mycobacterium tuberculosis, J. Exp. Med.*, 199, 649, 2004.

41. Duerring, M., Schmidt, G.B. and Huber, R., Isolation, crystallization, crystal structure analysis and refinement of constitutive c-phycocyanin from the chromatically adapting Cyanobacterium fremyella diplosiphon at 1.66 A resolution, *J. Mol. Biol.*, 217, 577, 1991.

42. Blinkova, L.P., Gorobets, O.B., and Baturo, A.P., Biological activity of *Spirulina, Zh. Mikrobiol Epidemiol Immunobiol.*, 2, 114, 2001.

12 *Spirulina* and Antibacterial Activity

Guven Ozdemir and Meltem Conk Dalay

CONTENTS

INTRODUCTION

Microbial natural products are the origin of most of the antibiotics on the market today. However, research in antibiotics and natural products has declined significantly over the past decade as a consequence of a variety of factors including lack of interest shown by industry in the field and the strong competition from collections of synthetic compounds as sources of drug leads.[1] In addition, owing to the increasing resistance of bacterial isolates for antibiotics more intense efforts are being made to find alternative antimicrobial compounds.[2] Against the growing problem of antibiotic-resistant bacteria, alternative sources which are nontoxic to humans must be found.

Natural antimicrobials will undoubtedly have an important role in protecting against infection. This new direction in research has been the subject of many studies on antimicrobial effect of various organism including cyanobacteria. Native people have harvested *Spirulina platensis* from Chad Lake in Africa and Texcoco Lake in Mexico for use as a source of food. Furthermore, *S. platensis* has been used by humans because of its nutritional and possibly medicinal effects.[3]

BIOACTIVE CHEMICALS IN CYANOBACTERIA

Cyanobacteria, sometimes still referred to as blue-green algae, have increasingly been shown to be producers of a diverse array of toxic, or otherwise biologically active,

243

compounds with potential applications in biomedicine, as well as implications for environmental health.[4-8]

Cyanobacteria are a diverse group of photosynthetic, prokaryotic organisms found in freshwater and marine environments. The origin of these organisms dates back 3 or 4 billion years[9] and their cell structure closely resembles that of other Gram negative bacteria, but as a rule they live photoautotrophically. Like higher plants they possess chlorophyll a and the water soluble red and blue phycobiliproteins as well as photosystem I and II producing oxygen, which is released to the atmosphere.

They are truly prokaryotic organisms having no nuclear membranes, internal organelles, and histone proteins associated with chromosomes. They are capable of using carbon dioxide as their sole carbon source employing the reductive pentose phosphate pathway or Calvin cycle.[10]

This group includes various edible and toxic species. Including about 2000 strains cyanobacteria are distributed all over the world. Some of them show a remarkable ecological diversity. Because of widespread eutrophication of lakes, ponds, and some parts of oceans cyanobacteria often form blooms, which lead to water hygiene problems.[11-13] They may cause unpleasant tastes and odors through excretion of volatile compounds.[14] Furthermore, animal poisonings and risks to human health are described and many of them which cause toxic water toxins produced have been characterized.[15-18] Possibly the synthesis of highly active toxins is a defense option of cyanobacteria against attack by other organisms like bacteria, fungi, zooplankton, and eukaryotic microalgae. Carmichael (1994) found that cyanobacterial toxins can be extremely harmful to zooplankters that feed on these cyanobacteria and may be lethal, or they may reduce the number of offspring.

In addition to the toxins a lot of active substances with antibacterial, antiviral, fungicide, enzyme inhibiting, immunosuppressive, cytotoxic, and algicide activity have been isolated from cyanobacterial biomass, or in some cases from the medium of laboratory cultures.[19-26] Producing active biocide components could be an important selective advantage. For example, in the 1970s a pronounced reduction of Gram-positive bacteria was observed in lakes during the occurrence of cyanobacterial blooms.[27] The production of antibacterial substances could be the reason for this phenomenon. In cyanobacterial blooms often only one species may account for >95% of the population. Though this has been interpreted as a result of competition between species, the dominance of one species could potentially hint at the formation of metabolites with cyanobactericidal activity. In addition, antibacterial, fungicidal and antiviral effective compounds formed by cyanobacteria could contribute to an improvement of the water quality in aquatic environment.[28]

Cyanobacteria have the appeal of being a raw unprocessed food, rich in carotenoid, chlorophyll, phycocyanin, amino acid, minerals, and many other bioactive components. The nutrient content depends on the location and environment in which the algae are grown. The environment includes altitude, temperature, and sun exposure, which can greatly affect the lipid and pigment content in algae.[29]

Cyanobacteria have been identified as one of the most promising group of organisms from which novel and biochemically active natural products are isolated. Cyanobacteria such as *Microcystis, Anabaena, Nostoc,* and *Oscillatoria* produce a great variety of secondary metabolites. The only comparable group of microorganisms

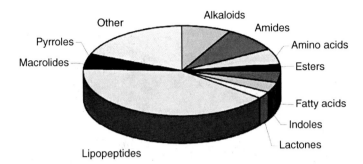

FIGURE 12.1 Types of chemical compounds isolated from marine Cyanobacteria[49] (From Burja, A.M., Banaigs, B., Abou-Mansour, E., Burgess, J.G., and Wright, P.C., *Tetrahedron.*, 57, 9347–9377, 2001.)

is *Actinomycetes*, which has yielded a large number of metabolites and include traditional microbial drug producers like *Actinomycetes* and *Hyphomycetes*, which have been the focus of pharmaceutical research for decades. As the rate of discovery of new compounds from these microorganisms is decreasing, it is time to turn to cyanobacteria and exploit their potential. This is of paramount importance to fight increasingly resistant pathogens and newly emergent diseases (Hayashi et al., 1996). Many agricultural and industrial materials have been obtained from cyanobacteria at laboratory, pilot, and commercial scales including: biomass,[30–33] restriction nucleases,[34] antifungal, antineoplastic,[35,36] antimicrobial,[37] antileukemia[38] and herbicidal compounds.[39] Some pigments have been produced from cyanobacteria[40,41] and other products include: amino acids,[42] and fertilizers.[43]

Bioactive molecules from cyanobacteria exhibit toxic effects against eukaryotes and antibiotic against prokaryotes. It is also reported that antibiotic effects are caused by distinct substances different from the cyanotoxins.[44–46]

Screening of cyanobacteria for antibiotics and pharmaceutically active compounds has received ever increasing attention for some time. The bioactive molecules isolated show a broad spectrum of biological activities including toxins, antibiotics, fungicides, and algaecides.[47]

Because cyanobacteria are largely unexplored, they represent a rich opportunity for discovery; the expected rate of rediscovery is far lower than for other better studied groups of organisms.[48] Cyanobacteria produce a wide variety of toxins and other bioactive compounds, these may be divided into the following chemical classes: 40% lipopeptides, 5.6% amino acids, 4.2% fatty acids, 4.2% macrolides, and 9% amides (Figure 12.1). Cyanobacterial lipopeptides include compounds that may be categorized as cytotoxic (41%), antitumor (13%), antiviral (4%), antibiotics (12%), and the remaining 18% activities include antimalarial, antimycotics, multidrug resistance reversers, antifeedant, herbicides, and immunosuppressive agents (Figure 12.2).[49] Cyanobacteria have a cholesterol-lowering effect in animals and humans. The level of the total cholesterol, LDL and VLDL cholesterol in rat serum was reduced when a high cholesterol diet was supplemented with cyanobacteria. Furthermore, it was found that adopohepatosis, caused by a high cholesterol diet, was "cured" by a diet

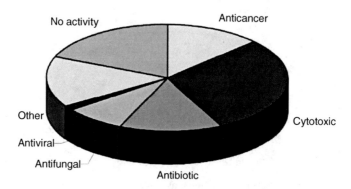

FIGURE 12.2   Reported biological activities of marine cyanobacterial compounds.[49] (From Burja, A.M., Banaigs, E.B., Abou-Mansour, Burgess, J.G., and Wright, P.C., *Tetrahedron.*, 57, 9347–9377, 2001.)

supplemented with algae owing to the activity of lipoprotein lipase, an enzyme for metabolism of triglyceride rich lipoproteins.[50] *Aphanizomenon flos-aquae* also shows a hypocholesterolemic effect, owing to its chlorophyll content, which stimulates the liver function and decreases blood cholesterol level.[51] *Aphanizomenon flos-aquae* inhibit the activity of a maltase and sucrase in the digestive tract of rats.[52] Valencia et al. presented evidence that *Aphanizomenon flos-aquae* accelerate recovery from mild traumatic brain injury.[53]

Many studies have assessed the antibacterial activity of some cyanobacteria and their extracts.[54–62,28] For example, Mian et al. (2003) investigated 22 terrestrial and freshwater cyanobacteria for antimicrobial activity. Of these, 54.5% of all extracts showed activity against Gram-positive bacteria, while 9.1% possessed antifungal activity against *Candida albicans*. However, no extract was obtained to be active against Gram-negative bacteria.

The above results demonstrated that terrestrial and freshwater cyanobacteria are still a promising source of new bioactive nature products.

Soltani et al. (2005) isolated 76 cyanobacteria strains from Iranian paddy fields. 22.4% of them (17 cyanobacteria) exhibited antimicrobial effects. The cyanobacteria with positive antimicrobial activity included members of the families Stigonemata-ceae, Nostocaceae, Oscillatoriaceae, and Chrococcaceae. Growth of *Bacillus subtilis* PTCC 1204 and *Staphylococcus epidermidis* PTCC 1114 was inhibited by 12 and 14 strains of cyanobacteria, respectively. In addition, eight cyanobacteria inhibited the growth of *Escherichia coli* PTCC 1047, and two species inhibited the growth of *Salmonella typhi* PTCC 1108.

Asthana et al. (2006)[63] demonstrated the effectiveness of 15–30 μl/mL of puri-fied bioactive molecule (active principle) from *Fischerella* sp., isolated from Neem (*Azadirachta indica*) tree bark, against *Mycobacterium tuberculosis*, *Enterobacter aerogenes*, *Staphylococcus aureus*, *Pseudomonas aeruginosa*, *Salmonella typhii*, multidrug resistant (MDR) strains of *E. coli*. Mundt et al. (2001) screened antibac-terial activities of lipophilic and hydrophilic extracts from cultured cyanobacteria, or "bloom" material, isolated from German lakes and the Baltic sea against some bacteria. In the above study antibacterial activity was found in the more lipophilic extracts and the aqueous extracts were ineffective.

In a recent study, Pahayokolide A was purified from *Lyngbya* sp. strain 15–2 biomass at yields of approximately 1.35% (w/v) of the crude extract. A lower yield (0.44%) was obtained when the strain was cultured without Na_2CO_3 supplemented medium. Samples of the purified Pahayokolide A isolated from the Na_2CO_3-supplemented cultures were used for toxicological and pharmacological evaluation. Pahayokolide A inhibited the growth of Gram-positive bacteria, *Bacillus megaterium* and *Bacillus cereus*, and the yeast, *Saccharomyces cerevisiae* as well as the green algae, *Ulothrix* Ev-17 and *Chlamydomonas* Ev-29. In addition, hormogonia development was inhibited within a zone around the Pahayokolide A treatment of a lawn of the cyanobacterium, *Nostoc* Ev-1, although growth of the organism was not otherwise affected.[58] Further examples of antimicrobial activity of cyanobacteria are listed in Table 12.1.

In another study, a total of 44 lipophilic and hydrophilic extracts obtained from 22 samples of cultured terrestrial and freshwater cyanobacteria were investigated for their biological activities. Of these, 54.5% of all extracts showed activity against Gram positive bacteria, while 9.1% possessed antifungal activity against *Candida albicans*; however, no extract was active against Gram-negative bacteria.[54]

SPIRULINA AND ITS ANTIBACTERIAL ACTIVITY

The spirally twisted filamentous cyanobacterium *Spirulina* has got a long history of human exploitation. An African tribe living on the lakeside of Chad in North Africa was collecting and eating the *Spirulina* (or Dihe) from the lake.[30]

Spirulina excretes variable quantities of products from its metabolism, such as organic acids, vitamins, and phytohormones, and extracts of *S. maxima* have shown antimicrobial activity against *Bacillus subtillis*, *Streptococcus aureus*, *Saccharomyces cerevisiae*, and *Candida albicans*. The presence of high quantities of acrylic acid in *Spirulina* was substantiated at the end of the seventies and this substance shows antimicrobial activity at 2 mg/L of biomass concentration. In addition, other bioactive compounds including propionic, benzoic, and mandelic organic acids were also found.[76]

Spirulina contains vitamin A, important in preventing eye diseases; iron and vitamin B_{12}, useful in treating hypoferric anemia and pernicious anemia; γ-linolenic acid, appropriate in treatment of atopic child eczema therapy, to alleviate premenstrual syndrome, and in immune system stimulation.[77] Edible microalgae such as *Spirulina* are rich in protein, lipid, polysaccharide, fiber, microelements, and bioactive substances.[78] It has also been reported to have health and pharmacological properties that can help to prevent and cure peptic ulcer and anemia, enhance immunity, as well as antitumor, antiradiation, antipathogenic activities against microorganisms, it can decrease blood lipid and some may act as antiarteroclerosis agents.[79–84]

To date, relatively few studies have been undertaken examining the antibacterial activity of *Spirulina* and its extracts.[65–67,85–88]. One of them, de Mule et al. (1996) tested crude methanolic and aqueous extracts of *S. platensis* on the growth of

TABLE 12.1

Compounds Isolated, Extracted from Cyanobacteria

Source	Compound	Class of compound	References
Order Chroococcales			
Gloeocapsa caldariorum	Methanol extracts		28
Chroococcus sp.	Dichloromethane/methanol 2 : 1 extract		54
Microcystis aeruginosa		Lipid complex, terpene fraction	64
Synechococcus elongatus	Dichloromethane/methanol 2 : 1 extract and methanol/water 7 : 3 extract		54
Gloeothece rupestris	Dichloromethane/methanol 2 : 1 extract and methanol/water 7 : 3 extract		54
Order Oscillatoriales			
S. platensis	Volatile components, methanol, dichloromethane, petroleum extracts		65
S. platensis	Ethanol, acetone, chloroform, hexane extracts		66
S. platensis	Ethanol, hexane and petroleum Ether extracts		67
Oscillatoria limosa	Methanol/water 7 : 3 extract		54
Oscillatoria redekei	Coriolic acid, α-dimorphecolic acid, linoleic acid	Fatty acid	54
Oscillatoria subtilissima strain Bo 62	Extracellular substances		68
Limnothrix redekei	*n*-hexane extracts		28
Lyngbyasp	Pahayokolide A	Peptide	58
Lyngbya majuscula	ApratoxinA 76	Cyclic depsipeptide	69
Lyngbya confervoides	Lobocyclamides A-C	Lipopeptide	70
Order Pleurocapsales			
Hyella caespitose	Carazostatin, chlorohyellazole	Alkaloids, carbazoles	49
Order Nostocales			
Gloeotrichia echinulata	Dichloromethane/methanol 2 : 1 extract		54

TABLE 12.1
Continued

Source	Compound	Class of compound	References
Petalonema alatum	Dichloromethane/methanol 2 : 1 extract and methanol/water 7 : 3 extract		54
Phormidium sp.	Methanol/water 7 : 3 extract		54
Hydrocoleus sp.	Dichloromethane/methanol 2 : 1 extract		54
Pseudanabaena sp.		Intracellular products	71
Pseudanabaena catenata	Methanol extracts		28
Anabaena sp. strain Hi 26	Extracellular substances		68
Anabaena flos-aquae	Dichloromethane/methanol 2 : 1 extract		54
Anabaena variabilis	Methanol extracts		28
Calothrix gracilis	*n*-hexane extracts		28
Nodularia harveyana	Norharmane (9H-pyrido(3,4-b)indole)	Alkaloids	(Volk and Furkert, 2006)
Nostoc sp.	Ethanol:water extracts and dichloromethane:isopropanol extracts		72(Piccardi et al., 2000)
Nostoc commune	Compound 1 and compound 2	a diterpenoid and an anthra-quinone,	73(Jaki et al., 2000)
Nostoc commune	Nostodione, microsporine	Lipopeptide, terpene	49
Nostoc sp. ex *Peltigera aphthosa* var. *variolosa*	Methanol/water 7 : 3 extract		54
Nostoc insulare	4,4′-dihydroxybiphenyl	Phenolic compound	57
Cylindrospermum	Dichloromethane/methanol 2 : 1 extract and methanol/water 7 : 3 extract		54
Cylindrospermum majus	*n*-hexane extracts		28
Rivularia haematites	Dichloromethane/methanol 2 : 1 extract and methanol/water 7 : 3 extract		54
Scytonema hofmanni	Hofmannolin	A cyan-opeptolin	74
Scytonema spirulinoides	Dichloromethane/methanol 2 : 1 extract and methanol/water 7 : 3		54
Tolypothrix byssoidea	Tolybyssidins A (1) and B (2),	Cyclic tride-capeptides	75

TABLE 12.1
Continued

Source	Compound	Class of compound	References
Order Stigonematales			
Hapalosiphon hibernicus	Petroleum ether extract; methanol extract; aqueous extract		56
Hapalosiphon fontinalis	Methanol extract; aqueous extract		56
Stigonema ocellatum	Metanol extracts		56
Fischerella sp.	Hapalindole T	Alkaloid	63
Fischerella sp.	γ-linolenic acid	Fatty acids	59
Fischerella muscicola	Fischerellin	Lipopeptide	49
Fischerella ambigua	Parsiguine	A cyclic polymer	61
Fischerella ambigua	Petroleum ether extract; methanol extract; aqueous extract		56
Order Chamaesi- phonaceae			
Chamaesiphon polonicus	Dichloromethane/methanol 2:1 extract and methanol/water 7:3 extract		54

Source: Data from literature search of January 2000–September 2006.

three microorganisms. In *Candida albicans*, growth was inhibited 17.6% by aqueous extracts and 7.8% by methanolic extracts; in *Staphylococcus aureus* and *Lactococcus lactis* there was growth promotion by both extracts, ranging from 7.5 to 14.7%. Ozdemir et al. (2004) demonstrated that extracts of *S. platensis* were active against four Gram-positive and six Gram-negative bacteria and a yeast, *Candida albicans* ATCC 10239 (Table 12.2).

In this study, the methanol extracts of *S. platensis* (comparable to tobramycin (10 μg/disc), especially against *S. faecalis*, *S. epidermidis*, and *C. albicans*) showed more potent antimicrobial activity than the ethanol, hexane, acetone, and chloroform extracts.

Generally, when compared with the standard, tobramycin, all extracts, except the methanol extracts, exhibited low antimicrobial activity. The methanol and ethanol extracts showed antifungal activity against *C. albicans*, but less than that of the standard nystatin.

Another study examined ethanol, acetone, chloroform, hexane extracts of *S. platensis* against some test microorganisms. Aceton, chloroform, and hexane extracts showed more potent antibacterial activity against *P. aeruginosa* and *S. typhimurium* than ethanol extracts, *S. faecalis*, and *E. coli* for acetone extracts *Mycobacterium*

TABLE 12.2
Antimicrobial Activity of *S. platensis* Extracts

	Diameter of zone of inhibition (mm)															
	Methanol extract (mg/mL)				Dichloromethane extract (mg/mL)				Petroleum ether extract (mg/mL)				Ethyl acetate extract (mg/mL)			
Microorganism	1	2	4	8	1	2	4	8	1	2	4	8	1	2	4	8
Streptococcusfaecalis	13	13	14	14	—	—	—	—	—	—	—	—	—	—	—	—
Bacillus subtilis	7	7	8	8	—	—	—	7	—	—	—	—	—	—	—	—
Staphylococcusaureus	7	7	7	7	—	—	—	7	—	—	—	—	—	—	—	—
S. epidermidis	13	14	15	16	—	—	7	8	—	—	—	—	—	—	—	—
Enterobacteraerogenes	—	7	7	7	—	—	9	10	—	—	—	—	—	—	—	—
E. cloacae	7	7	8	9	—	—	—	—	—	—	7	8	—	—	—	—
E. coli	—	—	7	7	—	—	—	—	—	7	7	8	—	—	—	—
Pseudomonas aeroginosa	—	7	7	7	—	—	—	7	—	—	—	—	—	—	—	—
Salmonella typhimurium	—	—	7	7	—	—	8	9	7	7	7	8	—	—	—	—
Proteus vulgaris	9	9	10	10	—	—	8	9	7	7	7	8	—	—	—	—
Candida albicans	10	11	12	13	—	—	—	—	—	—	—	—	—	—	—	—

Note: No activity.
Source: From Ozdemir et al. (2004).

smegmatis, P. aeruginosa and *S. aureus* for chloroform extracts, *Proteus vulgaris* for hexane extracts.[66] Antimicrobial activity of different pressure liquid extraction (PLE) fractions of *S. platensis* was tested against *S. aureus* ATCC 25923, *E. coli* ATCC 11775, *C. albicans* ATCC 60193, and *Aspergillus niger* ATCC 16404.[67]. Data obtained demonstrated that the hexane and petroleum ether extracts were slightly more active than ethanolic extracts. Furthermore, aqueous extracts were inactive against the microorganisms tested. However, *C. albicans* was the most sensitive micro-organism to all *Spirulina* PLE extracts.[67]

The results of studies on the detection of biologically active substances in biomass dilutions and culture fluid of *S. platensis* and algae (*Chlorella, Fucus, Laminaria*) by the agar diffusion method are presented. After the sterilization of the solutions with chloroform, a substance with lysozyme-like activity and two substances with antagonistic activity deep in agar and on its surface were detected with the use of the micrococcal indicator strain.[88]

EFFECTS OF FATTY ACIDS AND VOLATILE COMPONENTS ON ANTIBACTERIAL ACTIVITY OF *SPIRULINA*

It has been claimed that consumption of *Spirulina* is beneficial to health because of its chemical composition including compounds like essential amino acids, vitamins,

TABLE 12.3
Fatty Acid Composition of *S. platensis* Powder

Fatty acid	Fatty acids (%)
(C_{14}) Myristic acid	0.23
(C_{16}) Palmitic acid	46.07
($C_{16:1}$)Δ^9 Palmitoleic acid	1.26
($C_{18:1}$)Δ^9 Oleic acid	5.26
($C_{18:2}$)$\Delta^{9,12}$ Linoleic acid	17.43
($C_{18:3}$)$\Delta^{9,12,15}$ γ-Linolenic acid	8.87
Others	20.88

Source: From Otles and Pire, 2001[104].

natural pigments, and essential fatty acids, particularly γ-linolenic acid, a precursor of the body's prostaglandins.[89–92] It has also been reported that some cyanobacteria produce substances that can either promote or inhibit microbial growth.[93–95]

The fatty acid composition of *Arthrospira* (*Spirulina*) is influenced by the environmental factors and growth phase.[96–98] Although the total lipid content has been shown to decrease with decrease in temperature,[99] the proportion of desaturated fatty acids increases.[100–102] The predominant acids of *Spirulina* cultures grown under standard conditions of 30°C and low irradiance (10 μmol photon/m²/s) were palmitic, linoleic, and γ-linolenic acids (Table 12.3), which together may account for 88–92% total fatty acids.[103]

A decrease in temperature from 30 to 20°C, an increase in irradiance (at 30°C) from 10 to 70 μmol photon/m²/s and transfer to dark heterotrophy all favored an increase in polyunsaturated C_{18} fatty acids. The highest γ-linolenic acid content of any conditions was found for three strains grown heterotrophically on glucose in the dark at 30°C (Mühling et al., 2005). This is an adaptive response similar to that found in higher plants, where a temperature decrease generally leads to an increase in fatty acid desaturation of membrane lipids which is thought to compensate for the decrease in membrane fluidity at low temperatures,[105] thus providing the photosynthetic machinery with the ability to tolerate temperature stress (Wada et al., 1994). The desaturation to γ-linolenic acid involves three different desaturation enzymes, $\Delta 9$, $\Delta 12$, and $\Delta 6$ desaturases that are encoded by the *desC*, *desA*, and *desD* genes, respectively.[106] The $\Delta 9$ and $\Delta 12$ desaturases catalyze the desaturation of the first two double bonds in the fatty acids. Although it was thought that the amount of di-unsaturated fatty acids influences most the physiology of membranes at low temperatures[107] it has later been shown for *Arthrospira* strain C1 that the expression of *desC* and *desA* was almost constant within a temperature range of 22–40°C.[108] In contrast, the expression of the *desD* gene was strongly up-regulated upon a temperature shift from 35 to 22°C and led to an increase of γ-linolenic acid.[108]

TABLE 12.4
Volatile Components in *S. platensis*

Rt (min)	Compound	Area (%)
9.78	Tetradecane	34.61
11.06	α-Ionene	0.46
13.08	Pentadecane	3.20
13.84	2-Hexadecene	1.77
14.36	Hexadecane	2.18
14.58	Hexadecanenitrile (palmitonitril)	1.85
15.20	6(Z), 9(E)—Heptadecadiene	1.18
15.31	8-Heptadecene	1.06
15.60	Heptadecane	39.70
17.17	Neophytadiene	2.05
17.57	Pentadecanenitrile	2.15
17.70	9,12-Octadecadienoic acid (linoleic acid)	1.01
17.94	Hexadecanoic acid, methyl ester (palmitic acid)	0.84
18.64	Isophytol	1.14
19.94	Phytol	3.25
	Total	96.45

Source: From Ozdemir et al. (2004).

Spirulina lipids have been contained saturated, monounsaturated, and polyunsaturated fatty acids. It also contained hydrocarbons (Heptadecane as the major hydrocarbon, along with a minor amount of heptadecene) and phytol.[109]

A study on the antimicrobial effect of fatty acids showed the antimicrobial effect of volatile components of *S. platensis*.[65] Fifteen compounds from hydrodistillation for 4 h using a Clevenger-type apparatus were identified, constituting 96.45% of the total component. The components analyzed by GC and GC/MS are listed in Table 12.4. The major component was heptadecane (39.7%). Heptadecane has been reported to be a common major volatile component in many other cyanobacteria species.[65] In the study, it measured the antimicrobial activity of volatile components against ten bacteria and a yeast (Table 12.5).

Especially, 0.015 μg/disc volatile lipids had shown inhibitory activity against all test organisms. These results demonstrated that the activity could increase if the concentration gets higher.

EFFECTS OF LINOLENIC ACID AND LINOLEIC ACID ON ANTIMICROBIAL ACTIVITY OF *SPIRULINA*

γ-Linolenic acid (Figure 12.3), the long chain polyunsaturated fatty acid (LC-PUFA) has attracted attention worldwide because of its medicinal value with regard to cardiovascular diseases,[110] hypercholesterolaemia,[111] menstrual disorders,[112] skin diseases (atopic eczema),[113] and other disorders.[114]

TABLE 12.5

Antimicrobial Activity of *S. platensis* Volatile Components*

| | | | Inhibition zone (mm)[a] | | | |
| | | | μg/disc | | Standard | |
Microorganism	G	0.0075	0.015	Tob	Nys
Streptococcus faecalis ATCC 8043	+	—	7	9	nt
Bacillus subtilis ATCC 6643	+	—	8	24	nt
Staphylococcus aureus 6538/P	+	—	7.5	16	nt
Staphylococcus epidermidis ATCC 12228	+	—	8	7	nt
Enterobacter aerogenes CIP 6069	—	—	8	14	nt
Enterobacter cloacae ATCC 13047	—	—	7	13	nt
Escherichia coli ATCC 11230	—	7	8	10	nt
Pseudomonas aeroginosa ATCC 27853	—	—	7	12	nt
Salmonella typhimurium CCM 583	—	—	9	10	nt
Proteus vulgaris ATCC 6897	—	7	9	13	nt
Candida albicans ATCC 10239	—		7	nt	18

[a] Zone of inhibition, including the diameter of the filter paper disc (6 mm); mean value of three independent experiments; Tob,

tobramycin (10 μg/disc); Nys, nystatin (30 μg/disc); nt, not tested; G, gram reaction; —, no activity.

* Ozdemir et al., (2004)

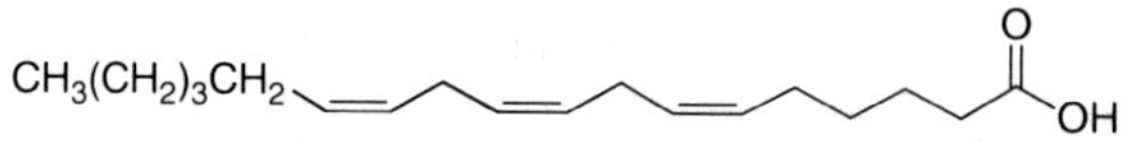

FIGURE 12.3 γ-Linolenic acid.

Microalgae are seen as a good γ-linolenic acid (GLA) resource; moreover, deciphering of gene sequences in cyanobacteria paved the way for biotechnological production of GLA. Whereas the antibacterial properties of α-linolenic acid from cyanobacteria are well established,[28] those of γ-linolenic acid have been little explored. Cohen et al. (1987) reported that the amount of total fatty acids is in the range 2.4–4.8% of dry weight and GLA content of the fatty acid varies from 8–31.7% in different *Spirulina* strains.

Asthana et al. (2006) revealed that the antibacterial activity of the GLA (25 μg/mL) from the cyanobacterium to different bacterial strains revealed the sequence of inhibition zones (mm) as: *Staphylococcus aureus* (18) >*E. coli* (16) >*Salmonella typhi* (14) >*Pseudomonas aeruginosa* (12) >*Enterobacter aerogenes* (7). However, this sequence was slightly altered with the equivalent dose (25 μg/mL) of GLA standard with reference to *P. aeruginosa* or *E. coli*, as both had almost the same sensitivity level. The apparent increase in sensitivity of the bacterial test strains

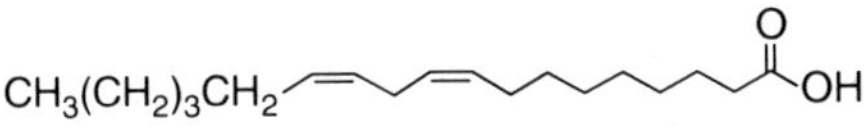

$$CH_3(CH_2)_3CH_2 \diagup\!\!\!=\!\!\!\diagdown\!\!\!\diagup\!\!\!\diagdown\!\!\!\diagup\!\!\!\diagdown\!\!\!\diagup\!\!\!\diagdown\!\!\!\diagup\overset{\displaystyle O}{\overset{\|}{\diagup}}OH$$

FIGURE 12.4 Linoleic acid.

is attributable mainly to the ultrapure GLA standard. Of the two linolenic acids, the antimicrobial activity has been established for α-linolenic acid (ALA) originating from *Limnothrix redekei* HUB 051 (*Oscillatoria redekei*),[28] while linolenic acid and linoleic acids excreted by cultures of *Phormidium tenue* caused autolysis of cells.[115,116] Mundt et al. (2001) determined that the minimal inhibition concentrations (MICs) of the isolated α-linolenic acid against *Staphylococcus aureus* SBUG 11 was 75 μg/mL and against *Micrococcus flavus* SBUG 16 was 25 μg/mL. A concentration of α-linolenic acid of 500 μg/filter disk was also effective against multiresistant *Staphylococcus* strains and inhibition zones from 10 to 20 mm were measured.

Mundt et al. (2003) reported that antimicrobial effect of linoleic acid (Figure 12.4) isolated from *Oscillatoria redekei* inhibited the growth of some Gram-positive bacteria. The minimal inhibition concentration (MIC) against *Staphylococcus aureus* SBUG 11 for linoleic acid was 100 μg/mL.

A study on the antimicrobial effect of fatty acids demonstrated that the antimicrobial effect is far more significant in those connected in straight chain fatty acids, rather than isomer fatty acids.[117] In the ester group of fatty acids composed with 6–18 carbons, a significant antimicrobial effect was observed in glycerol caprylate (C_{10}), glycerol laurate (C_{12}), and glycerol myristate (C_{14}) against bacteria, yeasts, and molds.[118–120] The strength of the antimicrobial effect of the fatty acids with 18 carbons and glycerol laurate (C_{12}) against *Bacillus cereus* was in the order of stearic < oleic < lauric < glycerol laurate < linolenic acid.[121] Also, ALA from the unicellular chlorophytes *Chlorococcum* sp. HS-101 and *Dunaliella primoluta* were active against methicillin resistant *Staphylococcus* strains.[122] Likewise, the relative MIC values with reference to the bacterial strains revealed antibacterial potential of the GLA. In such comparisons, ALA from *Limnothrix redekei* active against *S. aureus* (MIC 75 μg/mL)[28] is 18-fold less toxic than GLA from *Fischerella* sp. (MIC μg/mL), although, the bacterial strains were not the same in each study.

PROBIOTIC ACTIVITY OF *SPIRULINA*

Consumption of yoghurt and other fermented dairy products prepared with *Lactobacillus*, *Streptococcus*, and *Bifidobacteria* strains has increased all over the world in recent years. It is considered by both the general public and expert nutritionalist that they provide humans with major benefits: protection from infection of intestinal pathogen microorganisms,[123] stimulation of the immune system,[124] as well as better digestion, and absorption of lactose and minerals,[125] prevention of traveler's diarrhea,[126] (Alm, 1991), reduction of diarrhea and rotavirus infection in infants,[127] prevention of constipation in elderly people,[126] contribution to a faster recolonization of the intestinal microflora after administration of antibiotics,[128–131] improvement in lactose intolerance,[132] reduction of cholesterol level in the blood,[133] stimulation of the immune system,[134] and improvement in defense against cancer.[135] It has been demonstrated that *Lactobacillus* population in the human gastrointestinal tract is increased by *Spirulina* consumption. This has the potential to improve: food digestion and absorption improvement, intestinal protection against bacterial infections and immune system stimulation.[92,136] Immune system modulation is due to interference on production and NK cytotoxicity.[137] Because the human gut microbiota can play a major role in health, there is currently some interest in functional food ingredients that may stimulate endogenous or exogenous beneficial lactic acid bacteria (LAB).[138] It was established that biomass from *S. platensis* increased *Lactococcus lactis* subsp. *lactis* growth.[87]

Spirulina sp. among cyanobacteria is the best known genus because of its nutritional value. It contains 18 of the 20 known aminoacids; high-quality proteins; more calcium than milk; more vitamin B12 than cow liver; vitamins A, B2, B6, E, H, and K, and all essential minerals, trace elements, and enzymes.[89] *Spirulina* is one of the richest sources of iron among various organic health supplements. The fatty acid composition of *Spirulina* is characterized by high levels of the ω-6 series. Deficiency in linolenic acid is also associated with vision[139] and nervous system defects, regulation of blood pressure, cholesterol synthesis, infammation, and cell proliferation.

De Caire et al. (2000)[140] studied the effect of a natural additive, dry biomass from *S. platensis*, on the growth of LAB in milk. They showed that the addition of dry *S. platensis* to milk (6 mg/mL) stimulated growth of *Lactococcus lactis* by 27%. Recently, it was observed that growth of LAB in synthetic media was promoted by extracellular products of *S. platensis*.[141] Similarly, Varga et al. (2002)[142] studied the influence of a *S. platensis* biomass on the Microflora of Fermented *acidophilusbifidus-thermophilus* (ABT) Milks during storage (R1). In the study, *Spirulina*-enriched and control (plain) fermented ABT milks were produced using a fast fermentation starter culture (ABT-4) as the source of *Lactobacillus acidophilus* (A), bifidobacteria (B), and *Streptococcus thermophilus* (T). As for the cyanobacterial product, the *S. platensis* biomass was added to the process milk. Results showed that the counts of the starter organisms were satisfactory during the entire storage period at both temperatures applied in this research. The *S. platensis* biomass had a beneficial effect on the survival of ABT starter bacteria regardless of storage temperature. Postacidification was observed at 15°C, whereas pH remained stable during refrigerated storage at 4°C. Bifidobacteria were highly susceptible to acid injury and their counts fell more sharply than did those of lactobacilli and streptococci; however, the addition of *Spirulina* biomass was of beneficial effect on their viability.[142]

Varga et al. (1999a)[143] investigated that effect of a dried *S. platensis* cyanobacterial biomass enriched with iodine, zinc, and selenium on the growth and acid production of mixed starter cultures most commonly used for the manufacture of fermented dairy products. Five combinations of the single strains of *Streptococcus salivarius* subsp, *thermophilus* CH-1, *Lactobacillus delbrueckii* subsp, *bulgaricus* CH-2, *Lactobacillus acidophilus* La-5, and *Bifidobacterium bifidum* Bb-12 were tested. The stimulation of *L. bulgaricus* and *L. acidophilus* by the cyanobacterial biomass reduced the time needed for the manufacture of products containing lactobacilli considerably. The effect of a dried *S. platensis* cyanobacterial biomass enriched with trace elements on the rate of acid development by pure cultures of *Streptococcus salivarius* subsp.

thermophilus CH-I, *Lactobacillus delbrueckii* subsp. *bulgaricus* CH-2, L. *acidophilus* La-5 and *Bifidobacterium bifidum* Bb-12 was increased in milk. The *S. platensis* biomass that was rich in trace elements, vitamins, sulfur-containing amino acids, and unsaturated fatty acids also had a highly beneficial effect on the nutritional value of milk, thus providing a new opportunity for manufacture of functional dairy products.[144]

The *S. platensis* biomass stimulated the rod-shaped starter bacteria to a greater extent than the coccus-shaped one, and being rich in trace elements, vitamins, sulfur-containing amino acids and unsaturated fatty acids, it also had a beneficial effect on the nutritional value of cow's milk.

Nowadays, when the dairy industry is supplementing milk with minerals, vitamins, and antioxidants, it would be of interest to consider the possibility of adding *Spirulina biomass*, as a natural product, to fermented milk to induce a faster production of LAB and increase the number of viable cells in the product and in the gut.[140]

The abundance of bioactive substances in *S. platensis* is of great importance from a nutritional point of view because in this way the cyanobacterial biomass provides a new opportunity for the manufacture of functional dairy foods.

REGULATORY ACTIVITIES ON IMMUNE SYSTEM OF *SPIRULINA*

Certain species of *Spirulina* have shown to exhibit immunomodulating and biomodulating properties. Studies indicated immunoenhancing properties of *S. platensis* in animals and humans. Administration of this cyanobacterium has improved immunological resistance in subjects with various types of cancer, viral, and bacterial diseases (Figure 12.5).

It was reported[145] that *Spirulina* up-regulates key cells and organs of the immune system improving their ability to function in spite of stress from environmental toxins and infectious agents. Studies on animal models documented that phycocyanin of *Spirulina* stimulates hematopoiesis, especially erythropoiesis by inducing erythropoietin hormone (EPO). There is also evidence that c-phcocyanin and polysaccharides of *Spirulina* enhance white blood cell production [146,147] The percentage of phagocytic macrophages increased when cats were administered water-soluble extract of *S. platensis* (Qureshi and Ali, 1996). Increased phagocytic activity was also observed in other animals such as mice and chicken [146-148]

For example, Lee et al. (2003)[149] studied enhancing phagocytic activity of hemocytes and disease resistance in the prawn *Penaeus merguiensis* by feeding *S. platensis*. Cultured prawns are prone to infectious bacterial diseases, in particular *Vibrio* spp. [150,151] for they are often subjected to stressful conditions of high stocking density and waste concentration. Enhanced immune resistance to diseases in cultured prawns would be economically desirable. Prawns possess an immune system constituting phagocytic hemocytes and humoral factors;[152-154] however, they possess no immunological memory, as they do not have B and T lymphocytes and therefore do not have specific immune responses. Lee et al. (2003) found that exposing the

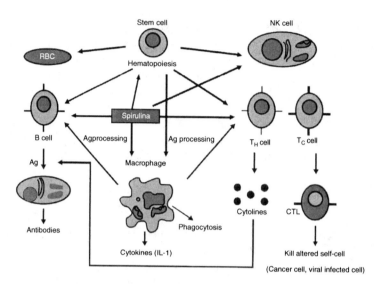

FIGURE 12.5 Effect of *Spirulina* on Immune system. *Spirulina* enhance rate of production of RBCs and WBCs by enhancing hematopoiesis. *Spirulina* also show direct effect on both innate and specific immunity *Spirulina* activate macrophage and Nk cells. *Spirulina* induce production of the antibodies. *Spirulina* also activate of T-cells, B cells and T cells, B and T lymphocytes; CTL, Cytotoxic T lymphocytes; NK cell, Natural Killer cells; L-1, Interleukin-1; Ag, Aggregation; Th, T helper; Tc, cytotoxic T cells (Khan et al., 2005).

prawn *Penaeus merguiensis* to the bacteria *Vibrio harveyi* and *E. coli* for an hour or feeding the prawns with *S. (Arthrospira) platensis* (0.3% w/w feed) enhanced the phagocytic activity of their hemocytes. Improvement of the phagocytic activity was primarily through the activation of the hemocytes. Furthermore, the activated phagocytic hemocytes had a higher capacity to engulf foreign agents, such as bacteria, and a higher rate of phagocytosis. The phagocytic enhancement effect peaked on the fourth day of feeding with *Spirulina*. In the *in vitro* study, the granular cells from prawns took 45–60 min to complete the process of degranulation. Preexposure to *Salmonella typhimurium* and *Bacillus subtilis* did not result in enhancement of phagocytic activity of hemocytes. Only 10% of the prawns fed with *Spirulina* died in the first 14 days when challenged by *V. harveyi* at a concentration of 1×104 CFUs mL^{-1}, while all control prawns (basal feed without *Spirulina*) died within 14 days.

Duncan and Klesius (1996)[155] have reported that *Spirulina* are also capable of enhancing nonspecific immune responses in fish. They demonstrated that peritoneal phagocytes from channel catfish (I. punctatus) fed *S. plantesis*, showed enhanced phagocytosis to zymosan and increased chemotaxis to *Edwardsiella ictaluri* exoantigen. In mice, *Spirulina* facilitated antibody production, increased the ratio of activated peritoneal macrophages, and induced spleen cells to grow better in response to Con A.[137] (Hirahashi, T. et al., 2002). Hayashi et al. (1994, 1998)[156,157] reported that *Spirulina* and its extracts enhanced immune responses in mice, mainly through increased production of interleukin-1(IL-1) in macrophages. They investigated antibody productions of IgA and other classes, such as IgE and IgG1, in mice as possible evidence of the protective effects of *Spirulina* toward food allergy and microbial infection. An increase of IgE antibody level in the serum was observed in the mice that were orally immunized with crude shrimp extract as an antigen (Ag group). The antibody level; however, was not further enhanced by treatment with *Spirulina* extract (SpHW). IgG1 antibody, on the other hand, which was increased by antigen administration, was further enhanced by *Spirulina* extract. It was noted that the ISA antibody level in the intestinal contents was significantly enhanced by treatment with *Spirulina* extract concurrently ingested with shrimp antigen, in comparison with that of the Ag group treated with shrimp antigen alone. It was reported that intraperitoneally injected polysaccharides of a hot-water extract of *Spirulina* increased the percentage of peritoneal phagocytic cells besides increasing the hemolysin contents in the blood of mice.[158]

Watanuki et al., 2006, studied immunostimulant effects of dietary *S. platensis* on carp, *Cyprinus carpi*. For this purpose, fish were fed with *Spirulina* and the parameters of non-specific defence mechanisms, including phagocytosis and production of superoxide anion were performed at 1, 3, and 5 days after *Spirulina* administration. The results demonstrated that *Spirulina* enhanced responses of phagocytic activity and superoxide anion production in kidney phagocytic cells. This activation of kidney cells was observed for at least 5 days post treatment. The expression of interleukin (IL)-1β and tumor necrosis factor (TNF)-α genes also increased in fish treated with *Spirulina*. On the other hand, the expression of IL-10 gene was decreased. Furthermore, the numbers of *Aeromonas hydrophila* were decreased in the liver and kidney of *Spirulina*-treated fish. The numbers of bacteria were lowed in the liver and kidney of carp treated with *Spirulina* than the control group. Sakai et al. (1993)[159] reported that fish treated with lactoferrin immediately decreased the number of bacteria in the blood, the kidney and the liver after artificial bacterial challenge and this elimination relates to the resistance of fish to these challenge pathogens. Thus, this result demonstrates the increased resistance to *A. hydrophila* infection on carp treated with *Spirulina*. This study indicate that oral administration of *Spirulina* to carp leads to (a) enhanced phagocytic activity and superoxide anion production by phagocytic cells, (b) augmented the expression of IL-1β and TNF-α genes in the kidney leucocytes, and (c) increased resistance against *A. hydrophila* infection.[160]

Recently, Liu et al. (2000)[161] reported that phycocyanin, a characteristic photosynthesis pigment protein in *Spirulina*, inhibited growth of human leukemia K562 cells and enhanced the arrest of the cell growth at G1 phase, suggesting enhancement of differentiation of the cells. Hayashi et al. (2006)[162] investigated effects of *Spirulina* and its extracts on the introduction of colony stimulating factor(s) and on their proliferation and differentiation activity for hematopoietic cells in mice. They show that the *Spirulina* extracts, phycocyanin, hot-water extract, phycocyanin, and cell-wall component extract, enhanced proliferation of bone-marrow cells and induced colony-forming activity in the spleen-cell culture supernatant. These findings suggest that *Spirulina*,and its components such as phycocyanin, affects immune functions by promoting immune component cell proliferation or differentiation in lymphoids.

REFERENCES

1. Pelaez, F., The historical delivery of antibiotics from microbial natural products—Can history repeat?, *Biochem. Pharmacol.*, 71 (7), 981, 2006.

2. Berkowitz, F.E., Antibiotic-resistance in bacteria, *South Med. J.*, 88 (8), 797, 1995.

3. Vonshak, A., *Spirulina platensis (Arthrospira), Physiology, Cell-biology and Biotechnology*, Taylor & Francis, London, 1997.

4. Moore, R.E., Cyclic peptides and depsipeptides from cyanobacteria: a review, *J. Ind. Microbiol.*, 134–143, 1996.

5. Gerwick, W.H., Tan, L.T., and Sitachitta, N., Nitrogen-containing metabolites from marine cyanobacteria, in: Cordell, G.A. Ed., *The Alkaloids*, vol. 57, Academic Press, New York, pp. 75–184, 2001

6. Osborne, N.J., Webb, P.M., and Shaw, G.R., The toxins of *Lyngbya majuscula* and their human and ecological health effects, *Environ. Int.*, 27, 381, 2001.

7. Mayer, A.M.S., and Gustafson, K.R., Marine pharmacology in 2000: antitumor and cytotoxic compounds, *Int. J. Cancer*, 105, 291–299, 2003.

8. Shimizu, Y., Microalgal metabolites, *Curr. Opin. Microbiol.*, 6, 236, 2003.

9. Schopf, W., and Packer, B., Early Archean (3.3 Billion to 3.5 Billion Year Old) microfossils from Warrawoona group, *Australia. Science*, 70–72, 1987.

10. Stal, L. J., and Moezelaar, R., Fermentation in cyanobacteria, *FEMS Microbiol Rev* 21, 179–211, 1997.

11. Henning, M., Kohl, J. G., Toxic blue-green algae blooms found in some lakes in the German Democratic Republic, *Int. Rev. Ges. Hydrobiol.*, 66, 553–561, 1981.

12. Skulberg, O.M., Codd, G.A., and Carmichael, W.W. 1984 Toxic blue-green algal blooms in Europe: a growing problem, *Ambio.*, 13, 244, 1984.

13. Duy, T. N., Lam, P. K., Shaw, G. R., and Connell, D.W., Toxicology and risk assessment of freshwater cyanobacterial (blue-green algal) toxins in water, *Rev. Environ. Contam. Toxicol.*, 163, 113–185, 2000.

14. Jones, G.J., and Korth, W., *In situ* production of volatile odour compounds by river and reservoir phytoplankton populations in Australia, *Water Sci. Technol.*, 31, 145–151, 1995.

15. Carmichael, W.W., Cyanobacterial secondary metabolites—the cyanotoxins, *J. Appl. Bacteriol.*, 72, 445, 1992.

16. Carmichael, W.W., The toxins of cyanobacteria, *Sci. Am.*, 1, 78, 1994.

17. Rinehart, K.L., Namikoshi, M., and Choi, B.W., Structure and biosynthesis of toxins from blue-green algae (cyanobacteria), *J. Appl. Phycol.*, 6, 159, 1994.

18. Hunter, P.R., Cyanobacterial toxins and their potential risk to drinking water supplies, *Microbiol. Eur.*, 3, 8–10, 1995.

19. Falch, B.S., Was steckt in Cyanobakterien?, *Pharmazie in unserer Zeit*, 25, 311–321, 1996.

20. Hayashi, K., Hamada, J., Hayashi, T., A screening strategy for selection of anti-HSV-1 and anti-HIV extracts form algae, *Phytother. Res.*, 10, 233–237, 1996.

21. Namikoshi, M., and Rinehart, K.L., Bioactive compounds produced by cyanobacteria, *J. Ind. Microbiol.*, 17, 373–384, 1996.

22. Banker, R., Carmeli, S., Tenuecyclamides A-D, cyclic hexapeptides from the cyanobacterium Nostoc spongiaeforme var. tenue, *J. Nat. Prod.*, 61, 1248, 1998.

23. Harrigan, G.G., Luesch, H., Yoshida, W.Y., Moore, R.E., Nagle, D.G., Paul, J., Mooberry, S. L., Corbett, T.H., and Valeriote, F.A., Symplostatin 1: a dolastatine 10 analogue from the marine cyanobacterium *Symploca hydnoides*, *J. Nat. Prod.*, 61, 1075–1077, 1998.

24. Harrigan, G.G., Luesch, H., Yoshida, W.Y., Moore, R.E., Nagle, D.G., and Paul, V.J., Symplostatin 2: a dolastatin 13 analogue from the marine cyanobacterium Symploca hydnoides, *J. Nat. Prod.*, 62, 655–658, 1999.

25. Jaki, B., Orjala, J., and Sticher, O., New extracellular diterpenoids with antibacterial activity from the cyanobacterium *Nostoc commune*, *In Symposium papers of the 45th Annual Congress of the Society of Medicinal Plant Research*, Vienna, G 51, 1998.

26. Jaki, B., Orjala J., and Sticher O., A novel extracellular diterpenoid with antibacterial activity from the cyanobacterium *Nostoc commune*, *J. Nat. Prod.*, 62, 502–503, 1999.

27. Chrost, R. J., Inhibitors produced by algae as an ecological factor affecting bacteria in water ecosystems, *Acta. Microbiol. Pol. Ser. B.*, 7, 125, 1975.

28. Mundt, S., Kreitlow, S., and Nowotny, A., Effmert, U., Biochemical and pharmacological investigations of selected cyanobacteria, *Int. J. Hyg. Environ. Health*, 203 (4), 327–334, 2001.

29. Singh, S., Kate, B.N., and Banerjee, U.C., Bioactive compounds from cyanobacteria and microalgae: An overview, *Crit. Rev. Biotechnol.*, 25, 73, 2005.

30. Ciferri, O., *Spirulina*, the edible microorganism, *Microbiol. Rev.*, 47, 551, 1983.

31. Richmond, A., and Becker, E.W., *Technological aspects of mass cultivation–a general outline*, in: Richmond, A., Ed., *Handbook of Microalgal Mass Culture*, CRC Press Inc, Boca Ratón, 245–263, 1984.

32. Shang-Hao, 1., Cultivation and application of microalgae in People's Republic of China, in: Stadler, T., Mollion, J., Verdus, M.C., Karamanos, Y., Morvan, H., and Christiasen, D., Eds., *Algal Biotechnology*, Proceedings of the 4th International Meeting of the SAA Elsevier Applied Science, London, New York, pp. 41–51, 1988.

33. Thein, M., Production of *Spirulina* in Myanmar, in: Doumengue, F., Durand-Chastel, H., Toulemont, A., Eds., *Spiruline algue de vie*. Musée Océanographique. *Bulletin de l'Institut Océanographique Monaco*, Numéro spécial 12, pp. 175–178, 1993.

34. Kawamura, M., Sakakibara, M., Watanabe, T., Kita, K., Hiraoka, N, and Abayashi, A., A new restriction endonuclease from *Spirulina platensis*, *Nucleic Acids Res.*, 14, 1985–1990, 1986.

35. Moore, R., Barchi, J., and Patterson, G., Acutiphicin and 20,21-didehydroacutiphicin, new antineoplastic agents from the cyanophyta *Oscillatoria acutissima*, *J. Am. Chem. Soc.*, 106, 8193–8197, 1984.

36. Clardy, J., Kato, Y., Brinen, L., Moore, B., Chen, J., Patterson, G., and Moore, R., Paracyclophanes from blue-green algae, *J. Am. Chem. Soc.*, 112, 4061–4063, 1990.

37. Gerwick, W., Reyes, S., and Alvarado, B., Two malyngamides from the Caribbean cyanobacterium *Lyngbya majuscule*, *Phytochem.*, 26, 1701–1704, 1987.

38. Moore, R., Mynderse, J., Kashiwagi, M., and Norton, T., Antileukemia activity in the oscillatoriaceae: isolation of debromoaplysiatoxin from *Lyngbya*, *Science*, 196, 538–539, 1977.

39. Entzeroth, M., Mead, D., Patterson, G., and Moore, R., A herbicidal fatty acid produced by *Lyngbya aestuarii*, *Phytochem.*, 24 (12), 2875–2876, 1985.

40. Jung, T., and Dailey, M., A novel and inexpensive source of allophycocyanin for multicolor flow cytometry, *J. Immunol. Meth.*, 121, 9–18, 1989.

41. Paniagua- Michel, J., and Sazón, A., Moléculas de microalgas de importancia económica, in: Alveal, K., Ferraio, M., Oliveila, E., Sar, E., Eds., *Manual de métodos ficológicos*, Universidad de Concepción, Chile, pp. 297–310, 1995.

42. Kerby, N., Niven, G., Rowell, P., and Steward, D., Ammonia and amino acid production by cyanobacteria, in: Stadler, T., Mollion, J., Verdus, M.C., Karamanos, Y., Morvan, H., and Christiasen, D., Eds., *Algal Biotechnology. Proceedings of the 4th International Meeting of the SAA.* Elsevier Applied Science, London, New York, pp. 277–283, 1988.

43. Boussiba, S., *Annabaena azollae* as a nitrogen biofertilizer, in: Stadler, T., Mollion, J., Verdus, M.C., Karamanos, Y., Morvan, H., and Christiasen, D., Eds., *Algal Biotechnology. Proceedings of the 4th International Meeting of the SAA*, Elsevier Applied Science, London, New York, pp. 169–171, 1988.

44. Campbell, D.L., Lawton, J.A., Beattie, K.A., and Codd, G.A., Comparative assessment of the specificity of the brine shrimp and Microtox assays to hepatotoxic (microcystin-LR-containing) cyanobacteria, *Env. Tox. Wat. Qual.*, 9, 71, 1994.

45. Lahti, K., Ahtiainen, J., Rapala, J., Sivonen, K., and Niemel,¨ a S.J., Assessment of rapid bioassays for detecting cyanobacterial toxicity, *Lett. Appl. Microbiol.*, 21, 109–114, 1995.

46. Østensvik, Ø., Skulberg, O.M., Underdal, B., and Hormazabal, V., Antibacterial properties of extracts from selected planktonic freshwater cyanobacteria—a comparative study of bacterial bioassays, *J. Appl. Microbiol.*, 84, 1117–1124, 1998.

47. Borowitzka, M.A., Microalgae as sources of pharmaceuticals and other biologically active compounds, *J. Appl. Phycol.*, 7, 3, 1995.

48. Olaizola, M., Commercial development of microalgal biotechnology: from the test tube to the marketplace, *Biomol. Eng.*, 20, 459–466, 2003.

49. Burja, A.M., Banaigs, B., Abou-Mansour, E., Burgess, J.G., and Wright, P.C., Marine cyanobacteria-a prolific source of natural products, *Tetrahedron.*, 57, 9347–9377, 2001.

50. Iwata, K., Inayama, T., and Kato, T., Effects of *Spirulina platensis* on plasma lipoprotein lipase activity in fructose-induced hyperlipidemic rats, *J. Nutr. Sci. Vitaminol.*, 36, 165–171, 1990.

51. Vlad, M., Bordas, E., Caseanu, E., Uza, G., Creteanu, E., and Polinicenco, C., Effect of cuprofilin on experimental atherosclerosis, *Biol. Trace. Elem. Res.*, 48, 99, 1995.

52. Kushak, R.I., VanCott, E., Drapeau, C., and Winter, H., Effect of algae *Aphanizomenon flos-aquae* on digestive enzyme activity and polyunsaturated fatty acids level in blood plasma, *Gastroenterol.*, 116, A559, 1999.

53. Valencia, A., and Walker, J., The ability of *Aphanizomenon flosaquae* from Klamath Lake to improve the outcome of the treatment for mild traumatic brain injury, *Presented at the 3rd World Congress on Brain Injury held in Quebec City*, 4, 1999.

54. Mian, P., Heilmann, J., Burgi, H.R., and Sticher, O., Biological screening of terrestrial and freshwater cyanobacteria for antimicrobial activity, brine shrimp lethality, and cytotoxicity, *Pharm. Biol.*, 41, 243, 2003.

55. Kreitlow, S., Mundt, S., and Lindequist, U., Cyanobacteria—a potential source of new biologically active substances, *J. Biotechnol.*, 70 (1–3), 61–63, 1999.

56. Soltani, N., Khavari-Nejad, R.A, Yazdi, M.T, Shokravi, S., and Fernandez-Valiente, E., Screening of soil cyanobacteria for antifungal and antibacterial activity, *Pharm. Biol.*, 43 (5), 455, 2005.

57. Volk, R.B., and Furkert, F.H., Antialgal, antibacterial and antifungal activity of two metabolites produced and excreted by cyanobacteria during growth, *Microbiol. Res.*, 161 (2), 180, 2006.

58. Berry, J.P., Gantar, M., Gawley, R.E., Wang, M.L., and Rein, K.S., Pharmacology and toxicology of pahayokolide A, a bioactive metabolite from a freshwater species of Lyngbya isolated from the Florida Everglades, *Comp Biochem. Phys. C.*, 139 (4), 231, 2004.

59. Asthana, R.K., Srivastava, A., Kayastha, A.M., Nath, G., and Singh, S.P., Antibacterial potential of c-linolenic acid from *Fischerella* sp colonizing Neem tree bark, *World J. Microb. Bio.technol.*, 22 (5), 443, 2006.

60. Schlegel, I., Doan, N.T., de Chazal, N., and Smith, G.D., Antibiotic activity of new cyanobacterial isolates from Australia and Asia against green algae and cyanobacteria, *J. Appl. Phycol.*, 10 (5), 471, 1998.

61. Ghasemi Y., Yazdi M.T., Shafiee A., Amini M., Shokravi S., Zarrini G., Parsiguine, a novel antimicrobial substance from *Fischerella ambigua*, *Pharmaceut.Biol.*, 42 (4–5): 318–322, 2004.

62. Mundt, S., Kreitlow, S., and Jansen, R., Fatty acids with antibacterial activity from the cyanobacterium *Oscillatoria redekei* HUB 051, *J. Appl. Phycol.*, 15 (2–3), 263–267, 2003.

63. Asthana, R.K., Srivastava, A., Singh, A.P., Deepali, Singh S.P., Nath, G., Srivastava, R., and Srivastava, B.S., Identification of an antimicrobial entity from the cyanobacterium *Fischerella* sp isolated from bark of Azadirachta indica (Neem) tree, *J. Appl Phycol.*, 18 (1), 33, 2006.

64. Gol'din, E.B., Antibacterial activity of pure cultures of cyanobacteria and algae, *Mikrobiolohichnyi zhurnal (Kiev, Ukraine : 1993)*, 65, 68, 2003.

65. Ozdemir, G., Karabay, N.U., Dalay, M.C., and Pazarbasi, B., Antibacterial activity of volatile component and various extracts of *Spirulina platensis*, *Phytother. Res.*, 18, 754, 2004

66. Özdemir, G., Conkdalay, M., Küçükakyüz, K., Pazarbaşi, B., Yilmaz, M., Türkiye Koşullarinda Üretimi Yapilan *Spirulina platensis*' in Çeşitli Ekstraktlarinin Antimikrobiyal Aktivite Kapasitesinin Belirlenmesi, Ege Üniversitesi Su ÜrÜnleri Fakültesi Su Ürünleri Dergisi, 18, 161, 2001.

67. Santoyo, S., Herrero, M., Senorans, F.J., Cifuentes, A., Ibanez, E., and Jaime, L., Functional characterization of pressurized liquid extracts of *Spirulina platensis*, *Eur. Food. Res. Technol.*, 224 (1), 75, 2006.

68. Heyduck-Söller, B., and Fischer, U., Extracellular cyanobacterial substances inhibit microbial growth. *Int. Microbiol.*, 3, 231, 2000.

69. Blunt, J.W., Copp, B.R., Munro, M.H., Northcote, P.T., Prinsep, M.R., Marine natural products, *Nat. Prod. Rep.*, 20, 1, 2003.

70. MacMillan, J.B., Ernst-Russell, M.A., de Ropp, J.S., and Molinski, T. F., Lobocyclamides A-C, lipopeptides from a cryptic cyanobacterial mat containing Lyngbya confervoides, *J. Org. Chem.*, 67, 8210, 2002.

71. Oufdou, K., Mezrioui, N., Oudra, B., Loudiki, M., Barakate, M., and Sbiyyaa, B., Bioactive compounds from Pseudanabaena species (Cyanobacteria), *Microbios*, 106, 21, 2001.

72. Piccardi, R., Frosini, A., Tredici, M. R., and Margheri, M.C., Bioactivity in free-living and symbiotic cyanobacteria of the genus Nostoc, *J. Appl. Phycol.*, 12, 543, 2000.

73. Jaki, B., Heilmann, J., and Sticher, O., New Antibacterial Metabolites from the Cyanobacterium *Nostoc commune*, (EAWAG 122b), *J. Nat. Prod.*, 63, 1283–1285, 2000.

74. Matern, U., Oberer, L., Erhard, M., Herdman, M., Weckesser, J., Hofmannolin, a cyanopeptolin from Scytonema hofmanni PCC 7110, *Phytochemistry*, 64, 1061, 2003.

75. Jaki, B., Zerbe, O., Heilmann, J., and Sticher, O.,Two novel cyclic peptides with antifungal activity from the cyanobacterium *Tolypothrix byssoidea*, (EAWAG 195), *J. Nat. Prod.*, 64, 154–158,2001.

76. Balloni, W., Tomaselli, L., Giovannetti, Ls., and Margheri, M.C., Biologia fondamentale del genere *Spirulina*, in: Cantarelli, C., Ciferri, O., Florenzano, G., Kapsiotis, G., Materassi, R., and Treccani, U., Eds., Progetto finalizzato *"Ricerca di nuove fonti proteiche e di nuove formulazioni alimentari"*. Atti del Convegno: Prospettive della coltura di *Spirulina* in Italia. Consiglio Nazionale delle Richerche. Firenze-Academia dei Georgofili, CNR, Tipografia Coppini, pp. 49–82, 1980.

77. Pascaud, M., The essential polyunsaturated fatty acids of *Spirulina* and our immune response, in Doumengue, F., Durand-Chastel, H., and Toulemont, A., Eds., *Spiruline* algue de vie, Musée Océanographique, Bulletin de l'Institut Océanographique Monaco, Numéro spécial 12, pp. 49–57, 1993.

78. Li, S.W., and Li, H. Q., Nutriological and toxicological analysis of the Chlorella dry powder, *Food Science*, 18, 48, 1997. (in Chinese).

79. Sonoda, M., Effect of *Chlorella* extract on pregnancy anemia, *Jpn. J. Nutr.*, 30, 218, 1972.

80. Sano, T., and Tanaka, Y., Effect of dried, powdered *Chlorella vulgaris* on experimental arterosclerosis and alimentary hypercholesterolemia in cholesterol-fed rabbits,*Artery*, 14 (2), 76, 1987.

81. Hasegawa T., Okuda, M., Makino, M., Hiromatsu, K., Nomoto, K., and Yoshikai, Y., Hot water extracts of *Chlorella vulgaris* reduce opportunistic infection with *Listeria* monocytogenes in C57BL/6 mice infected with LP-BM5 murine leukemia viruses, *Int. J. Immunopharmacol.*, 17, 505–512, 1995.

82. Singh, S.P., Tiku, A.B., and Kesavan, P.C., Post-exposure radioprotection by *Chlorella vulgaris* (E-25) in mice, *Indian J. Exp. Biol.*, 33, 612, 1995.

83. Hayashi, T., and Hayashi, K., Calcium Spirulan, an inhibitor of enveloped virus replication, from a blue-green alga *Spirulina*, *J. Nat. Prod.*, 59, 83–87, 1996.

84. Tanaka, K., Yamada, A., Noda, K., Hasegawa, T., Okuda, M., Shoyama Y., and Nomoto, K., A novel glycoprotein from *Chlorella vulgaris* strain CK22 shows antimetastatic immunopotentiation, *Cancer Immunol. Immunother.*, 45, 313, 1998.

85. Martinez-Nadal, N.G., Antimicrobial activity of *Spirulina*. Paper presented at X Intl Cong. of Microbiology, Mexico City, Aug. 1970.

86. Jorjani, G., and Amirani, P., Antibacterial activities of *Spirulina platensis*, *Maj. Iimy Puz. Danisk. Jundi. Shap.*, 1, 14–18, 1978.

87. de Mule,' M.C.Z., de Caire, G.Z., and de Cano, M.S., Bioactive substances from *Spirulina platensis* (Cyanobacteria), *Phyton.*, 58, 93–96, 1996.

88. Blinkova, L.P., Gorobets, O.B., and Baturo, A.P., Detection of biologically active substances with antagonistic and stimulating activity in *Spirulina platensis*, *Zhurnal mikrobiologii, epidemiologii, immunobiologii*, 5, 11, 2002.

89. Fox, R.D., Algaculture: la *Spirulina*, un espoir pour le characterization of these bioactive substances. monde de la faim, Edisud, France, 1986, 319.

90. Richmond, A., *Spirulina*, in: Borowitzka, M.A., and Borowitzka L.J., Eds., *Microalgal Biotechnology*, Cambridge University Press, 85–121, 1988.

91. Doumenge, F., Durand-Chastel, E., and Toulemont, A., *Spirulina* algue de vie, *Bull. Inst. Oceanogr.*, Monaco, 222, 1993.

92. Henrikson, R., *Microalga Spirulina, superalimento del futuro*, 2nd Ed. Ediciones Urano, Ronore Enterprises, Barcelona, España, 1994, p. 222.

93. de Caire, G.Z., de Cano, M.S., de Mule', M.C.Z., de Halperin, D.R., and Galvagno, M.A., Action of cell-free extracts and extracellular products of *Nostoc muscorum* on growth of *Sclerotinia sclerotiorum*, *Phyton.*, 47, 43–46, 1987.

94. de Cano, M.S., de Mule', M.C.Z., de Caire, G.Z., and de Halperin, D.R., Inhibition of *Candida albicans* and *Staphylococcus aureus* by phenolic compounds from the terrestrial cyano bacterium *Nostoc muscorum*, *J. Appl. Phycol.*, 2, 79, 1990.

95. Kulik, M.M., The potential for using cyanobacteria (blue–green algae) and algae in the biological control of plant pathogenic bacteria and fungi, *Eur. J. Plant Pathol.*, 101, 585–599, 1995.

96. Cohen, Z., Vonshak, A., Richmond, A., Fatty acid composition of. *Spirulina* strains grown under various environmental conditions, *Phytochemistry*, 26, 2255, 1987.

97. Cohen, Z., Reungj?tchachawal?, M., S?angdung,W.,Tant?charoen, M., Production and partial purification of gammalinolenic acid and some pigments from *Spirulina Platensis*, *J. Appl. Phycol.*, 5, 109, 1993.

98. Olguin, E.J., Galicia, S., Angulo-Guerrero, O., and Hernandez, E., The effect of low light flux and nitrogen deficiency on the chemical composition of *Spirulina* sp. (*Arthrospira*) grown on digested pig waste, *Biores. Technol.*, 77, 19–24, 2001.

99. Tedesco, M., and Duerr, E., Light, temperature and nitrogen starvation effects on the total lipid and fatty acid content and composition of *Spirulina platensis* UTEX 1928, *J. Appl. Phycol.*, 1, 201, 1989.

100. Murata, N., Ono, T.A., and Sato, N., Lipid phase of membrane and chilling injury in the blue-green alga, *Anacystis nidulans*, in: Lyons, J.M., Graham, D., and Radison, J.K., Eds., *Low Temperature Stres in Crop Plants: The Role of the Membrane*, Academic Press, New York, pp. 337–345, 1979.

101. Wada, H., Gombos, Z., and Murata, N., Contribution of membrane lipids to the ability of the photosynthetic machinery to tolerate temperature stress, *Proc. Natl. Acad. Sci., USA* 91, 4273–4277, 1994.

102. Colla, L.M., Bertolini, T.E., Vosta, and J.A.V., Fatty acids profile of *Spirulina platensis* grown under different temperatures and nitrogen concentrations, *Z. Naturforsch*, 59c, 55–59, 2004.

103. Mühling, M., Belay, A., and Whitton, B.A., Variation in fatty acid composition of *Arthrospira* (*Spirulina*) strains, *J. Appl. Phycol.*, 17 (2), 137–146, 2005.

104. Otles, S., and Pire, R., Fatty acid composition of Chlorella and *Spirulina* microalgae species, *Journal of AOAC International*, 84, 1708, 2001.

105. Murata, N., and Nishida, I., Lipids of blue-green algae (cyanobacteria), in: Stumpf, P.K., Ed., *The Biochemistry of Plants*, vol. 9., Academic Press, San Diego, USA, pp. 315–347, 1987.

106. Murata, N., Deshnium, P., and Tasaka, Y., Biosynthesis of γ-linolenic acid in the cyanobacterium *Spirulina platensis*, in Huang, Y.S., and Mills, D.E., Eds., γ-*Linolenic Acid—Metabolism and its Role in Nutrition and Medicine*, AOCS Press, Champaign, Illinois, USA, pp. 22–32, 1996.

107. Coolbear, K.P., Berde, C.B., and Keough, K.M.W., Gel to liquid crystalline phase transition of aqueous dispersions of polyunsaturated mixed-acid phosphatidylcholines, *Biochemistry* 22, 1466–1473, 1983.

108. Deshnium, P., Paithoonrangsarid, K., Suphatrakul, A., Meesapyodsuk, D., Tanticharoen, M., and Cheevadhanarak, S., Temperature independent and -dependent expression of desaturase genes in filamentous cyanobacterium *Spirulina platensis* strain C1 (*Arthrospira* sp. PCC9438), *FEMS Microbiol. Letts* 184, 207–213, 2000.

109. Pinkart, H. C., Devereux, R., and Chapman, P. J., Rapid separation of microbial lipids using solid phase extraction columns, *J. Microbiol. Meth.*, 34 (1), 9, 1998.

110. Horrobin, D.F., and Huang, Y.S., The role of linolenic acid and its metabolites in the lowering of plasma cholesterol and the prevention of cardiovascular disease, *Int. J. Cardiol.*, 17, 241–255, 1987.

111. Horrobin, D.F., and Manku, M.S., How do polyunsaturated fatty acids lower plasma cholesterol levels? *Lipids*, 18, 558, 1983.

112. Puolakka, J., Makarainen, L., Viinikka, L., and Ylikorkala, O., Biochemical and clinical effects of treating the premenstrual syndrome with prostaglandin synthesis precursors, *J. Reprod. Med.*, 30, 149, 1985.

113. Schalin-Karrila, M., Mattila, L., Jansen, C.T., and Uotila, P., Evening primrose oil in the treatment of atopic eczema: effect on clinical status, plasma phospholipid fatty acid and circulating blood prostaglandins, *Brit. J. Dermatol.*, 117, 11, 1987.

114. Carter, J.P., Gamma-linolenic acid as a nutrient, *Food Tech.*, 42, 72, 1988.

115. Murakami, N., Yamada, N., and Sakakibara, J., An autolytic substance in a fresh water cyanobacterium Phormidium tenue, *Chem. Pharm. Bull. (Tokyo)*, 38, 812, 1990.

116. Yamada, N., Murakami, N., Motimoto, T., and Sakakibara, J., Auto-growth inhibitory substance from the fresh water cyanobacterium Phormidium tenue. *Chem. Pharm. Bull. (Tokyo)*, 41, 1863, 1993.

117. Bistline, R.G., Maurer, F.E., Smith, F.D.,and Linfield, W.M., Fatty acid amides and anilides, syntheses and antimicrobial properties, *J. Am. Oil Chem. Soc.*, 57, 98–103, 1980.

118. Kabara, J.J., Antimicrobial agent derived from fatty acid, *J. Am. Oil Chem. Soc.*, 61, 397–403, 1984.

119. Oh, D.H., and Marshall, D.L., Influence of temperature, pH, and glycerol monolaurate on growth and survival of *Listeria monocytogenes*, *J. Food Prot.*, 56, 744–749, 1993.

120. Wang, L.L., Yang, B.K., Parkin, K.L., and Johnson, E.A., Inhibition of *Listeria monocytogenes* by monoacylglycerols synthesized from coconut oil and milk fat by lipase-catalyzed glycerolysis, *J. Agric. Food Chem.*, 41, 1000–1009, 1993.

121. Ababouch, H.L., Bouqartacha, F., and Busta, F.F., Inhibition of *Bacillus cereus* spores and vegetative cells by fatty acids and glyceryl monododecanoate, *Food Microbiol.*, 11, 327–336, 1994.

122. Ohta, S., Shiomo, Y., Kawashima, A., Aozasa, O., and Teruyuki, N., Antibiotic effect of linolenic acid from the *Chlorococcum* strain HS-101 and *Dunaliella primolecta* onmethicil lin-resistant *Staphylococcus aureus*, *J. Appl. Phycol.*, 7, 121–127, 1995.

123. Nader de Macias, M.E., Romero, N.C., Apella, M.C., González, S.N., and Oliver, G., Prevention of infections produced by *Escherichia coli* and *Listeria monocytogenes* feeding milk fermented with lactobacilli, *J. Food Protect.*, 56, 401–405, 1993.

124. Perdigón, G., Alvarez, S., and Medici, M., Systemic and local augmentation of the immune response in mice by feeding with milk fermented with *Lactobacillus acidophilus* and/or *Lactobacillus casei*, in: Paubert-Braquet, M., Dupont, C. and Paoletti, R., Eds., *Foods Nutrition and Immunity* (Dynamic Nutrition Research), Karger ISBN 3-80555605-5, Basel, p. 66, 1992.

125. Hove, H., Norgaard, H., and Mortensen, P.B., Lactic acid bacteria and the human gastrointestinal tract, *Eur. J. Clin. Nutr.*, 53, 339–350, 1999.

126. Alm, L., The therapeutic effects of various cultures - an overview. In: R.K. Robinson, Ed., Therapeutic Effects of Fermented Milk. Elsevier Applied Food Science Series. London,UK, pp. 45–64, 1991.

127. Saavedra, J.M., Bauman, N.A., Oung, I., Perman, J.A., and Yolken, R.H., Feeding of *Bifidobacterium bifidum* and *Streptococcus thermophilus* to infants in hospital for prevention of diarrhoea and shedding of rotavirus, *Lancet.*, 344, 1046, 1994.

128. Black, F.T., Einarsson, K., Lidbeck, A., Orrhage, K., and Nord, C.E., Effect of lactic acid producing bacteria on the human intestinal microflora during ampicillin treatment, *Scand. J. Infect. Dis.*, 23, 247, 1991.

129. Henning, S., Metz, R., and Hammes, W.P., New aspects for the application of nisin to food products based on its mode of action, *Int. J. Food Microbiol.*, 33, 135–141, 1986.

130. Parada, J. L., and Pamies de Giacchi, M., Resistance of *Streptococcus lactis* mutants to b-lactam antibiotics, *J. Dairy Sci.*, 69, 2033, 1986.

131. Fernandes, C.F., Shahani, K.M., and Amer, M.A., Therapeutic role of dietary lactobacilli and lactobacillic fermented dairy products, *FEMS Microbiol. Rev.*, 4646, 343–356, 1987.

132. Lin, M.Y., Savaiano, D., and Harlander, S., Influence of nonfermented dairy products containing bacterial starter cultures on lactose maldigestion in humans, *J. Dairy Sci.*, 74, 87–95, 1991.

133. Agerbaek, M., Gerdes, L.V., and Richelsen, B., Hypocholesterolaemic effect of a new fermented milk product in healthy middle-aged men, *Eur J Clin Nutr.*, 49, 346, 1995.

134. Schiffrin, E. J., Rochat, F., Link-Amster, H., Aeschlimann, J. M., and Donnet-Hughes, A., Immunomodulation of human blood cells following the ingestion of lactic acid bacteria, *J. Dairy Sci.*, 78, 491, 1995.

135. Krishnakumar, V., and Gordon, I. R., Probiotics: Challenges and opportunities, *Dairy Ind. Int.*, 66, 38, 2001.

136. Schiffrin, E., Brassart, D., Servin, A., Rochat, F., and Donnet-Hughes, A., Immune modulation of blood leukocytes in humans by lactic acid bacteria: criteria for strain selection, *Am. J. Clin. Nutr.*, 66, 515S–520S, 1997.

137. Hirahashi, T., Matsumoto, M., Hazeki, K., Saeki, Y., Ui, M., and Seya, T., Activation of the human innate immune system by *Spirulina* augmentation of interferon production and NK cytotoxicity by oral administration of hot water of *Spirulina platensis*, *Int. Immunopharmacol.*, 2, 423–434, 2002.

138. Gibson, G.R., and Roberfroid, M.B., Dietary modulation of the human colonic microbiota: introducing the concept of pre biotics, *J. Nutr.*, 125, 1401–1412, 1995.

139. Neuringer, M., and Connor, W.E., n-3(W3) fatty acids in the brain and retina: evidence for their essentiality, *Nutr. Rev.*, 44(9), 285–294, 1986.

140. de Caire, G.Z., Parada, J.L., Zaccaro, M.C., and de Cano, M.M.S., Effect of *Spirulina platensis* biomass on the growth of lactic acid bacteria in milk, *World J. Microb. Biot.*, 16 (6), 563–565, 2000.

141. Parada, J.L., Zulpa de Caire, G., Zaccaro de Muleâ , M.C., and Storni de Cano, M.M., Lactic acid bacteria growth promoters from *Spirulina platensis*, *Int. J. Food Microbiol.*, 45, 222, 1998.

142. Varga, L., Szigeti, J., Kovacs, R., Foldes, T., and Buti, S., Influence of a *Spirulina platensis* biomass on the microflora of fermented ABT milks during storage (R1), *J. Dairy Sci.*, 85 (5), 1031, 2002.

143. Varga, L., Szigeti, J., and Ordog, V., Effect of a *Spirulina platensis* biomass enriched with trace elements on combinations of starter culture strains employed in the dairy industry, *Milchwissenschaft*, 54 (5), 247, 1999.

144. Varga, L., Szigeti, J., and Ordog, V., Effect of a *Spirulina platensis* biomass and that of its active components on single strains of dairy starter cultures, *Milchwissenschaft*, 54 (4), 187, 1999.

145. Khan, Z., Bhadouria, P., Bisen, P.S., Nutritional and therapeutic potential of *Spirulina*, *Curr. Pharm. Biotechnol.*, 6, 373, 2005.

146. Qureshi, M.A., and Ali R.A., *Spirulina platensis* exposure enhances macrophage phagocytic function in cats, *Immunopharm. Immunot.*, 18 (3), 457, 1996.

147. Qureshi, M.A, Garlich, J.D., and Kidd, M.T., Dietary *Spirulina platensis* enhances humoral and cell-mediated immune functions in chickens, *Immunopharm. Immunot.*, 18 (3), 465, 1996.

148. Al-Batshan, H.A., Al-Mufarrej, S.I., Al-Homaidan, A.A., and Qureshi, M.A., Enhancement of chicken macrophage phagocytic function and nitrite production by dietary *Spirulina platensis*, *Immunopharm Immunot.*, 23 (2), 281, 2001.

149. Lee, Y.K., Chew, P.F., Soh, B.S., and Tham, L.Y., Enhancing phagocytic activity of hemocytes and disease resistance in the prawn *Penaeus merguiensis* by feeding *Spirulina platensis*, *J. Appl. Phycol.*, 15 (4), 279–287, 2003.

150. Brock J.A., and Lightner D.V., Diseases of Crustacea. Diseases caused by microorganisms. In: Kinne O. Ed., *Diseases of Marine Animals*, John Wiley & Sons, New York, pp. 245–260, 1990.

151. Johnson S.K., Handbook of Shrimp Diseases. Texas A and M University Sea Grant College, pp. 4–24, 1990.

152. Gupta, A.P., (ed.) Hemocytic and Humoral Immunity in Arthropods. John Wiley & Sons, New York, 535, 1986.

153. Holmblad, T., and Soderhall K., Cell adhesion molecules and antioxidative enzymes in a crustacean, possible role in immunity, *Aquaculture*, 172, 111, 1999.

154. Thornqvist P.-O., and Soderhall K., Crustacean immune reactions, a short review, in: Flegel T.W. and Macrae I.H. Eds., *Diseases in Asian Aquaculture III*, Fish Health Section, Asian Fisheries Society, Manila, pp. 203–217, 1997.

155. Duncan, P.L., and Klesius, P.H., Effects of feeding *Spirulina* on specific and nonspecific immune responses of channel catfish, *J. Aquat. Anim., Health*, 8, 308–313, 1996.

156. Hayashi, O., Katoh, T., and Okuwaki, Y., Enhancement of antibody production in mice by dietary *Spirulina platensis*, *J. Nutr. Sci. Vitaminol.*, 40, 431–441, 1994.

157. Hayashi, O., Hirahashi, T., Katoh, T., Miyajima, H., Hirano, T., and Okuwaki, Y., Class specific influence of dietary *Spirulina platensis* on antibody production in mice, *J. Nutr. Sci. Vitaminol.*, 44 (6), 841–851, 1998.

158. Liu, L., Guo, B., Ruan, J., Dai, X., Chen, L., and Wu, B., Study on effect and mechanism of polysaccharides on *Spirulina platensis* on body immune functions improvement, *Marine Sci.*, 6, 44–49, 1991.

159. Sakai, M., Otubo, T., Atsuta, S., and Kobayashi, M.,. Enhancement of resistance to bacterial infection in rainbow trout, Oncorhynchus mykiss (Walbaum) by oral administration of bovine lactoferrin. *J. Fish Dis.* 16, 239, 1993.

160. Watanuki, H., Ota, K., Tassakka, A.C.M.A.R., Kato, T., and Sakai, M., Immunostimulant effects of dietary Spirulina platensis on carp, Cyprinus carpio, *Aquaculture*, 258, 157, 2006.

161. Liu, Y., Xu, L., Cheng, N., Lin, L., and Zhang, C., Inhibitory effect of phycocyanin from *Spirulina platensis* on the growth of human leukemia K562 cells, *J. Appl. Phycol.*, 12, 125–130, 2000.

162. Hayashi, O., Ono, S., Ishii, K., Ishii, K., Shi, Y.H., Hirahashi, T., and Katoh, T., Enhancement of proliferation and differentiation in bone marrow hematopoietic cells by *Spirulina* (*Arthrospira*) *platensis* in mice, *J. Appl. Phycol.*, 18 (1), 47–56, 2006.

163. Gasson, M.J., Progress and potential in the biotechnology of lactic acid bacteria, *FEMS Microbiol. Rev.*, 12, 3–19, 1993.

164. Gerwick, W.H., Jianga, Z.D., Agarwala, S.K., and Farmer, B.T., Total structure of hormothamnin A, A toxic cyclic undecapeptide from the tropical marine cyanobacterium hormothamnion enteromorphoides, *Tetrahedron.*, 48, 2313–2324, 1992.

165. Guililand, S.E., Health and nutritional benefits from lactic acid bacteria, *FEMS Microbiol. Rev.*, 87, 175–188, 1990.

166. Koehn, F.E., Longley, R.E., and Reed, J.K., Microcolins A & B, new immunosuppressive peptides from the blue green alga *Lyngbya majuscule*, *J. Nat. Prod.*, 55, 613–619, 1992.

167. Lai, J.-Y., Yu, J., Mekonnen, B., and Falck, J.R., Synthesis of curacin A, an antimitotic cyclopropane-thiazoline from a marine cyanobacterium *Lyngbya majuscule*, *Tetrahedron Lett.*, 37, 7167–7170, 1996.

168. Orjala, J., Nagle, D.G., Hsu, V.L., and Gerwick, W.H., Antillatoxin: An exceptionally ichthyotoxic cyclic lipopeptide from the tropical cyanobacterium *Lyngbya majuscule*, *J. Am. Chem. Soc.*, 117, 8281–8282, 1995.

169. Piard, J.C., and Desmazeaud, M., Inhibiting factors produced by lactic acid bacteria, bacteriocins and other antibacterial substances, *Lait*, 72, 113, 1992.

170. Özdemir, G., Conk Dalay, M., Kücükakyüz, K., Pazarbaþı, B., and Yılmaz, M., Türkiye Koþullarında Üretimi Yapılan *Spirulina platensis*'in Çeþitli Ekstraktlarının Antimikrobiyal Aktivite Kapasitesinin Belirlenmesi, *J. Fish. Aqua. Sci.*, 18(1), 161–166, 2001.

171. Rajab, M.S., Cantrell, C.L., Franzblau, S.G., and Fisher, N. H., Antimycobacterial activity of (E)-phytol and derivatives: a preliminary structure-activity study, *Planta Med*, 64, 2, 1998.

172. Volk, R.B., Antialgal activity of several cyanobacterial exometabolites, *J. Appl. Phycol.*, 18, (2), 145, 2006.

13 *Spirulina*, Aging, and Neurobiology

Jennifer Vila, Carmelina Gemma,
Adam Bachstetter, Yun Wang, Ingrid Strömberg,
and Paula C. Bickford

CONTENTS

Normal aging, an unavoidable fact of life, results in, manageable changes for most; yet, others encounter aging with immense changes in neurobiology and disease. To understand the spectrum of changes that accompany age, we must first understand the neurobiology of aging, in order to develop therapeutic or lifestyle interventions that extend the functional lifespan. There are numerous theories that assess the natural aging process. Consequentially, there are several ways to evaluate the neurobiology of aging. Currently inflammation and oxidative stress are the predominate theories of aging in the central nervous system (CNS).

THE ROLE OF INFLAMMATION IN AGING

In aging, a series of unchecked inflammatory events can lead to exaggerated proin-flammatory cytokine levels; such as, increases in interleukin 1 (IL-1), IL-1 receptor agonists, tumor necrosis factor (TNF), and transforming growth factor-β.[1,2] When functioning correctly, cytokines send the appropriate amount of the correct signal to assist in resolving the immune stimulus; such as, IL-4, IL-10, and IL-13, which act to suppress inflammation, or IL-1, IL-6, IL-8, IL-11, and IL-12, which act to stimulate inflammation. In a healthily immune system both pro- and anti-inflammatory cytokine are used to acutely handle the immune stimulus. In the aged system, the profile of cytokine activation does not resemble acute activation; instead a chronic inflammation state is seen. This chronic pattern of activation can change the microenvironment within the CNS leading to detrimental outcomes. A growing body of evidence has linked age-dependent alterations in cognitive ability with an altered inflammatory response in the brain.[3,4] Increased levels of the proinflammatory cytokine IL-1β have been correlated with natural aging and with the development of cognitive dysfunction.[5-7] A great deal of evidence suggests that IL-1β plays an important role in neuronal plasticity, as revealed by the fact that this cytokine is implicated in the age-related impairment in long-term potentiation (LTP), a model system for the neural mechanism underlying hippocampus-dependent memory.[2,8] Consistent with this finding it has been demonstrated that, IL-1β inhibits LTP in dentate gyrus,[9] CA1, and CA3[10,11] and that such effect is associated with a decrease in glutamate release, a neurotransmitter that mediates LTP.[11] In addition, intraperitoneal injection of lipopolysaccride (LPS) also leads to an inhibition of glutamate release and a compromise in LTP, which is accompanied by increases in IL-1β concentration in hippocampus.[12] In spite of a general agreement concerning the impairment in the maintenance of LTP in aged rats, it is still questioned whether or not the induction of LTP is impaired in aged rats. Induction of LTP *in vitro* and *in vivo* caused a long lasting increase in IL-1β gene expression, which was prevented by blockade of potentiation with *N*-methyl-D-aspartate (NMDA) receptor antagonist.[13] NMDA receptor binding and density have been reported to decrease with increasing age.[14,15] We have recently shown that the nonsteroidal anti-inflammatory drug (NSAID) sulindac reversed age-related deficits in radial arm water maze performance and contextual fear conditioning and attenuated age-related decreases in hippocampal NMDA receptor subunits NR1 and NR2B at the same time we observed a decline in IL-1β.[16] A recent study using a genome-scale screening has shown a distinct temporal gene expression profile associated with spatial learning and memory of rats in Morris water maze in young rats. Among other changes the authors have shown a reduction in IL-1β gene expression in water maze trained animals, and this data was consistent with the finding that central administration of IL-1β impairs the consolidation of memories that depend on the hippocampal formation.[17]

THE ROLE OF OXIDATIVE STRESS IN AGING

A second focus of aging in the CNS is oxidative stress and the mitochondrion. Reactive oxygen species (ROS) are oxidants that, if unrestricted, can cause oxidative damage to the mitochondria, cellular proteins, lipids, and nucleic acids. ROS are the normal byproducts of cellular metabolism in the mitochondrion. Free radicals are chemical species with a single unpaired electron, which is highly reactive. The majority of free radicals that damage biological systems are oxygen radicals and other ROS, which are byproducts formed in the cells of aerobic organisms. The generation of mitochondrial ROS is a consequence of oxidative phosphorylation, a process that occurs in the inner mitochondrial membrane and one that involves the oxidation of NADH to produce energy. Under normal circumstances our natural antioxidant defense systems detoxify the superoxide anion by the mitochondrial manganese (Mn) superoxide dismutase

(MnSOD) to yield hydrogen peroxide (H_2O_2), and the H_2O_2 is then converted to H_2O by catalase. H_2O_2 in the presence of reduced transition metals can also be converted to hydroxyl radical.

In the aging brain as well as in the case of several neurodegenerative diseases, there is a decline in the normal antioxidant defense mechanisms that increase the vulnerability of the brain to the deleterious effects of oxidative damage.[18] The antioxidant enzymes superoxide dismutase (SOD), catalase, glutathione peroxidase, and glutathione reductase, for example, display reduced activities in the brain of patients with Alzheimer's disease.[19] It is believed that free radicals of mitochondrial origin are one of the primary causes of mitochondrial DNA (mtDNA) damage. Several studies have found increased levels of 8- hydroxy-2′-deoxyguanosine (8-OHdG), a biomarker of oxidative DNA damage, in mtDNA in the aged brain.[20] Other studies have shown that the age-related increase in oxidative damage to mtDNA is greater than the oxidative damage that occurs to nuclear DNA in rodents.[21,22] For instance, oxidative DNA damage has been detected in human brain mtDNA and in rat liver at levels more than 10 times higher than in nuclear DNA from the same tissue.[20,23−25]

Aging is also accompanied by changes in membrane fatty acid composition, including a decrease in the levels of polyunsaturated fatty acids (PUFAs) and an increase in monosaturated fatty acids. PUFAs, such as arachidonic acid (AA), are abundant in the aging brain and are highly susceptible to free radical attack. A correlation between the concentration of AA and LTP has been shown,[8,26] suggesting that oxidative depletion of AA levels may relate to a cognitive deficit in rats. For example, levels of AA are decreased in the hippocampus of aged rats with impaired ability to sustain LTP. Oxidative damage to lipids can also occur indirectly through the production of highly reactive aldehydes. Peroxidation of AA forms malondialdehyde (MDA), which induces DNA damage by reacting with amino acids in protein to form adducts that disrupt DNA base-pairing. Increased levels of MDA have been found in the aged canine brain.[27] In the aged human brain, MDA has been found to be increased in inferior temporal cortex and in cytoplasm of neurons and astrocytes,[28] as well as in the hippocampus and cerebellum of aged rodents.[29] Peroxidation of linoleic acid forms 4-hydroxy-2-nonenal (HNE). HNE is more stable than free radicals and it is able to migrate to sites that are distant from its formation, resulting in greater damage. The most damaging effect of HNE is its ability to form covalent adducts with histidine, lysine, and cysteine residues in proteins enabling a modification in their activity.[30] It has been shown that the HNE-modified proteins, along with neurofibrillary tangles, are present in the senile plaques in aged dogs.[31] Increased levels of HNE have also been found in Alzheimer's and Parkinson's disease.[32] This finding gave support to the hypothesis that lipid peroxidation contributes to the deterioration of CNS function. Most of the studies conducted to assess the role of protein oxidation in aging brains conclude that there is an increase of oxidized proteins. An increase in the oxidation of mitochondrial proteins with age has been demonstrated by measuring the levels of protein carbonyl groups in the human cerebral cortex along with age.[33] Carbonyl formation can occur through a variety of mechanisms including direct oxidation of amino acid side chains and oxidation-induced peptide cleavage. Increasing evidence suggests that protein oxidation may be responsible for the gradual decline in physiological functioning that accompanies aging. Elevated protein carbonyls have been shown to be present in the hippocampus of aged rats with memory impairment.[34] Increased protein carbonyl levels were found in the frontal and occipital cortex of aged humans.[33,35] and rats.[36] Measuring protein 3-nitrotyrosine (3-NT) levels is another way to assess the oxidative modification of proteins. Increased 3-NT levels have been identified in the hippocampus and the cerebral cortex of aged animals as well as in the CSF of aged human and in the white matter of aging monkeys.[37–39] 3-NT immunoreactivity has been observed in the cerebellum in the Purkinje cell layer, the molecular layer, and in the cerebellar nuclei of aged rats.[40] However, contradictory findings of decreased protein 3-NT levels of brain homogenate were reported in aged Wistar rats . Recently, proteomics studies enabled the identification of specific proteins that undergo oxidative stress in Alzheimer's disease (AD) patients.[41,42]

THE ROLE OF MICROGLIA IN AGING

Throughout our lives when inflammation occurs in the CNS microglia are activated to quickly deal with the source of inflammation much like the peripheral macrophages deal with inflammation throughout the rest of the body. Microglial cells are the resident immune cells of the CNS, which constitutively express surface receptors that trigger or amplify the innate immune response. These include complement receptors, cytokine receptors, chemokine receptors, major histocompatibility complex II, and others. In the case of cellular damage, they respond promptly by inducing a protective immune response, which consists of a transient up regulation of inflammatory molecules as well as neurotrophic factors.[43] This innate immune response usually resolves potential pathogenic conditions.

It has been proposed that the increase in brain microglial activation may be one of the early events that leads to oxidative damage. Activated microglia release radicals such as superoxide and nitric oxide.[44] Microglia derived radicals, as well as their reaction products hydrogen peroxide and peroxynitrite, can harm cells and these products have been shown to be involved in oxidative damage and neuronal cell death in neurological diseases.[45] Microglial cells are equipped with efficient antioxidative defense mechanisms. They contain high concentrations of gluthatione, the antioxidative SOD enzymes, catalase, glutathione peroxidase, and glutathione reductase, as well as nicotinamide adenine dinucleotide phosphate (NADPH)-regenerating enzymes.[45] When the production of ROS is prolonged, the endogenous reserves of antioxidants become exhausted and result in cell damage.

It has been proposed that at least two activation states of peripheral macrophages can be identified[46] and as microglia are the macrophages of the brain it is likely that these phenotypes apply to microglia as well. The state induced by TH1 cytokines such as IL-1, IL-6, TNFα, and CD40 ligand is referred to as the classical inflammation state by Duffield (2003) and M1 by others.[47] This is a proinflammatory state that is associated with further production of these proinflammatory cytokines, ROS, chemokines, and matrix metalloproteases, resulting in cell death of invading cells and further inflammation. A second state of activation, the alternative activation state is associated with the TH2 cytokine profile of IL-4, IL-10, and TGFβ-1.

When macrophages/microglia are in this state there is little release of proinflammatory cytokines and resistance to activation by agents such as LPS. In this alternative state macrophages promote extracellullar matrix formation and angiogenesis. Duffield (2003) suggests that a major difference between beneficial resolving inflammation and detrimental chronic inflammation is a failure to transition between classical and alternative states of activation, leading to tissue destruction and organ failure. It is possible that in the aged brain, microglia are primarily in the classical activation state as reflected by high levels of tumor necrosis factor alpha (TNFα) and other TH1 cytokines and low levels of Il-10 and other TH2 cytokines. As a result of chronic inflammation, prolonged activation of microglia triggers a release of a wide array of neurotoxic products[48] and proinflammatory cytokines such as IL-1β, IL-6, TNFα. Aged brains seem to be in this state of chronic inflammation; as seen by, elevated protein levels of proinflammatory molecules such as, IL-1β, TNFα, and IL-6.[29,49,50] Microglia have been attributed to some of these increases. Animal studies have shown that increased levels of IL-6 in the hippocampus and cerebral cortex are primarily from microglia.[51]

Patients with diseases such as AD and Parkinson's disease (PD) show signs of microglia in the chronic inflammatory state and this may be one of the predisposing factors that leads to the development of these neurodegenerative diseases.[52–54]

THE ROLE OF NEUROGENESIS IN AGING

Another process impaired in normal aging is neurogenesis within the granule cell layer (GCL) in the hippocampus. Neurogenesis continues to occur throughout the life predominantly in the subgranular zone (SGZ) of the dentate gyrus in the hippocampal formation and in the subventricular zone (SVZ). Neural stem cells in the SGZ give rise to progenitor cells that migrate in the granule cell layer and differentiate into neuronal or glial phenotype. Progenitors in the SVZ migrate into the olfactory bulb through the rostral migratory stream and differentiate into interneurons. Newly generated hippocampal granule cells acquire the morphological and biochemical properties of neurons, develop synapses on their cell bodies and dendrites, and extend axonal projection along the mossy fibers into the hippocampal CA3 region.[55] Newborn granule neurons are electrically active and capable of firing action potentials and receive synaptic inputs.[56] However, the functional significance of adult neurogenesis is still unclear. The finding that increased hippocampal neurogenesis occurs in the brain of patients with Alzheimer's disease and after cerebral ischemia, have suggested that new neurons may integrate into existing brain circuitry and contribute to repair.[57,58]

An increasing amount of evidence suggests that neurogenesis is involved in hippocampal-dependent learning and memory. The Shors laboratory has shown a strong correlations between the number of new neurons and performance on some forms of hippocampal-dependent memory tasks, such as the trace eye-blink conditioning task,[59] as well as, observing a deficit in a hippocampal-dependent memory task by reducing the generation of new neurons with an anti-mitotic agent.[60] The correlation between neurogenesis and learning is not without controversy as other reports, either failed to find a correlation between the number of newly generated neurons and performance on a memory task, or observed that aged animals who perform better on a hippocampal-dependent memory task have fewer new neurons compared with animals that perform worse.[61,62] The precise reasons for age-related decreases in neurogenesis are unknown, as the production of new neurons in adult hippocampus depends on multiple factors. The above observations suggest that the age-related decrease in neurogenesis is due to the overall age-related alteration in the microenvironment of the brain. The importance of the microenvironment was supported in a study that showed that the subgranuler zone of the dentate gyrus of a young Fisher 344 rats contains around 50,000 Sox-2+ progenitor cells and that this population of cells is intact in the aged animal.[63] The decrease in hippocampal neurogenesis during aging appears to be an outcome of increased quiescence of neural stem cells due to changes in neural stem cell environment.[63] Indeed, a recent report suggests that stem cells in aged animals can be rejuvenated. In this study parabiosis between aged and young mice demonstrated that muscle satellite cells from the aged mice increased proliferative rates when exposed to serum of young rats.[64] This report suggests that the environment in aged animals may play a significant role in the reduced proliferative capacity of stem cells. A decrease in multiple stem/progenitor cell proliferation factors, insulin growth factor-1, fibroblast growth factor -2, and brain derived neurotrophic factor has been identified as important facts for the alteration of the microenvironment of the aged brain. Inflammation within the brain is also a potent inhibitor of neurogenesis.[65] Inflammation in the brain, as well as increased oxidative stress, have been indicated as factors responsible for the alteration in the aged brain microenvironment. It has been shown that nutritional treatments that aim to decrease oxidants and inflammation, such as feeding with blueberry, can improve cognitive function[66] and can also increase neurogenesis.[67,68] Preliminary studies from our laboratory have indicated that pretreatment with *Spirulina* may have the potential to combat inflammation caused by LPS in the young hippocampus of the rat.[69] In addition, *Spirulina* may also have the ability to assist with neurogenesis in the aged rat hippocampus.[70]

THERAPEUTIC INTERVENTIONS FOR INFLAMMATION AND OXIDATIVE STRESS IN AGING

The incidence of neurodegenerative diseases increases with age and may be a result of changes in the aged microenvironment that make the brain more susceptible to insults and genetic predispositions of these disease processes. Taking into consideration the above descriptions of oxidative stress and inflammation that occur with age, it becomes evident that bolstering the immune system or finding therapeutic interventions that would shift the balance away from the chronic inflammatory state and towards the alternative inflammatory response maybe a useful strategy. Dietary supplements, as well as, pharmaceuticals have been extensively investigated for their potential as anti-inflammatories and anti-oxidants. With respect to pharmaceuticals, researchers have investigated the potential of NSAIDs in aging. While promising results were initially found with Alzheimers disease,[71−73] they were overshadowed by the implications of long-term NSAID usage on the digestive and cardiac system.[74] A possible result of this finding was a shift away from manufactured pharmaceuticals and a shift towards a natural occurring source of supplementation. Supplementation of diets with antioxidants can be viewed as a way to support the internal antioxidant system in order to help deter an exacerbation of proinflammatory cytokines. A great natural source of antioxidants are fruits and vegetables. Researchers have used an *in vitro* assay of oxygen radical absorbance capacity (ORAC) to determine which fruits and vegetables contain the highest oxidative fighting capacity.[75] Experiments using dietary interventions with fruit and vegetable supplements (blueberry, strawberry, spinach, and vitamin E) high in ORAC activity have resulted in successful amelioration of such age-related declines as muscarinic receptor sensitivity, noradrenergic modulation of cerebellar Purkinje neurons, calcium regulation, and Morris water maze performance, among others.[66,76,77]

SPIRULINA AS A NATURAL THERAPEUTIC INTERVENTION FOR INFLAMMATION AND OXIDATIVE STRESS IN AGING

Spirulina, is a very interesting and promising source of phytochemicals that has also shown hopeful results in dealing with age-related changes. With both antioxidant and anti-inflammatory actions, *Spirulina* has the ability to supplement our internal anti-oxidant defense systems as well as control any excessive inflammation. The first known use of *Spirulina* as a dietary supplement came from the Aztecs more than 400 years ago. The Spanish conquistadors found the Aztecs drying the green growth, called tecuitlatl, from Lake Texcoco located near Mexico city. Today, Lake Texcoco is still plentiful in *Spirulina*. It has also been speculated that the Mayans specifically farmed *Spirulina* as a crop. Likewise, the Kanembu who live along lake Chad were found to be taking the growth form the lake and drying it for food (Ciferri and Tiboni, 1985).

Classified as a cynobacteria (blue-green algae) *Spirulina* is abundant in phycocyanin, which gives it a blue pigmentation. The large amount of chlorophyll accounts for the vivid green color. Other additional carotenoids present contribute to the rich pigmentation of *Spirulina*. Interestingly, in nature, fruits and vegetables that have brighter and deeper hues often supply more antioxidants per serving then their paler cohorts.[78] A familiar example is found in the blueberry. The deep pigmentation of the blueberries produces a high ORAC value. The ORAC of blueberries is 2600 μmol Trolox equivalents/gram, whereas the ORAC for *Spirulina* is 13,000.[29] *Spirulina* has demonstrated that it has antioxidant activity, which scavenges peroxyl radicals.[79] It also contains components that act as inhibitors of cylooxygenase (COX), one of the main biological activities of nonsteroidal anti-inflammatory drugs.[80]

As mentioned earlier, with aging there are normal age-related changes occurring in the CNS in the absence of diseased states. These include increases in markers of oxidative stress and inflammation as well as changes in learning and memory as well as fundamental aspects of communications between neurons in the brain, such as changes in neurotransmitter receptor function. One study examined the significant decrease in β-adrenergic receptor function in aged rats. These age-related changes in β-adrenergic receptor function occur in the cerebellum and could underlie motor learning impairments with age.[81] In the cerebellum there is a correlation between the loss of function of β-adrenergic receptors in the aged brain and a loss in the ability to learn complex motor skills.[81] Feeding aged F344 rats a diet rich in spinach improves cerebellar β-adrenergic receptor function and improves motor learning that is associated with a decrease in oxidized glutathione and the proinflammatory cytokine TNFα.[82] Further studies have attempted to correlate the ability to improve cerebellar β-adrenergic receptor function with the *in vitro* antioxidant capacity of the foods added into the diet. This study examined dietary supplementation with apple, *Spirulina* or cucumber for 14 days in aged (18 months) and young (4 months) Fisher 344 rats. Using this paradigm aged rats on the *Spirulina* and apple enriched diet (both high in ORAC) but not on the cucumber diet, which is low in ORAC showed improvement in β-adrenergic receptor function as measured by electrophysiology (Figure 13.1a). In addition, a down regulation of proinflammatory cytokines (TNF-α and TNF-β) was observed in the aged animals on the *Spirulina* and apple enriched diet, but not the cucumber diet (Figure 13.1c). This is important because the reduced function of the beta-adrenergic receptor in the aged rat could be attributed to the elevated cytokine levels. In addition, there was a decrease in MDA in the cerebellum of the aged rats fed the high ORAC diets of *Spirulina* and apple (Figure 13.1b). MDA is a measure of oxidative lipid peroxidation. These results suggested that even in the aged rat cerebellum, an area high in oxidative damage and proinflammatory cytokines, *Spirulina* and apple were able to down regulate markers of inflammation and oxidative stress and improve the function of the β-adrenergic receptor. This study showed the potential of *Spirulina* to decrease markers of inflammation and oxidative stress in the CNS even after these processes had begun.[29]

There are many active components that contribute to the biological activity seen with *Spirulina*. In the case of aging, ingesting the whole compound may be the most beneficial. It is likely that the complete profile may work synergistically to delay oxidative insults and inflammation that are occurring with age. However, it is important to understand the combinations of different components that are driving the therapeutic effects of the whole compound. This is the key to comprehending why *Spirulina* could be beneficial in aging. This cyanobacteria has a powerful combination of fatty acids, proteins, vitamins, essential amino aids, minerals, and antioxidants that can aid in overall health. One important health benefit of *Spirulina* is to activate the innate immune system.[83] The innate immune system is the first line of defense in our bodies. Inflammation, caused by the innate immune system, is one of the first signs of infection. Thus, the possibility that *Spirulina* can assist in innate immunity holds the potential for this compound to exhibit widespread effects throughout the body.

Certain fractions of *Spirulina* have been investigated in depth to observe innate immune system activation. One such fraction is Immulina, a high molecular weight polysaccharide fraction obtained from crude dried extract. Immulina polysaccharide activates NF-kappa B through a CD14- and TLR2-dependent pathway.[84] Toll-like receptors (TLRs) are transmembrane proteins that are essential in the innate immune response because they identify pathogen-associated molecular patterns that are highly

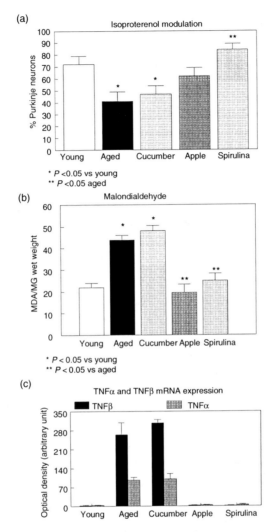

FIGURE 13.1 *Spirulina*, apple, or cucumber diets were administered to rats for 14 days before electrophysiolgical examination of β-adrenergic receptor function followed by analysis of MDA and TNF mRNA levels in cerebellar tissues from young and aged rats. (a) Bargraph showing the response of Purkinje neurons in the cerebellar cortex to locally applied isoproterenol. In young rats close to 70% of neurons recorded respond to isoproterenol with an augmentation of GABA responses. In aged rats the β-adrenergic receptor looses function and only 40% of neurons respond to isoproterenol. Following a diet enriched in either apple or *Spirulina* the Purkinje cells respond to isoproterenol and are not significantly different from young rats. However, cucumber a food low in ORAC, was not capable of altering the response to isorproterenol in aged rats. (b) Malondialdehyde (MDA) levels were measured by HPLC in cerebellar tissues from young and aged animals studied in 1a. Both the apple and *Spirulina* diets reduced the increase is MDA observed with age, cucumber had no effect on MDA levels in the aged cerebellar tissue, (1c) mRNA levels of TNFα, and TNFβ were measured by the RNA polymerase assay. As can be seen in the bar graph, levels of these two cytokines increase in the cerebellar tissue of the aged rats. Both the cucumber and *Spirulina* diets decreased the levels of TNFα and TNFβ, however the cucumber diet did not have any significant effect on cytokine levels.

conserved antigenic structures. TLRs are essential in the first stages of detecting infection and triggering host defenses. TLR2 is generally associated with identifying Gram-positive bacteria and Mycobacteria and its function is enhanced by CD14. CD14 is a membrane-associated glycosylphosphatidylinositol-linked protein expressed at the surface of cells. This pattern recognition receptor is especially associated with macrophages. CD14 acts by assisting in the transfer of bacterial ligands from circulation to TLRs. This complex then activates innate host defense mechanisms, such as release of inflammatory cytokines.[85] In addition, human data has shown the effects of *Spirulina* on monocytes and NK cells with the possibility that it may act on monocytes that induce IFN-gamma production in natural killer (NK) cells.[86] NK cells execute a major role in the host-rejection of both tumors and virally infected cells.[87] NK cells receive a signal before activation, importantly, cytokines, in particular IFNα/β aids in NK-cell activation.

An important essential fatty acid gamma linolenic acid (GLA) is present in *Spirulina*. GLA is also found in nuts green and leafy vegetables. This essential fatty acid is said to contain anti-inflammatory properties because of its metabolism to dihomogamma linolenic acid (DGLA).[88] DGLA is a competitive inhibitor of 2-series prostaglandins (PGs). PGs are, transient hormone-like chemicals that regulate cellular activities. They are comprised of unsaturated carboxylic acids, consisting of a 20 carbon skeleton that also contains a five member ring. PGs are biochemically synthesized from the fatty acid, arachidonic acid (AA) and executing various actions depending on the series type. PGs fall into 3 series—PG_1, PG_2, and PG_3. Series 1 and 3 execute anti-inflammatory effects as they decrease inflammation, increase oxygen flow, prevent cell aggregation, and decrease pain. Series 2, conversely, have proinflammatory effects. DGLA has also been shown to be a competitive inhibitor of 4-series leukotrienes (LTs). Leukotrienes are synthesized in the cell from AA by 5-lipoxygenase and function to sustain inflammatory reactions. Dietary GLA has the potential to prevent the formation and therefore the negative inflammatory effects of AA. In addition, a DGLA 15-hydroxyl derivative blocks the transformation of AA to LTs. In order to convert GLA to DGLA, instead of AA, nutrients including magnesium, zinc, and vitamins C, B3, and B6 are necessary with the exception of vitamin C all are present in *Spirulina*. Supplementation with fatty acids to the aged system can be of use in fortifying degenerating cell walls. Another prominent health concern in the aged population is cancer. The *Spirulina* component calcium spirulan, a sulfated polysaccharide chelating calcium, has shown promising results in studies. *In vitro* it has shown tumor migration and adhesion inhibition suggesting a therapeutic agent to reduce metastasis of tumor cells.[89] Because the aged individual has a compromised immune system, anything that can help defend the body from future viral infections can be useful. *Spirulina* has been investigated for its anti-viral activity. In one such study investigators isolated intracellular and extracellular polysaccharide fractions from the *A. platensis* species. These spirulan-like molecules showed pronounced antiviral activity in the absence of cytotoxic effects. There was inhibition of human cytomegalovirus, herpes simplex virus type 1, human herpes virus type 6, and human immunodeficiency virus type 1. Also, cells that were preincubated with the polysaccharide fraction showed lowered expression of the herpes viruses, pointing to inhibiting the entry of this virus. Other viruses were affected at other points of the viral process.[90] In addition to these findings, *Spirulina* extracts have shown antioxidant effects *in vitro* and *in vivo*.[79] Furthermore, c-phycocyanin found in *Spirulina* inhibits COX-2, which leads to a reduction in the inflammatory process.[91] Both of these findings are quite beneficial in the aged CNS and can help explain the mechanisms of action with in the system.

Neuroprotection from ischemic brain damage is another area where nutritional and herbal approaches may be of benefit as there is much evidence that oxidative stress and inflammation play a role in the neurodegeneration following ischemic injury. One study sought to investigate the potential of *Spirulina* to protect the CNS before a focal ischemic stroke and reperfusion injury.[92] The experiment involved feeding adult Sprague-Dawley rats a blueberry, spinach or *Spirulina* enriched diet for 4 weeks before a 60 min right middle cerebral artery occlusion (MCAO) followed by reperfusion. MCAO normally causes a substantial umbra and penumbra owing to multiple causes. Those animals that received the enriched diets showed a significant reduction in the volume of the infarction with *Spirulina* being the most effective showing a close to 70% reduction in infarct size (Figure 13.2). The rats that received the diets also showed improved motor behavior following the stroke as demonstrated by an increase in locomotor activity after the stroke. There was a reduction in apoptosis as shown by reduced caspase 3 and tunnel in the animals fed *Spirulina* before stroke. The data from Wang et al. (05) shows that a diet enriched in spriulina can help in the prevention of damage to brain tissue following an ischemic insult.

The neuroprotective effects of *Spirulina* have also been investigated in models of neurodegenerative disease. In one model of PD the neurotoxin 6-hydroxydopamine (6-OHDA) is injected into the striatum to induce a slowly progressive degeneration of dopamine neurons in the substantia nigra.[93] The death of the dopamine neurons is accompanied by an increase in proinflammatory cytokines, in particular TNF-α and can be modulated by altering TNFα levels.[94] This also occurs in the brains of PD patients. In the study by Strömberg et al. (05), Fischer 344 rats were given a diet supplemented with either blueberry or *Spirulina* for 28 days before the 6-OHDA lesion into the dorsal striatum.[95] Seven days or 4 weeks following the lesion, rats were euthanized for analysis of the dopamine neurons by immunohistochemistry. Results from this study indicated that the enriched diets led to an increase in recovery from the PD like insult 1 month following the 6-OHDA lesion, but did not prevent the damage from the initial insult when examined 1 week after the lesion. This was measured as the amount of area in the striatum where dopamine terminals were missing (the tyrosine hydroxylase (TH) negative zone (Figure 13.3). This was accompanied by a significant increase in activated microglia that express OX-6- (MHC class II) in the striatum and the globus pallidus at 1 week following the lesion and a reduced number of microglia at the 1 month time point, an event that was opposite of what was observed in the control animals (Figure 13.4). This early, transient increase in OX-6-positive microglia in the diet-treated animals is likely a beneficial action of the response to the injury where the microglia are phagocytocing the damaged tissues and secreting trophic factors and anti-inflammatory cytokines. Later on in the response to injury the microglial response becomes harmful and the blueberry and *Spirulina* diets reduced this later harmful phase of inflammation thus promoting regeneration of the dopamine nerve terminals back into the damaged striatum.[95]

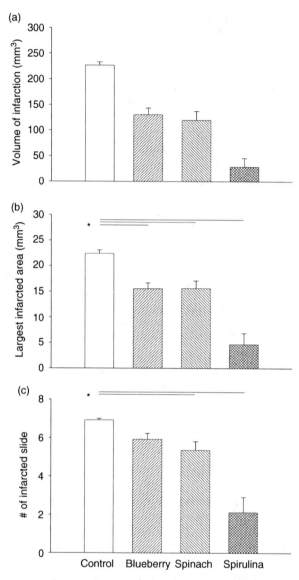

FIGURE 13.2 Bar graph demonstrating that pretreatment with either blueberry, spinach or *Spirulina* enriched diets significantly reduced the cortical infarction induced by middle cerebral artery occlusion/reperfusion. The right middle cerebral artery was ligated for 60 min. Animals were euthanized for TTC staining 48 h after ischemia/reperfusion, this is a marker of mitochondrial function. Marked infarction in the right cerebral cortex was found in animals receiving the control diet. Pretreatment with blueberry, spinach, or *Spirulina* significantly reduced the amount of infarction. Bar graph demonstrates that the infarcted area was significantly reduced compared with control diet in the blueberry spinach and *Spirulina* pretreated groups. This was observed when the infarcted area was measured using either (a) volume of infarcted area, (b) largest infarcted area, or (c) number of infarcted slides. This data can be seen in full in Reference 92.

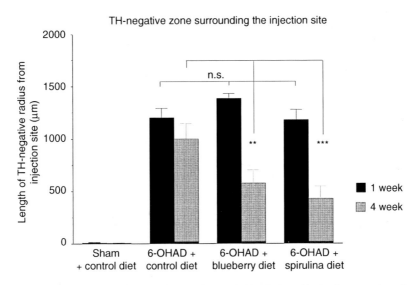

FIGURE 13.3 Bargraph showing the size of the 6-OHDA induced lesion in rats at 1 week and 4 weeks following the lesion. The size of the lesion was measured as the tyrosine hydroxylase (TH) negative zone. TH is a marker of dopamine neurons. Following a sham lesion there is not loss of TH as shown in the bar graph. In all groups there was a large loss of TH at 1 week following the lesion and at this time there was no significant difference between the control and blueberry or *Spirulina* pretreated groups. The decrease in TH negative zone observed in the blueberry and *Spirulina* groups at 4 weeks after the lesion indicates a regrowth of dopamine fibers into the lesioned area. There was no significant decrease in the size of the TH negative zone in the control lesioned animals.

In another animal model that mimics the neurodegeneration seen in PD is the 1-methyl-4-phenyl-1,2,3,6-tetrahydropyridine (MPTP) model. In this model MPTP is injected and it selectively targets the dopamine neurons in the striatum causing necrosis. A recently published study failed to see a large beneficial effect of *Spirulina* to improve dopamine levels 1 week following the MPTP lesion. One possible reason for the difference in the two studies could be the time frame of the examination of dopamine levels. In fact, in the study referred to above, there was no difference in dopamine levels as measured by immunohistochemistry at 1 week following the 6-OHDA injury, but only at 1 month, suggesting that the primary effect was to promote regeneration of the dopamine neurons following injury, rather than an initial protection from the insult itself.[96]

The above compilation of data highlights recent publications pertaining to *Spirulina* in the CNS. These findings demonstrate that *Spirulina* has many beneficial actions in animal models of aging and neurodegernerative disease. Its combination of proteins, vitamins, essential amino aids, minerals, fatty acids, and antioxidants undoubtedly aid in overall health. This, has been known for many years and utilized by ancient civilizations. Its anti-inflammatory effects peripherally have lead researchers into investigating the potential of *Spirulina* to decrease inflammation in the aged brain and following insults to the brain. The idea that *Spirulina* can affect

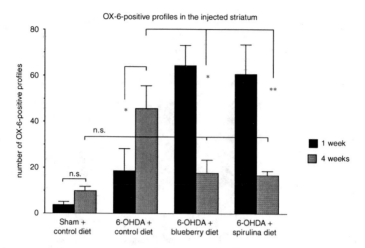

FIGURE 13.4 Bar graph depicting the number of OX-6 positive microglia in the striatum of rats following either sham of 6-hydroxydopamine (6-OHDA) lesions into the corpus striatum. This quantification of MHC class II receptors on microglia demonstrates that in rats treated with 6-OHDA and fed the control diet with normal levels of vitamins and minerals the inflammatory process continues to increase over the 4 weeks following the 6-OHDA insult. In rats that were fed the blueberry or *Spirulina* diet before the insult, there was initially a much larger response to the 6-OHDA at 1 week; however at 1 month following the insult there was a significant reduction in the numbers of OX-6 positive microglia observed in the striatum. $* = p < .05$, $p < .01$ One way ANOVA (see Reference 95 for full description).

the brain is stimulating as science is constantly pioneering novel natural compounds for innovative new therapies and drug formulations. Importantly, unlike many manufactured therapeutics *Spirulina* extracts have not shown toxic effects in experimental animals.[97,98] Human studies have shown beneficial results through TLRs using a dose of 2 grams a day.[83] Animal studies indicate that oral dosing of *Spirulina* can have effects within the CNS such as enhancing antioxidant activity.[79] Since other antioxidants such as fruits like apples and blueberries have shown protective mechanisms in the aging brain, it opens the way for *Spirulina* to be considered as a therapeutic intervention for the aging brain. *Spirulina*'s effects are widespread, which states that general mechanisms may be mediating some of its effects. It appears as though many beneficial outcomes of *Spirulina* can be linked to the activation of the innate immune system. The innate immune system is a first-line defense in our bodies and inflammation is a result of the innate immune system activation. Therefore, the enhancement of inflammation seen with normal aging could be down regulated by *Spirulina*. These widespread effects of *Spirulina* are also present in the periphery as seen with the benefits of *Spirulina* administration in arthritis.[99,100] These exclusively peripheral effects cannot be discounted as another possibility for CNS benefit. For example, *Spirulina* has been shown to have an effect in the spleen. Peripherally, the spleen is vital to the immune system to regulate inflammation because it disperses macrophages peripherally. There is evidence that when we age our blood brain barrier acquires small tears and openings through which macrophages and other immune regulatory cells can infiltrate. This is particularly pertinent in situations of inflammation.[101] There are data that support that *Spirulina* can promote spleen activation.[84,102] Furthermore, recent data investigates the potential involvement of the spleen in CNS repair after stroke.[103] In this manner, *Spirulina* and its' metabolites could then affect the CNS without physically crossing to blood brain barrier. Combining these data unveils the possibility that *Spirulina* may work directly in the CNS with its antioxidants and also peripherally by assisting in peripheral dispersal of macrophages into the aging CNS. Although some studies have focused on components of *Spirulina.* It is most likely a synergistic effect of all components within *Spirulina* that are supporting the aging brain. Importantly, studies that reveal the antioxidant activity[79] and anti-inflammatory activity[91] of *Spirulina* highlight global mechanisms that are needed in the aging CNS.

An inescapable truth of life is aging. Some complete this challenge with few setbacks while others encounter many struggles including disease. Some of the differences encountered while aging undoubtedly has to do with genetics. However, it is doubtful that the quality of life in old age is wholly dependant on genes. More likely, diet and exercise play a role in how the CNS functions with aging. Studies outlined here show the prospect of supporting the aging CNS with diet such as fruits and vegetables including blue-green algae. *Spirulina* is an interesting candidate for supporting the health of the aging CNS because it contains antioxidants and can modulate the innate immune system. In conclusion, *Spirulina* is a potent food that has many actions in the CNS to counteract oxidative stress and inflammation that occur as a consequence of aging and to aid regeneration of the brain following injury or neurodegenerative disease.

REFERENCES

1. Lynch, M. A. Age-related impairment in long-term potentiation in hippocampus: a role for the cytokine, interleukin-1 beta? *Prog. Neurobiol.* **1998,** 56 (5), 571–589.
2. Balschun, D., Randolf, A., Pitossi, F., Schneider, H., del Rey, A., Besedovsky, H. O. Hippocampal interleukin-1 beta gene expression during long-term potentiation decays with age. *Ann. N. Y. Acad. Sci.* **2003,** 992, 1–8.
3. Gahtan, E., Overmier, J. B. Inflammatory pathogenesis in Alzheimer's disease: biological mechanisms and cognitive sequeli. *Neurosci. Biobehav. Rev.* **1999,** 23 (5), 615–633.
4. Peterson, P. K., Hu, S., Anderson, W. R., Chao, C. C. Nitric oxide production and neurotoxicity mediated by activated microglia from human versus mouse brain. *J. Infect. Dis.* **1994,** 170 (2), 457–460.
5. Lynch, M. A. Interleukin-1 beta exerts a myriad of effects in the brain and in particular in the hippocampus: analysis of some of these actions. *Vitam. Horm.* **2002,** 64, 185–219.
6. Pugh, C. R., Fleshner, M., Watkins, L. R., Maier, S. F., Rudy, J. W. The immune system and memory consolidation: a role for the cytokine IL-1beta. *Neurosci. Biobehav. Rev.* **2001,** 25 (1), 29–41.
7. Yirmiya, R., Winocur, G., Goshen, I. Brain interleukin-1 is involved in spatial memory and passive avoidance conditioning. *Neurobiol. Learn. Mem.* **2002,** 78 (2), 379–389.

8. Lynch, M. A. Age-related impairment in long-term potentiation in hippocampus: a role for the cytokine, interleukin-1 beta? [Review] [187 refs]. *Prog. Neurobiol.* **1998,** 56 (5), 571–589.

9. Cunningham, A. J., Murray, C. A., O'Neill, L. A., Lynch, M. A., O'Connor, J. J. Interleukin-1 beta (IL-1 beta) and tumour necrosis factor (TNF) inhibit long-term potentiation in the rat dentate gyrus *in vitro. Neurosci. Lett.* **1996,** 203 (1), 17–20.

10. Katsuki, H., Nakai, S., Hirai, Y., Akaji, K., Kiso, Y., Satoh, M. Interleukin-1 beta inhibits long-term potentiation in the CA3 region of mouse hippocampal slices. *Eur. J. Pharmacol.* **1990,** 181 (3), 323–326.

11. Murray, C. A., McGahon, B., McBennett, S., Lynch, M. A. Interleukin-1 beta inhibits glutamate release in hippocampus of young, but not aged, rats. *Neurobiol. Aging* **1997,** 18 (3), 343–348.

12. Vereker, E., O'Donnell, E., Lynch, M. A. The inhibitory effect of interleukin-1beta on long-term potentiation is coupled with increased activity of stress-activated protein kinases. *J. Neurosci.* **2000,** 20 (18), 6811–6819.

13. Schneider, H., Pitossi, F., Balschun, D., Wagner, A., del Rey, A., Besedovsky, H. O. A neuromodulatory role of interleukin-1beta in the hippocampus. *Proc. Natl. Acad. Sci. U. S. A* **1998,** 95 (13), 7778–7783.

14. Clayton, D. A., Mesches, M. H., Alvarez, E., Bickford, P. C., Browning, M. D. A hippocampal NR2B deficit can mimic age-related changes in long-term potentiation and spatial learning in the Fischer 344 rat. *J. Neurosci.* **2002,** 22 (9), 3628–3637.

15. Clayton, D. A., Browning, M. D. Deficits in the expression of the NR2B subunit in the hippocampus of aged Fisher 344 rats. *Neurobiol. Aging* **2001,** 22 (1), 165–168.

16. Mesches, M. H., Gemma, C., Veng, L. M., Allgeier, C., Young, D. A., Browning, M. D., Bickford, P. C. Sulindac improves memory and increases NMDA receptor subunits in aged Fischer 344 rats. *Neurobiol. Aging* **2004,** 25 (3), 315–324.

17. Cavallaro, S., D'Agata, V., Manickam, P., Dufour, F., Alkon, D. L. Memory-specific temporal profiles of gene expression in the hippocampus. *Proc. Natl. Acad. Sci. U. S. A.* **2002,** 99 (25), 16279–16284.

18. Finkel, T., Holbrook, N. J. Oxidants, oxidative stress and the biology of ageing. *Nature* **2000,** 408 (6809), 239–247.

19. Zemlan, F. P., Thienhaus, O. J., Bosmann, H. B. Superoxide dismutase activity in Alzheimer's disease: possible mechanism for paired helical filament formation. *Brain Res.* **1989,** 476 (1), 160–162.

20. Richter, C., Park, J. W., Ames, B. N. Normal oxidative damage to mitochondrial and nuclear DNA is extensive. *Proc. Natl. Acad. Sci. U. S. A.* **1988,** 85 (17), 6465–6467.

21. Agarwal, S., Sohal, R. S. Aging and protein oxidative damage. *Mech. Ageing Dev.* **1994,** 75 (1), 11–19.

22. Ames, B. N., Shigenaga, M. K., Hagen, T. M. Oxidants, antioxidants, and the degenerative diseases of aging. *Proc. Natl. Acad. Sci. U. S. A.* **1993,** 90, 7915–7922.

23. Richter, C. Do mitochondrial DNA fragments promote cancer and aging? *FEBS Lett.* **1988,** 241 (1–2), 1–5.

24. Richter, C., Suter, M., Walter, P. B. Mitochondrial free radical damage and DNA repair. *Biofactors* **1998,** 7 (3), 207–208.

25. Richter, C. Do mitochondrial DNA fragments promote cancer and aging? *FEBS Lett.* **1988,** 241 (1–2), 1–5.

26. Ulmann, L., Mimouni, V., Roux, S., Porsolt, R., Poisson, J. P. Brain and hippocampus fatty acid composition in phospholipid classes of aged-relative cognitive deficit rats. *Prostaglandins Leukot. Essent. Fatty Acids* **2001,** 64 (3), 189–195.

27. Head, E., Liu, J., Hagen, T. M., Muggenburg, B. A., Milgram, N. W., Ames, B. N., Cotman, C. W. Oxidative damage increases with age in a canine model of human brain aging. *J. Neurochem.* **2002,** 82 (2), 375–381.

28. Dei, R., Takeda, A., Niwa, H., Li, M., Nakagomi, Y., Watanabe, M., Inagaki, T., Washimi, Y., Yasuda, Y., Horie, K., Miyata, T., Sobue, G. Lipid peroxidation and advanced glycation end products in the brain in normal aging and in Alzheimer's disease. *Acta Neuropathol. (Berl)* **2002,** 104 (2), 113–122.

29. Gemma, C., Mesches, M. H., Sepesi, B., Choo, K., Holmes, D. B., Bickford, P. C. Diets enriched in foods with high antioxidant activity reverse age-induced decreases in cerebellar beta-adrenergic function and increases in proinflammatory cytokines. *J. Neurosci.* **2002,** 22 (14), 6114–6120.

30. Butterfield, D. A., Howard, B. J., Yatin, S., Allen, K. L., Carney, J. M., Aging, Membrane proteins, Anti-aging agents. Free radical oxidation of brain proteins in accelerated senescence and its modulation by n-tert-butyl-alpha-phenylnitrone. *Proc. Natl. Acad. Sci. U. S. A.* **1997,** 94 (2), 674–678.

31. Papaioannou, N., Tooten, P. C., van Ederen, A. M., Bohl, J. R., Rofina, J., Tsangaris, T., Gruys, E. Immunohistochemical investigation of the brain of aged dogs. I. Detection of neurofibrillary tangles and of 4-hydroxynonenal protein, an oxidative damage product, in senile plaques. *Amyloid* **2001,** 8 (1), 11–21.

32. Yoritaka, A., Hattori, N., Uchida, K., Tanaka, M., Stadtman, E. R., Mizuno, Y. Immunohistochemical detection of 4-hydroxynonenal protein adducts in Parkinson disease. *Proc. Natl. Acad. Sci. U. S. A.* **1996,** 93 (7), 2696–2701.

33. Smith, M. A., Rudnicka-Nawrot, M., Richey, P. L., Praprotnik, D., Mulvihill, P., Miller, C. A., Sayre, L. M., Perry, G. Carbonyl-related posttranslational modification of neurofilament protein in the neurofibrillary pathology of Alzheimer's disease. *J. Neurochem.* **1995,** 64 (6), 2660–2666.

34. Nicolle, M. M., Gallagher, M., McKinney, M. No loss of synaptic proteins in the hippocampus of aged, behaviorally impaired rats. *Neurobiol. Aging* **1999,** 20 (3), 343–348.

35. Hensley, K., Hall, N., Subramaniam, R., Cole, P., Harris, M., Aksenov, M., Aksenova, M., Gabbita, S. P., Wu, J. F., Carney, J. M. Brain regional correspondence between Alzheimer's disease histopathology and biomarkers of protein oxidation. *J. Neurochem.* **1995,** 65 (5), 2146–2156.

36. Aksenova, M. V., Aksenov, M. Y., Carney, J. M., Butterfield, D. A. Protein oxidation and enzyme activity decline in old brown Norway rats are reduced by dietary restriction. *Mech. Ageing Dev.* **1998,** 100 (2), 157–168.

37. Shin, C. M., Chung, Y. H., Kim, M. J., Lee, E. Y., Kim, E. G., Cha, C. I. Age-related changes in the distribution of nitrotyrosine in the cerebral cortex and hippocampus of rats. *Brain Res.* **2002,** 931 (2), 194–199.

38. Sloane, J. A., Hollander, W., Moss, M. B., Rosene, D. L., Abraham, C. R. Increased microglial activation and protein nitration in white matter of the aging monkey. *Neurobiol. Aging* **1999,** 20 (4), 395–405.

39. Tohgi, H., Abe, T., Yamazaki, K., Murata, T., Ishizaki, E., Isobe, C. Alterations of 3-nitrotyrosine concentration in the cerebrospinal fluid during aging and in patients with Alzheimer's disease. *Neurosci. Lett.* **1999,** 269 (1), 52–54.

40. Chung, H. Y., Kim, H. J., Kim, K. W., Choi, J. S., Yu, B. P. Molecular inflammation hypothesis of aging based on the anti-aging mechanism of calorie restriction. *Microsc. Res. Tech.* **2002,** 59 (4), 264–272.

41. Butterfield, D. A., Perluigi, M., Sultana, R. Oxidative stress in Alzheimer's disease brain: new insights from redox proteomics. *Eur. J. Pharmacol.* **2006,** 545 (1), 39–50.

42. Butterfield, D. A., Poon, H. F., St, C. D., Keller, J. N., Pierce, W. M., Klein, J. B., Markesbery, W. R. Redox proteomics identification of oxidatively modified hippocampal proteins in mild cognitive impairment: insights into the development of Alzheimer's disease. *Neurobiol. Dis.* **2006,** 22 (2), 223–232.

43. Batchelor, P. E., Liberatore, G. T., Wong, J. Y., Porritt, M. J., Frerichs, F., Donnan, G. A., Howells, D. W. Activated macrophages and microglia induce dopaminergic sprouting in the injured striatum and express brain-derived neurotrophic factor and glial cell line-derived neurotrophic factor. *J. Neurosci.* **1999,** 19 (5), 1708–1716.

44. Chang, J. Y., Liu, L. Z. Manganese potentiates nitric oxide production by microglia. *Brain Res.* **1999,** *Mol. Brain Res. 68* (1–2), 22–28.

45. Dringen, R. Oxidative and antioxidative potential of brain microglial cells. *Antioxid. Redox. Signal.* **2005,** 7 (9–10), 1223–1233.

46. Duffield, J. S. The inflammatory macrophage: a story of Jekyll and Hyde. *Clin. Sci. (Lond)* **2003,** 104 (1), 27–38.

47. Mantovani, A., Sica, A., Sozzani, S., Allavena, P., Vecchi, A., Locati, M. The chemokine system in diverse forms of macrophage activation and polarization. *Trends Immunol.* **2004,** 25 (12), 677–686.

48. Colton, C. A. Microglial oxyradical production: causes and consequences. *Neuropathol. Appl. Neurobiol.* **1994,** 20 (2), 208–209.

49. Terao, I. Effects of once-daily low-dose administration of sustained-release theophylline on airway inflammation and airway hyperresponsiveness in patients with asthma. *Arerugi* **2002,** 51 (4), 364–370.

50. Lee, C. K., Allison, D. B., Brand, J., Weindruch, R., Prolla, T. A. Transcriptional profiles associated with aging and middle age-onset caloric restriction in mouse hearts. *Proc. Natl. Acad. Sci. U. S. A.* **2002,** 99 (23), 14988–14993.

51. Ye, S. M., Johnson, R. W. Increased interleukin-6 expression by microglia from brain of aged mice. *J Neuroimmunol.* **1999,** 93 (1–2), 139–148.

52. McGeer, P. L., Itagaki, S., Boyes, B. E., McGeer, E. G. Reactive microglia are positive for HLA-DR in the substantia nigra of Parkinson's and Alzheimer's disease brains. *Neurology* **1988,** 38 (8), 1285–1291.

53. Nagatsu, T., Mogi, M., Ichinose, H., Togari, A. Cytokines in Parkinson's disease. *J. Neural Transm.* **2000,** 58 (Suppl), 143–151.

54. Hirsch, E. C., Hunot, S., Damier, P., Faucheux, B. Glial cells and inflammation in Parkinson's disease: a role in neurodegeneration? *Ann. Neurol.* **1998,** 44 (3 Suppl 1), S115–S120.

55. Stanfield, B. B., Trice, J. E. Evidence that granule cells generated in the dentate gyrus of adult rats extend axonal projections. *Exp. Brain Res.* **1988,** 72 (2), 399–406.

56. van Praag, H., Schinder, A. F., Christie, B. R., Toni, N., Palmer, T. D., Gage, F. H. Functional neurogenesis in the adult hippocampus. *Nature* **2002,** 415 (6875), 1030–1034.

57. Greenberg, D. A., Jin, K. Neurodegeneration and neurogenesis: focus on Alzheimer's disease. *Curr. Alzheimer Res.* **2006,** 3 (1), 25–28.

58. Parent, J. M., Yu, T. W., Leibowitz, R. T., Geschwind, D. H., Sloviter, R. S., Lowenstein, D. H. Dentate granule cell neurogenesis is increased by seizures and contributes to aberrant network reorganization in the adult rat hippocampus. *J. Neurosci.* **1997,** 17 (10), 3727–3738.

59. Shors, T. J., Townsend, D. A., Zhao, M., Kozorovitskiy, Y., Gould, E. Neurogenesis may relate to some but not all types of hippocampal-dependent learning. *Hippocampus* **2002,** 12 (5), 578–584.

60. Shors, T. J., Miesegaes, G., Beylin, A., Zhao, M., Rydel, T., Gould, E. Neurogenesis in the adult is involved in the formation of trace memories. *Nature* **2001,** 410 (6826), 372–376.
61. Bizon, J. L., Lee, H. J., Gallagher, M. Neurogenesis in a rat model of age-related cognitive decline. *Aging Cell* **2004,** 3 (4), 227–234.
62. Merrill, D. A., Karim, R., Darraq, M., Chiba, A. A., Tuszynski, M. H. Hippocampal cell genesis does not correlate with spatial learning ability in aged rats. *J. Comp. Neurol.* **2003,** 459 (2), 201–207.
63. Hattiangady, B., Shetty, A. K. Aging does not alter the number or phenotype of putative stem/progenitor cells in the neurogenic region of the hippocampus. *Neurobiol. Aging* **2006.**
64. Conboy, I. M., Conboy, M. J., Wagers, A. J., Girma, E. R., Weissman, I. L., Rando, T. A. Rejuvenation of aged progenitor cells by exposure to a young systemic environment. *Nature* **2005,** 433 (7027), 760–764.
65. Ekdahl, C. T., Claasen, J. H., Bonde, S., Kokaia, Z., Lindvall, O. Inflammation is detrimental for neurogenesis in adult brain. *Proc. Natl. Acad. Sci. U. S. A.* **2003,** 100 (23), 13632–13637.
66. Joseph, J. A., Shukitt-Hale, B., Denisova, N. A., Bielinski, D., Martin, A., McEwen, J. J., Bickford, P. C. Reversals of age-related declines in neuronal signal transduction, cognitive, and motor behavioral deficits with blueberry, spinach, or strawberry dietary supplementation. *J. Neurosci.* **1999,** 19 (18), 8114–8121.
67. Casadesus, G., Shukitt-Hale, B., Stellwagen, H. M., Zhu, X., Lee, H. G., Smith, M. A., Joseph, J. A. Modulation of hippocampal plasticity and cognitive behavior by short-term blueberry supplementation in aged rats. *Nutr. Neurosci.* **2004,** 7 (56), 309–316.
68. Cuppini, R., Ciaroni, S., Cecchini, T., Ambrogini, P., Ferri, P., Cuppini, C., Ninfali, P., Del, G. P. Tocopherols enhance neurogenesis in dentate gyrus of adult rats. *Int. J. Vitam. Nutr. Res.* **2002,** 72 (3), 170–176.
69. Vila, J. L., Gemma, C., Hudson, C., Cole, M. J., Bickford, P. C. *Spirulina* protects against LPS-induced decrease in neurogenesis. Society for Neuroscience Abstracts online. 2005.
70. Vila, J. L., Gemma, C., Hudson, C., Cole, M. J., Bickford, P. C. Effect of long-term spriulina administration on hippocampal neurogenesis in the aged rat. Society for Neuroscience Abstracts online. 2006.
71. McGeer, E. G., McGeer, P. L. Brain inflammation in Alzheimer disease and the therapeutic implications. *Curr. Pharm. Des* **1999,** 5 (10), 821–836.
72. McGeer, P. L., McGeer, E. G. Inflammation of the brain in Alzheimer's disease: implications for therapy. *J. Leukoc. Biol.* **1999,** 65 (4), 409–415.
73. In't Veld, B. A., Ruitenberg, A., Hofman, A., Launer, L. J., van Duijn, C. M., Stijnen, T., Breteler, M. M., Stricker, B. H. Nonsteroidal antiinflammatory drugs and the risk of Alzheimer's disease. *N. Engl. J. Med.* **2001,** 345 (21), 1515–1521.
74. Sanghi, S., MacLaughlin, E. J., Jewell, C. W., Chaffer, S., Naus, P. J., Watson, L. E., Dostal, D. E. Cyclooxygenase-2 inhibitors: a painful lesson. *Cardiovasc. Hematol. Disord. Drug Targets.* **2006,** 6 (2), 85–100.
75. Cao, G., Giovanoni, M., Prior, R. L. Antioxidant capacity in different tissues of young and old rats. *Proc. Soc. Exp. Biol. Med.* **1996,** 211 (4), 359–365.
76. Bickford, P. C., Gould, T., Briederick, L., Chadman, K., Pollock, A., Young, D., Shukitt-Hale, B., Joseph, J. Antioxidant-rich diets improve cerebellar physiology and motor learning in aged rats. *Brain Res.* **2000,** 866 (1–2), 211–217.

77. Joseph, J. A., Shukitt-Hale, B., Denisova, N. A., Prior, R. L., Cao, G., Martin, A., Taglialatela, G., Bickford, P. C. Long-term dietary strawberry, spinach, or vitamin E supplementation retards the onset of age-related neuronal signal-transduction and cognitive behavioral deficits. *J. Neurosci.* **1998,** 18 (19), 8047–8055.

78. Cao, G., Alessio, H. M., Cutler, R. G. Oxygen-radical absorbance capacity assay for antioxidants. *Free. Radic. Biol. Med.* **1993,** 14 (3), 303–311.

79. Miranda, M. S., Cintra, R. G., Barros, S. B., Mancini, F. J. Antioxidant activity of the microalga *Spirulina* maxima. *Braz. J. Med. Biol. Res.* **1998,** 31 (8), 1075–1079.

80. Reddy, M. C., Subhashini, J., Mahipal, S. V., Bhat, V. B., Srinivas, R. P., Kiranmai, G., Madyastha, K. M., Reddanna, P. C-Phycocyanin, a selective cyclooxygenase-2 inhibitor, induces apoptosis in lipopolysaccharide-stimulated RAW 264.7 macrophages. *Biochem. Biophys. Res. Commun.* **2003,** 304 (2), 385–392.

81. Bickford, P. Motor learning deficits in aged rats are correlated with loss of cerebellar noradrenergic function. *Brain Res.* **1993,** 620, 133–138.

82. Cartford, M. C., Gemma, C., Bickford, P. C. Eighteen-month-old Fischer 44 rats fed a spinach-enriched diet show improved delay classical eyeblink conditioning and reduced expression of tumor necrosis factor alpha (TNFalpha) and TNFbeta in the cerebellum. *J. Neurosci.* **2002,** 22 (14), 5813–5816.

83. Hirahashi, T., Matsumoto, M., Hazeki, K., Saeki, Y., Ui, M., Seya, T. Activation of the human innate immune system by *Spirulina*: augmentation of interferon production and NK cytotoxicity by oral administration of hot water extract of *Spirulina platensis*. *Int. Immunopharmacol.* **2002,** 2 (4), 423–434.

84. Balachandran, P., Pugh, N. D., Ma, G., Pasco, D. S. Toll-like receptor 2-dependent activation of monocytes by *Spirulina* polysaccharide and its immune enhancing action in mice. *Int. Immunopharmacol.* **2006,** 6 (12), 1808–1814.

85. Dziarski, R., Gupta, D. Peptidoglycan recognition in innate immunity. *J. Endotoxin. Res.* **2005,** 11 (5), 304–310.

86. Khan, Z., Bhadouria, P., Bisen, P. S. Nutritional and therapeutic potential of *Spirulina*. *Curr. Pharm. Biotechnol.* **2005,** 6 (5), 373–379.

87. Arnon, T. I., Markel, G., Mandelboim, O. Tumor and viral recognition by natural killer cells receptors. *Semin. Cancer Biol.* **2006,** 16 (5), 348–358.

88. Fan, Y. Y., Chapkin, R. S. Importance of dietary gamma-linolenic acid in human health and nutrition. *J. Nutr.* **1998,** 128 (9), 1411–1414.

89. Mishima, T., Murata, J., Toyoshima, M., Fujii, H., Nakajima, M., Hayashi, T., Kato, T., Saiki, I. Inhibition of tumor invasion and metastasis by calcium spirulan (Ca-SP), a novel sulfated polysaccharide derived from a blue-green alga, *Spirulina platensis*. *Clin. Exp. Metastasis* **1998,** 16 (6), 541–550.

90. Rechter, S., Konig, T., Auerochs, S., Thulke, S., Walter, H., Dornenburg, H., Walter, C., Marschall, M. Antiviral activity of Arthrospira-derived spirulan-like substances. *Antiviral Res.* **2006,** 72 (3), 197–206.

91. Reddy, C. M., Bhat, V. B., Kiranmai, G., Reddy, M. N., Reddanna, P., Madyastha, K. M. Selective inhibition of cyclooxygenase-2 by C-phycocyanin, a biliprotein from *Spirulina platensis*. *Biochem. Biophys. Res. Commun.* **2000,** 277 (3), 599–603.

92. Wang, Y., Chang, C. F., Chou, J., Chen, H. L., Deng, X., Harvey, B. K., Cadet, J. L., Bickford, P. C. Dietary supplementation with blueberries, spinach, or *spirulina* reduces ischemic brain damage. *Exp. Neurol.* **2005,** 193 (1), 75–84.

93. Sauer, H., Oertel, W. H. Progressive degeneration of nigrostriatal dopamine neurons following intrastriatal terminal lesions with 6-hydroxydopamine: a combined retrograde tracing and immunocytochemical study in the rat. *Neuroscience* **1994,** 59 (2), 401–415.

94. Gemma, C., Catlow, B., Cole, M., Hudson C., Samec, A., Shah, N., Vila, J., Bachstetter, A., Bickford, P. C. Early inhibition of TNFalpha increases 6-hydroxydopamine-induced striatal degeneration. *Brain Res.*, in press.

95. Stromberg, I., Gemma, C., Vila, J., Bickford, P. C. Blueberry- and *spirulina*-enriched diets enhance striatal dopamine recovery and induce a rapid, transient microglia activation after injury of the rat nigrostriatal dopamine system. *Exp. Neurol.* **2005,** 196 (2), 298–307.

96. Chamorro, G., Perez-Albiter, M., Serrano-Garcia, N., Mares-Samano, J. J., Rojas, P. *Spirulina maxima* pretreatment partially protects against 1-methyl-4-phenyl-1,2,3,6-tetrahydropyridine neurotoxicity. *Nutr. Neurosci.* **2006,** 9 (5–6), 207–212.

97. Chamorro, G., Salazar, M. Teratogenic study of *Spirulina* in mice. *Arch. Latinoam. Nutr.* **1990,** 40 (1), 86–94.

98. Salazar, M., Martinez, E., Madrigal, E., Ruiz, L. E., Chamorro, G. A. Subchronic toxicity study in mice fed *Spirulina maxima*. *J. Ethnopharmacol.* **1998,** 62 (3), 235–241.

99. Remirez, D., Gonzalez, R., Merino, N., Rodriguez, S., Ancheta, O. Inhibitory effects of *Spirulina* in zymosan-induced arthritis in mice. *Mediators. Inflamm.* **2002,** 11 (2), 75–79.

100. Rasool, M., Sabina, E. P., Lavanya, B. Anti-inflammatory effect of *Spirulina fusiformis* on adjuvant-induced arthritis in mice. *Biol. Pharm. Bull.* **2006,** 29 (12), 2483–2487.

101. Engelhardt, B. Regulation of immune cell entry into the central nervous system. *Results Probl. Cell Differ.* **2006,** 43, 259–280.

102. Hayashi, O., Katoh, T., Okuwaki, Y. Enhancement of antibody production in mice by dietary *Spirulina platensis*. *J. Nutr. Sci. Vitaminol. (Tokyo)* **1994,** 40 (5), 431–441.

103. Vendrame, M., Gemma, C., Pennypacker, K. R., Bickford, P. C., Davis, S. C., Sanberg, P. R., Willing, A. E. Cord blood rescues stroke-induced changes in splenocyte phenotype and function. *Exp. Neurol.* **2006,** 199 (1), 191–200.

14 *Spirulina* Interactions

Andrea T. Borchers, Carl L. Keen, and M. Eric Gershwin

CONTENTS

INTRODUCTION

In recent years, there has been much interest in interactions between botanicals and drugs, that is, the ability of medicinal "herbs" to influence the pharmacokinetics (absorption, metabolism, or excretion) of pharmaceuticals. This interest was sparked by the rising awareness that the prevalence of herbal supplement use was high in the general population and higher yet in patients with chronic diseases requiring regular intake of a variety of medications. Reports of life-threatening consequences resulting from herb–drug interactions further underscored the urgent need for a better understanding of these interactions.

The metabolism or biotransformation of drugs and many other chemicals and environmental pollutants ultimately results in their excretion and is, therefore, referred to as detoxification. Detoxification is at least a two-step process and is mediated by phase I and phase II enzymes. Phase I reactions are catalyzed by members of the cytochrome P450 system, which are located mainly in the liver, but are also present in gut wall, lung, and kidney. The cytochrome P450 enzymes are monooxygenases, that is, they use oxygen in order to add a reactive group. The metabolite resulting from this activation can be more reactive or toxic than the parent compound and can cause damage unless phase II enzymes further metabolize it. Phase II enzymes catalyze conjugation reactions, that is, they conjugate the metabolites arising from phase I reactions with molecules like glutathione, glucuronic acid, sulfate, or a variety of amino acids. The effect of medicinal botanicals on cytochrome P450 enzymes has been the focus of extensive research. It is, therefore, rather surprising that the interaction of *Spirulina* (now called *Arthrospira*) with this large family of enzymes has rarely been investigated.

EFFECTS OF *SPIRULINA* ON CYTOCHROME P450, CYTOCHROME P450 REDUCTASE, AND GLUTATHIONE TRANSFERASE

In Swiss albino mice, oral administration of *Spirulina fusiformis* at a dose of 800 mg/kg body weight for 10 days resulted in a significant decrease in hepatic cytochrome P450 content, whereas cytochrome b5 content was not significantly affected.[1,2] Cytochrome b5 is a group of electron transport hemoproteins that enhance the efficiency of certain P450 isoforms. In contrast, the activity of the phase II enzyme glutathione *S*-transferase (GST) was increased in the liver of these mice. However, according to the p value of <0.1, this increase was at best marginally significant in both of these studies, although the actual data in one of them suggest a very marked elevation with little standard deviation.[1] GST was not increased in any of the other tissues examined, which included kidney, lung, and intestine.[1] Glutathione reductase activity and concentrations of reduced glutathione were not significantly altered.[1,2]

The same group of researchers obtained somewhat different results in another investigation of phase I and phase II enzymes in the same strain of mice, treated with 250 or 500 mg/kg body weight of *S. platensis* orally for 15 days.[3] The liver of these animals contained similar levels of cytochrome P450 and cytochrome b5 as untreated controls, whereas cytochrome P450 reductase, and b5 reductase activities were significantly up-regulated. GST and DT diaphorase, which is considered a detoxification enzyme, also exhibited significantly higher activity after *Spirulina* treatment. Interestingly, the lower dose frequently resulted in greater stimulation than the higher dose. In the same study, oral administration of *Spirulina* to Swiss albino mice significantly reduced tumor incidence and tumor burden after treatment with two different carcinogens. Unfortunately, the effect of *Spirulina* on detoxifying enzymes was only examined in healthy mice, but not in those exposed to tumor-inducing chemicals. The reasons for these discrepancies are not immediately obvious, but may involve differences in the dosage and duration of *Spirulina* administration.

Another group of researchers did not observe a significant effect of orally administered *S. fusiformis* at doses of 250 and 500 mg/kg per day for 5 days on GST activity in liver of mice.[4] At the highest dose (1000 mg/kg), however, *Spirulina* significantly induced GST activity. In the same study, *Spirulina* was found to dose dependently reverse the inhibition of GST activity seen after treatment with cyclophosphamide or mitomycin-C, with the highest dose resulting in complete normalization. Similarly, *Spirulina* significantly attenuated the inhibition of GST activity induced by cisplatin and urethane, and again the highest dose essentially normalized the activity of this enzyme.[5] Of note, urethane undergoes metabolic activation through cytochrome P450, and part of the protective effect of *Spirulina* could be due to inhibiting this process.

There is also one investigation of the ability of phycocyanin to influence cytochrome P450 enzymes. Phycocyanin is a major protein of *Spirulina*, making up 15–20% of algal dry weight. It consists of the apoprotein and covalently attached phycocyanobilin chromophores, which are responsible for the blue coloring of these cyanobacteria. Phycocyanin by itself did not significantly affect hepatic cytochrome P450 activity in rats when administered intraperitoneally.[6] However, when injected 1 h before treatment with a single dose of a compound known to cause liver toxicity (R-(+)-pulegone or carbon tetrachloride) phycocyanin significantly, but not completely, reversed the depression of cytochrome P450 activity induced by these hepatotoxins. Interestingly, phycocyanin increased the urinary excretion of one of the major R-(+)-pulegone metabolites, a precursor of more toxic intermediates. Since both the metabolite and the more toxic intermediates arise from P450-mediated reactions, this suggests that phycocyanin inhibited specific components of the P450 system, while possibly inducing others and at the same time reversing the inhibition of overall P450 activity associated with R-(+)-pulegone treatment.

DRUG TOXICITY STUDIES

Drug-induced toxicity is almost invariably associated with oxidative stress in the target organ or tissue. This stems from a variety of sources, including increased generation of reactive oxygen species as an inevitable consequence of certain enzyme activities, the conversion of the drug itself into a radical or a compound able to generate radicals, and drug-induced inhibition of antioxidant enzyme activities. *Spirulina* contains a variety of antioxidants, including ascorbic acid (vitamin C), α-tocopherol (vitamin E), β-carotenes, and phenolic compounds.[7] Various aqueous or alcoholic extracts of this alga can scavenge a variety of radicals *in vitro* and exhibit antioxidant activity in vivo.[7–10] Another constituent of *Spirulina*, phycocyanin, has been demonstrated to scavenge peroxyl,[11] hydroxyl,[12,13] alkoxyl,[12] and superoxide radicals[10] as well as peroxynitrite.[14] There are also results suggesting that phycocyanin is capable of chelating iron,[11] which can be a powerful pro-oxidant. It has been proposed that much of the radical scavenging and antioxidant activity of *Spirulina* is attributable to phycocyanin, particularly its chromophore, phycocyanobilin.[15] Note, however, that phycocyanin was more effective than phycocyanobilin in scavenging peroxynitrite.[14]

In addition to antioxidant molecules, a variety of antioxidant enzymes protect humans and animals from oxidative stress. These include superoxide dismutase (SOD), glutathione peroxidase (GPx), and catalase. There have been several investigations of the effects of *Spirulina* on the activity of these enzymes, but the results have been somewhat controversial. In mice treated with 250 or 500 mg/kg of *S. platensis* orally for 15 days, the activities of hepatic SOD, GPx, and catalase along with reduced glutathione levels were significantly increased compared to saline-treated controls.[3] In contrast, another group of researchers did not observe a significant effect of orally administered *S. fusiformis* at doses of 250 and 500 mg/kg per day for 5 days on the activities of these antioxidant enzymes in mouse liver.[4] At the highest dose (1000 mg/kg), however, *Spirulina* significantly induced SOD, but not GPx and catalase, activity. There are also several studies that examined the effect of *Spirulina* treatment on antioxidant enzymes in the kidneys, since the major focus was the prevention of drug-induced nephrotoxicity. Neither *S. platensis* nor *S. fusiformis* alone markedly altered the activities of any of these enzymes in kidney tissue of rats treated for between 5 and 17 days, even though treatment with these algae reversed the inhibition of SOD, GPx, and catalase activities induced by cisplatin or cyclosporine.[16–18] The ability of *Spirulina* to act as an antioxidant and, possibly, induce endogenous antioxidant enzymes prompted several groups of researchers to investigate the effectiveness of this alga in ameliorating drug-induced toxicities. The results of these studies are summarized below. The study design and the effects of *Spirulina* on antioxidant enzyme activity in the various studies are summarized in Table 14.1.

STUDIES OF *SPIRULINA* IN DRUG-INDUCED TOXICITIES

Cisplatin is a highly effective chemotherapy drug. Unfortunately, it can be associated with kidney toxicity, resulting in severe and often irreversible renal failure. Several recent studies have investigated the ability of *Spirulina* to protect rats from cisplatin-induced nephrotoxicity. In one of these studies *S. fusiformis* was given orally at doses of 500, 1000, or 1500 mg/kg body weight from 2 days before until 3 days after the injection of cisplatin.[18] Administration of this alga was associated with marked amelioration of the cisplatin-induced changes in kidney morphology and significant, dose-dependent reduction of markers of renal dysfunction, such as serum creatinine and blood urea nitrogen. In addition, *Spirulina* reduced lipid peroxidation in the kidney and partially reversed the cisplatin-induced decrease in the levels of reduced glutathione and the activity of the antioxidant enzymes SOD and catalase.

Similar results were obtained in another investigation, where rats received *S. platensis* orally at a dose of 1000 mg/kg for 4 days before until 4 days after cisplatin injection.[16] This treatment significantly reduced the severity of histological changes in the kidney and ameliorated plasma and urinary markers of renal dysfunction. In this study, administration of the alga completely inhibited lipid peroxidation not only in the kidney but also in plasma and restored the activities of SOD, GPx, and catalase to the levels seen in control animals. It is possible that the selenium content of *Spirulina* played a role in the induction of GPx, which is a selenium-containing enzyme. The somewhat greater effectiveness in preventing oxidative stress in this compared to the previous study may have been due to the longer duration of *Spirulina* administration.

Gentamicin is an antibiotic used for the treatment of serious gram-negative infections.[19] It also is associated with significant nephrotoxicity. Oral administration of *S. fusiformis* at doses of 500, 1000, or 1500 mg/kg for 2 days before and 8 days concurrently with gentamicin resulted in a dose-dependent restoration of renal function. The highest dose largely prevented the gentamicin-induced changes in renal morphology. All three doses significantly inhibited the increase in kidney lipid peroxidation following gentamicin treatment, with the highest dose providing complete protection. *Spirulina* also dose dependently reversed the gentamicin-induced inhibition of antioxidant enzyme activity in the kidney. Animals treated with the highest

TABLE 14.1
Effect of *Spirulina* on Antioxidant Enzymes in the Target Tissues of Drug Toxicities

Drug	Drug dose	Affected tissue	Animals	*Spirulina* species	Dose and duration of *Spirulina*	GPx	CAT	SOD	Ref
Cyclosporine	50 mg/kg, d 0–d 13	Kidney	Wistar rats	*S. platensis*	500 mg/kg, d 2–d 14[a]	Norm.[b]	Norm.	Norm.	17
Cisplatin	6 mg/kg, d 0	Kidney	Wistar rats	*S. platensis*	1000 mg/kg, d 3–d 4	Norm.	Norm.	Norm.	16
Cisplatin	5 mg/kg, d 0	Kidney	Wistar rats	*S. fusiformis*	500, 1000, or 1500 mg/kg, d 1–d 3	—	Sign. rev.[c]	Sign. rev.	18
Cisplatin	5 mg/kg, d 0	DNA[d]	Swiss albino mice	*S. fusiformis*	250, 500, or 1000 mg/kg, d 4–d 0	Sign. rev.	Sign. rev.	Sign. rev.	5
Gentamicin	100 mg/kg, d 0–d 7	Kidney	Wistar rats	*S. fusiformis*	500 or 1000 mg/kg, d 1–d 8	—	Sign. rev.	Sign. rev.	19
					1500 mg/kg, d 1–d 8				
Doxorubicin	4 mg/kg, d 0, 6, 13, 20	Heart	Swiss albino mice	*S. platensis*	250 mg/kg, d 2–d 48	Norm.	—	Norm.	9
Cyclophosphamide	40 mg/kg, d 0	DNA[d]	Swiss albino mice	*S. fusiformis*	250, 500, or 1000 mg/kg, d 4–d 0	Sign. rev.	Sign. rev.	Sign. rev.	4
Mitomycin-C	1 mg/kg, d 0	DNA[d]	Swiss albino mice	*S. fusiformis*	250 mg/kg, d 4–d 0	No effect	Sign. rev.[e]	No effect	4
					500 or 1000 mg/kg, d 4–d 0	Sign. rev.[e]	Sign. rev.[e]	Sign. rev.[d]	

[a] A minus sign indicates that treatment with *Spirulina* began before the drug treatment, which was given starting on Day 0
[b] Norm. = normalized, that is, not significantly different from control levels.
[c] Sign. rev. = significant reversal of drug-induced inhibition.
[d] Antioxidant enzymes were measured in the liver.
[e] The highest dose appeared to normalize these enzyme activities, but no statistical comparison was performed between controls and animals treated with drugs plus *Spirulina*.

dose exhibited essentially normal SOD and catalase activity and levels of reduced glutathione.

Cyclosporine is an immunosuppressive agent used to prevent rejection of transplanted organs. It is associated with considerable renal toxicity in up to 30% of patients. When rats were given *S. platensis* at a dose of 500 mg/kg for 3 days before and 14 days concurrently with cyclosporine treatment, drug-induced changes in renal morphology were largely prevented.[17] Markers of renal dysfunction were essentially normalized, including plasma urea and creatinine levels and creatinine and lithium clearance. In addition, *Spirulina* treatment almost completely reversed the cyclosporine-induced rise in the levels of lipid peroxidation not only in the kidney but also in plasma. It also normalized SOD, GPx, and catalase activity in the kidney.

Doxorubicin (DOX) is a potent antitumor agent used for the treatment of a variety of malignancies. It can induce significant and dose-dependent damage to the heart, leading to congestive heart failure. In a recent study, *S. platensis* was administered twice daily for 3 days before the first injection of DOX and for 7 weeks thereafter, while DOX was injected once a week for 4 weeks.[9] Compared to animals given DOX plus saline, mice that had received the alga exhibited markedly fewer and less severe morphological and ultrastructural changes in the heart and this was associated with significantly reduced levels of lipid peroxidation in this tissue. DOX treatment resulted in a decline in plasma antioxidant activity, and this was partially reversed by *Spirulina*. In addition, the alga completely restored SOD activity, and GPx activity was also similar to that seen in controls.

Pretreatment with *S. fusiformis* for 5 days before cisplatin, urethane, cyclophosphamide, or mitomycin-C injection significantly decreased drug-induced hepatic lipid peroxidation in a dose-dependent manner.[4,5] The highest dose (1000 mg/kg per day) provided complete protection against lipid peroxidation induced by cyclophosphamide and mitomycin-C, but not by cisplatin or urethane. All of these drugs significantly inhibited the activity of hepatic GPx, SOD, and catalase and decreased the reduced glutathione content of the liver. *Spirulina* treatment dose dependently reversed this inhibition, though not to the levels seen in untreated controls. It also provided partial protection from the chromosomal damage associated with these drugs.

Similar results have been obtained when *Spirulina* or phycocyanin was administered to animals treated with chemicals that simulate certain human diseases. Oral pretreatment with *S. maxima* for 14 days provided some protection from the neurotoxic effects of 1-methyl-4-phenyl-1,2,3,6-tetrahydropyridine, a chemical used as a model of Parkinson's disease.[20] This was evidenced by complete prevention of the drug-induced rise in lipid peroxidation in the brain striatum. In addition, phycocyanin partially restored striatal dopamine levels, but this effect was dose-independent.

Kainic acid is a chemical used to model epileptic seizures. Phycocyanin given orally before administration of kainic acid resulted in a significant reduction in tremors and seizures, particularly in the groups that received several doses of phycocyanin over the 24-h period before treatment with kainic acid.[21] Neuronal damage was also significantly attenuated by phycocyanin treatment, suggesting that a component of this protein was able to cross the blood-brain barrier. This suggests that the same component may also have participated in the neuroprotective effects in the previously described model of Parkinson's disease.

Phycocyanin has also been investigated in a model of toxic liver injury using either carbon tetrachloride or R-(+)-pulegone as hepatotoxic agents.[6,11] When injected intraperitoneally 3 h before treatment with a single dose of carbon tetrachloride, phycocyanin completely inhibited the rise in hepatic lipid peroxidation associated with this chemical.[11] This was seen at all doses, which ranged from 50 to 200 mg/kg. A single intraperitoneal dose of phycocyanin 1 or 3 h before injection of either carbon tetrachloride or R-(+)-pulegone completely reversed the drug-induced changes in the activity of all liver enzymes tested.[6]

In summary, the results of the presented studies clearly show that oral administration of the various species of *Spirulina* can significantly inhibit lipid peroxidation in the tissue that is the main target of the drug toxicity. Similar effects have been reported for phycocyanin. The findings of these studies also demonstrate that *Spirulina* and its major biliprotein are able to reverse drug-induced inhibition of the antioxidant enzymes, SOD, catalase, and GPx. From the available data, it cannot be established whether this restoration of endogenous antioxidant enzyme activity is the major antioxidative mechanism by which *Spirulina* and phycocyanin protect from drug-induced oxidative stress and the resulting tissue damage. It seems rather likely that the direct radical scavenging and antioxidant activities of *Spirulina* and phycocyanin also contribute.

OTHER MECHANISMS

Reactive nitrogen species: Nitric oxide is an inflammatory mediator produced by the inducible form of nitric oxide synthase (iNOS). It is converted into a variety of reactive nitrogen species, which eventually yield nitrite as a stable product that can be measured in serum and tissues. There are indications that reactive nitrogen species are involved in the toxicity of a variety of drugs, including the renal toxicity of gentamicin and cisplatin and the nephrotoxicity of cyclosporine. When *S. fusiformis* was given orally to mice 2 days before and 8 days concomitantly with gentamicin a dose-dependent inhibition of the gentamicin-induced increase in serum nitrite concentrations was observed.[19] Similar results were obtained in animals that were treated orally with *S. fusiformis* for 2 days before and 3 days during administration of cisplatin.[18] In this study, *Spirulina* was somewhat less effective in decreasing serum nitrite concentrations, possibly because it was given for a shorter duration than in the gentamicin study. Other investigators showed that *Spirulina* was able to inhibit hepatic iNOS activity,[22] and this ability may account for the observed reduction in serum nitrite levels in the above studies.

Prevention of apoptosis: As discussed earlier, *Spirulina* significantly attenuated DOX-induced cardiomyopathy.[9] In vitro results obtained by the same group of researchers suggest that one of the mechanisms involved in the cardioprotective effect of *Spirulina* is the prevention of cardiomyocyte apoptosis, a tightly regulated cellular suicide program.[10] Both *Spirulina* and phycocyanin were able to markedly inhibit apoptosis. Oxidative stress is well known to induce this form of cell death, and the radical scavenging and antioxidant activities of *Spirulina* and phycocyanin may have contributed to the inhibition of DOX-induced apoptosis in cardiomyocytes.

In addition, however, both *Spirulina* and phycocyanin reversed the DOX-induced increase in the activity of caspase-3. Caspases are central mediators of apoptosis, and caspase-3 is indispensable for several steps within the apoptotic process. Furthermore, phycocyanin was able to significantly inhibit the drug-induced increase in the expression of the proapoptotic Bax protein. It also induced the expression of Bcl-2, an antiapoptotic molecule. No results were reported for *Spirulina*.

OTHER TOXICITIES

Lead: As in drug toxicities, *Spirulina* or its bioactive constituent, phycocyanin, has been found to protect from heavy metal poisoning. Again, this protection seems to be mediated mostly by the prevention of oxidative damage through direct antioxidant actions and through induction of endogenous antioxidant enzymes. For example, in rats treated with lead acetate, dietary *S. fusiformis* (1500 mg/kg) reversed the lead-induced inhibition of SOD and catalase activity in liver, lung, heart, and kidney to levels that were only slightly, but not significantly, lower than those of untreated controls.[23] Lead did not induce significant decreases in the activities of these anti-oxidant enzymes in the brain, and *Spirulina* did not markedly alter them either. Interestingly, brain was the only tissue in which *Spirulina* feeding resulted in a significant reduction in lead concentrations compared to the lead-treated unsupplemented group. Dietary *S. fusiformis* was also associated with a pronounced decrease in the levels of lipid peroxidation in liver, lung, heart, and kidney, although they remained higher than in control animals that had not received lead acetate.

Mercury: When mice were given *S. fusiformis* orally for 10 days before and 30 days after mercury chloride administration, they exhibited significantly decreased levels of lipid peroxidation in the liver, reduced histological damage, and lower liver enzyme activities than animals that received only mercury chloride.[24] In mice treated according to the same protocol, kidney tissue of *Spirulina*-treated animals also showed markedly fewer and less severe lesion in association with reduced lipid peroxidation. In addition, *Spirulina* partially inhibited mercury-induced changes in the activities of several kidney enzymes.

Arsenic poisoning: In a recent randomized placebo-controlled study, the efficacy of an ethanol extract of *Spirulina* in combination with zinc against chronic arsenic poisoning was examined in a total of 41 patients.[25] Filtered water was provided to all the patients and resulted in decreased urinary excretion of arsenic. Between second week and sixth week of treatment, the urinary arsenic concentration rose sharply in the group treated with *Spirulina* plus zinc, but not in the placebo group. This strongly suggests that *Spirulina* plus zinc enhanced the urinary excretion of this toxin. It is not immediately obvious why this effect was no longer evident after 4–6 weeks of treatment. From that time until the end of the study after 16 weeks, the urinary excretion remained slightly and nonsignificantly higher in the group treated with *Spirulina* plus zinc compared to the placebo group. At the end of 16 weeks of treatment, arsenic concentrations in hair of patients in the placebo group had decreased only slightly. In contrast, a marked decline (47%) occurred in the *Spirulina* plus zinc-treated group. Significant clinical improvements in the skin manifestations of arsenic poisoning, that is, hyperpigmentation primarily of the upper chest and arms and keratosis, were seen only in patients treated with *Spirulina* plus zinc, but not in the placebo group.

Once absorbed, arsenic is enzymatically or nonenzymatically reduced to arsenite and then methylated. Note that, while methylation enhances arsenic excretion, the resulting metabolites exhibit significant toxicities of their own.[26] Approximately 60–80% of ingested arsenic is excreted in urine, while the remainder is secreted into bile, which results in fecal elimination. It has been shown that glutathione plays an important role in biliary arsenic excretion.[27] Arsenic triglutathione and methylarsenic diglutathione have also been detected in urine of mice and these two species were found to represent ~60–70% of urinary arsenic.[28] This suggests that the ability of *Spirulina* to restore drug- or chemical-induced levels of reduced glutathione may be a factor in the enhanced arsenic excretion in the above study. It is as yet unknown whether the glutathione conjugation of arsenic metabolites is catalyzed by GST or occurs nonenzymatically. If mediated by GST, the ability of *Spirulina* to upregulate GST activity—as seen in liver,[3,4] though not in kidney[1]—may also have contributed to the observed higher urinary excretion of arsenic and the significant reduction in hair arsenic levels and presumably body burden.

CONCLUDING REMARKS

The available literature contains little information about the potential of *Spirulina* to influence the metabolism of pharmaceuticals. Given the widespread use of this alga for the purpose of enhancing immune function, studies addressing this issue are urgently needed. There are data showing that *Spirulina* can provide considerable protection from the renal toxicity associated with cyclosporine, gentamicin, and cisplatin, the cardiotoxicity of DOX, and the genotoxicity of cyclophosphamide and mitomycin-C in mice and rats. This protective effect seems to be mediated mostly by the ability of this alga to act as an antioxidant and to reverse the drug-induced inhibition of endogenous antioxidant enzymes. Other mechanisms involve the ability to reduce the levels of reactive nitrogen species, possibly by inhibiting inducible nitric oxide synthase, and the ability to prevent apoptosis by altering the expression of proteins that regulate the apoptotic process. Although these results are promising, their applicability to humans remains to be established.

REFERENCES

1. Mittal, A., Kumar, P.V., Banerjee, S., et al., Modulatory potential of *Spirulina fusiformis* on carcinogen metabolizing enzymes in Swiss albino mice. *Phytother Res* 13, 111, 1999.
2. Mittal, A., Kumar, A., and Rao, A.R., Modulatory influence of *Spirulina fusiformis* on 7, 12-dimethylbenz(*a*)anthracene induced papillomagenesis in the skin of mice. *Pharmaceutical Biol* 36, 341, 1998.
3. Dasgupta, T., Banerjee, S., Yadav, P.K., et al., Chemomodulation of carcinogen metabolising enzymes, antioxidant profiles and skin and forestomach papillomagenesis by *Spirulina platensis. Mol Cell Biochem* 226, 27, 2001.

4. Premkumar, K., Pachiappan, A., Abraham, S.K., et al., Effect of *Spirulina fusiformis* on cyclophosphamide and mitomycin-C induced genotoxicity and oxidative stress in mice. *Fitoterapia* 72, 906, 2001.
5. Premkumar, K., Abraham, S.K., Santhiya, S.T., et al., Protective effect of *Spirulina fusiformis* on chemical-induced genotoxicity in mice. *Fitoterapia* 75, 24, 2004.
6. Vadiraja, B.B., Gaikwad, N.W., and Madyastha, K.M., Hepatoprotective effect of C-phycocyanin: protection for carbon tetrachloride and R-(+)-pulegone-mediated hepatotoxicty in rats. *Biochem Biophys Res Commun* 249, 428, 1998.
7. Miranda, M.S., Cintra, R.G., Barros, S.B., et al., Antioxidant activity of the microalga *Spirulina maxima*. *Braz J Med Biol Res* 31, 1075, 1998.
8. Wu, L.-C., Ho, J.A., Shieh, M.-C., et al., Antioxidant and antiproliferative activities of *spirulina* and chlorella water extracts. *J Agric Food Chem* 53, 4207, 2005.
9. Khan, M., Shobha, J.C., Mohan, I.K., et al., Protective effect of *Spirulina* against doxorubicin-induced cardiotoxicity. *Phytother Res* 19, 1030, 2005.
10. Khan, M., Varadharaj, S., Shobha, J.C., et al., C-phycocyanin ameliorates doxorubicin-induced oxidative stress and apoptosis in adult rat cardiomyocytes. *J Cardiovasc Pharmacol* 47, 9, 2006.
11. Bhat, V.B., and Madyastha, K.M., C-phycocyanin: a potent peroxyl radical scavenger *in vivo* and *in vitro*. *Biochem Biophys Res Commun* 275, 20, 2000.
12. Romay, C., Armesto, J., Remirez, D., et al., Antioxidant and anti-inflammatory properties of C-phycocyanin from blue-green algae. *Inflamm Res* 47, 36, 1998.
13. Romay, C., and González, R., Phycocyanin is an antioxidant protector of human erythrocytes against lysis by peroxyl radicals. *J Pharm Pharmacol* 52, 367, 2000.
14. Bhat, V.B., and Madyastha, K.M., Scavenging of peroxynitrite by phycocyanin and phycocyanobilin from *Spirulina platensis*: protection against oxidative damage to DNA. *Biochem Biophys Res Commun* 285, 262, 2001.
15. Hirata, T., Tanaka, M., Ooike, M., et al., Antioxidant activities of phycocyanobilin prepared from *Spirulina platensis*. *J Appl Phycol* 12, 435, 2000.
16. Mohan, I.K., Khan, M., Shobha, J.C., et al., Protection against cisplatin-induced nephrotoxicity by *Spirulina* in rats. *Cancer Chemother Pharmacol* 58, 802, 2006.
17. Khan, M., Shobha, J.C., Mohan, I.K., et al., *Spirulina* attenuates cyclosporine-induced nephrotoxicity in rats. *J Appl Toxicol* 26, 444, 2006.
18. Kuhad, A., Tirkey, N., Pilkhwal, S., et al., Renoprotective effect of *Spirulina* fusiformis on cisplatin-induced oxidative stress and renal dysfunction in rats. *Ren Fail* 28, 247, 2006.
19. Kuhad, A., Tirkey, N., Pilkhwal, S., et al., Effect of *Spirulina*, a blue green algae, on gentamicin-induced oxidative stress and renal dysfunction in rats. *Fundam Clin Pharmacol* 20, 121, 2006.
20. Chamorro, G., Pérez-Albiter, M., Serrano-García, N., et al., *Spirulina maxima* pretreatment partially protects against 1-methyl-4-phenyl-1,2,3,6-tetrahydropyridine neurotoxicity. *Nutr Neurosci* 9, 207, 2006.
21. Rimbau, V., Camins, A., Romay, C., et al., Protective effects of C-phycocyanin against kainic acid-induced neuronal damage in rat hippocampus. *Neurosci Lett* 276, 75, 1999.
22. Remirez, D., Fernández, V., Tapia, G., et al., Influence of C-phycocyanin on hepatocellular parameters related to liver oxidative stress and Kupffer cell functioning. *Inflamm Res* 5, 351, 2002.
23. Upasani, C.D., and Balaraman, R., Protective effect of *Spirulina* on lead induced deleterious changes in the lipid peroxidation and endogenous antioxidants in rats. *Phytother Res* 17, 330, 2003.

24. Kumar, M., Sharma, M.K., and Kumar, A., *Spirulina fusiformis*: a food supplement against mercury induced hepatic toxicity. *J Health Sci* 51, 424, 2005.

25. Misbahuddin, M., Islam, A.Z., Khandker, S., et al., Efficacy of *spirulina* extract plus zinc in patients of chronic arsenic poisoning: a randomized placebo-controlled study. *Clin Toxicol* (Phila) 44, 135, 2006.

26. Kenyon, E.M., Del Razo, L.M., and Hughes, M.F., Tissue distribution and urinary excretion of inorganic arsenic and its methylated metabolites in mice following acute oral administration of arsenate. *Toxicol Sci* 85, 468, 2005.

27. Kala, S.V., Neely, M.W., Kala, G., et al., The MRP2/cMOAT transporter and arsenic-glutathione complex formation are required for biliary excretion of arsenic. *J Biol Chem* 275, 33404, 2000.

28. Kala, S.V., Kala, G., Prater, C.I., et al., Formation and urinary excretion of arsenic triglutathione and methylarsenic diglutathione. *Chem Res Toxicol* 17, 243, 2004.

Index

Note: Page numbers in *italics* refer to figures and tables.

305